PDxMD
Dermatology

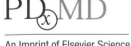

An Imprint of Elsevier Science

Philadelphia ■ St Louis ■ London ■ Sydney ■ New York ■ Toronto

PDxMD
An imprint of Elsevier Science

Publisher:	Steven Merahn, MD
Project Managers:	Caroline Barnett, Lucy Hamilton, Zak Knowles
Programmer:	Narinder Chandi
Production:	Aoibhe O'Shea – GMS UK, Alan Palfreyman – PTU
Designer:	Jayne Jones
Layout:	The Designers Collective Limited

Printed in China by RDC Group

PDxMD
Elsevier Science
The Curtis Center
625 Walnut Street,
Philadelphia, PA 19106

The
Publisher's
policy is to use
**paper manufactured
from sustainable forests**

ISBN 1-932141-02-2

Contents

Introduction

Editorial Faculty and Staff   xi

MediFiles

Contents

Introduction

What is PDxMD?

PDxMD is a new, evidence-based primary care clinical information system designed to support your judgment with practical clinical information. The content is continuously updated by expert contributors with the latest on evaluation, diagnosis, management, outcomes and prevention – all designed for use at the point and time of care.

First and foremost, PDxMD is an electronic resource. This book gives you access to just a fraction of the content available on-line. At www.pdxmd.com, you will find:

- Over 1400 differential diagnoses for you to search for information according to your patient's chief complaint via a unique signs and symptoms matrix
- Information on more than 450 medical conditions and more than 750 drugs and other therapies, organised in condition-specific 'MediFiles'
- Patient information sheets on 300 topics for you to customize and hand to your patient during consultation

About This Book

The PDxMD Medical Conditions Series is a print version of the comprehensive approach offered on line. Concise information on medical conditions is systematically organized in a consistent MediFile format, our electronic equivalent of chapters.

Each MediFile covers summary information and background on each condition, and comprehensive information on diagnosis, treatment, outcomes, and prevention, and other resources, especially written and designed for use in practice. Each MediFile is organized identically to allow you to find information consistently and reliably for every condition. See the MediFile 'Road Map' inside the back cover for more information.

Ranging from epidemiology to risk assessment and reduction, from diagnostic evaluation and testing to therapeutic options, prognosis and outcomes – you'll find the information that you need is easier to locate with this methodical approach.

How to Use This Book

Find the MediFile for any specific medical condition in the Contents list. Familiarize yourself with the MediFile Road Map (see inside back cover) to rapidly find the precise information you require.

Information on drugs and tests are found within the MediFiles for the specific conditions. For an overview, see the 'Summary of options' sections under DIAGNOSIS and under TREATMENT in the relevant MediFile. Details of tests, drugs and other therapies then follow.

PDxMD believes that physician clinical judgment is central to appropriate diagnostic and therapeutic decision-making. The information is designed to support professional judgment and, accounting for individual patient differences, does not provide direct answers or force specific practices or policies.

Introduction

How is PDxMD created?

PDxMD is created through Collaborative Authoring. This process allows medical information to be reviewed and synthesized from multiple sources – including but not limited to peer-reviewed articles, evidence databases, guidelines and position papers – and by multiple individuals. The information is organized around and integrated into a template that matches the needs of primary care physicians in practice.

Professional medical writers begin the process of reviewing and synthesizing information for PDxMD, working from core evidence databases and other expert resources and with the guidance of Editorial Advisory Board (EAB) members. This first draft is sent to a physician 'clinical reviewer', who works with the writer to make sure the information is accurate and properly organized. A second review by the physician clinical reviewer ensures that appropriate changes are in place.

After these first two levels of clinical review, the files are reviewed and edited by the relevant specialist member of the Editorial Advisory Board. A primary care member of the EAB, who has final sign-off authority, then conducts the final review and edit. Editorial checks are conducted between all review stages and, after primary care sign-off, a pharmacist double checks the drug recommendations prior to a final editorial review.

There are a minimum of three and as many as five physicians involved in each MediFile, and additional clinical reviewers and/or EAB members are added when appropriate (e.g., alternative/complementary medicine experts, or conditions requiring multi-disciplinary approaches). The contributor team for each MediFile is listed in the Resources section.

A complete list of Editorial Faculty and staff of PDxMD is provided below. All Editorial Faculty, and specifically the Editorial Advisory Board members, participate in PDxMD as individuals and not as representatives of, or on behalf of, their affiliated institutions or associations and any indication of their affiliation with a specific institution or association should not be taken as an endorsement of PDxMD or any participation of their institution or association with PDxMD.

Continuous Product Improvement

PDxMD is committed to continuous quality improvement and welcomes any comments, suggestions and feedback from the professional community. Please send any ideas or considerations regarding this volume or any other volume in the PDxMD series via e-mail to feedback.pdxmd@elsevier.com or to PDxMD, Elsevier Science, The Curtis Center, 625 Walnut Street, Philadelphia, PA 19106.

Introduction

Evidence-Based Medicine Policies

PDxMD is committed to providing available and up-to-date evidence for the diagnostic and therapeutic recommendations provided in our knowledge base. All MediFiles begin with a core set of evidence-based references from recognized sources. These are supplemented with extensive searches of the literature and reviews of reference books, peer-reviewed journals, association guidelines and position papers, among others.

Criteria for Evidence-Based Medicine
Evidence Sources

PDxMD has taken the best evidence currently available from the following:

Published Critically Evaluated Evidence

- Cochrane Systematic Reviews – respected throughout the world as one of the most rigorous searches of medical journals with highly structured systematic reviews and use of meta-analysis to produce reliable evidence
- Clinical Evidence – produced jointly by the British Medical Journal Publishing Group and the American College of Physicians–American Society of Internal Medicine. Clinical Evidence provides a concise account of the current state of knowledge on the treatment and prevention of many clinical conditions based on the search and appraisal of the available literature
- The National Guideline Clearinghouse – a comprehensive database of evidence-based clinical practice guidelines and related documents produced by the Agency for Healthcare Research and Quality in partnership with the American Medical Association and the American Association of Health Plans

Evidence Published in Peer-Reviewed Journals

- Association Guidelines and Position Papers

Where evidence exists that has not yet been critically reviewed by one of the sources listed above, for example randomized controlled trials and clinical cohort studies, the evidence is summarized briefly, categorized, and fully referenced.

Clinical Experience

While recognizing the importance of these evidence-based resources, PDxMD also highlights the importance of experience in clinical practice. Therefore, our Editorial Advisory Board also provide advice from their own clinical experience, within Clinical Pearl sections of the MediFiles and elsewhere. Contributing expert physicians are identified in the Resources section of every MediFile.

Introduction

Evaluation of Evidence

PDxMD evaluates all cited evidence according to the AAFP Recommended Basic Model for Evaluating and Categorizing the Clinical Content of CME, based on the model used by the University of Michigan:

Level M   Evidence from either:
Meta-analysis or
Multiple randomized controlled trials

Level P   Evidence from either:
A well-designed prospective clinical trial or
Several prospective clinical cohort studies with consistent findings (without randomization)

Level S   Evidence from studies other than clinical trials, such as:
Epidemiological studies
Physiological studies

References

The information provided by PDxMD is concise and action-oriented. As a result, our editorial policy is to cite only essential reference sources. References and evidence summaries are provided in four areas:

1.   In the Diagnostic Decision section under Diagnosis
2.   In the Guidelines and Evidence sections under Treatment
3.   In the Outcomes section under Evidence
4.   In the Key Reference Section under Resources

Where on-line references to the Cochrane Abstracts, BMJ Clinical Evidence and National Guideline Clearinghouse are cited in the text, the internet addresses of the home pages are given. The internet addresses of individual reports are not given.

When references are to association guidelines and position papers, the internet address of the association home page is generally provided. When possible, the internet address of the specific report is provided.

Editorial Faculty and Staff

Executive Committee

Fred F Ferri, MD, FACP
Editorial Board & Medical Chair, Executive Committee Family Medicine
Clinical Professor
Brown University of Medicine, Chief
Division of Internal Medicine
Fatima Hospital, St Joseph's Health Services
Providence, RI

George T Danakas, MD, FACOG
Editorial Board & Executive Committee Obstetrics, Gynecology
Clinical Assistant Professor
SUNY at Buffalo
Williamsville, NY

David G Fairchild, MD, MPH
Editorial Board & Executive Committee Primary Care, Signs & Symptoms
Brigham and Women's Hospital
Boston, MA

Russell C Jones, MD, MPH
Editorial Board & Executive Committee Family Medicine
Dartmouth Medical School
New London, NH

Kathleen M O'Hanlon, MD
Editorial Board & Executive Committee Primary Care
Professor, Marshall University School of Medicine
Department of Family & Community Health
Huntington, WV

John L Pfenninger, MD, FAAFP
Editorial Board & Executive Committee Primary Care, Procedures
President and Director
The National Procedures Institute
Director, The Medical Procedures Center, PC
Clinical Professor of Family Medicine
Michigan State University
Midland, MI

Joseph E Scherger, MD, MPH
Editorial Board & Executive Committee Primary Care, Site Search
Dean, College of Medicine
Florida State University
Tallahassee, FL

Myron Yanoff, MD
Editorial Board & Executive Committee Ophthalmology, Otolaryngology
Professor & Chair, Department of Ophthalmology
MCP Hahnemann University
Philadelphia, PA

Editorial Board

Philip J Aliotta, MD, MHA, FACS
Editorial Board, Urology
Attending Urologist and Clinical Research
Director Center for Urologic Research of
Western New York
Main Urology Associates, PC
Williamsville, NY

Gordon H Baustian, MD
Editorial Board, Family Medicine
Director of Medical Education and Residency
Cedar Rapids Medical Education Foundation
Cedar Rapids, IA

Editorial Faculty and Staff

Editorial Faculty and Staff

Editorial Faculty and Staff

Gary M White, MD
Editorial Board, Dermatology Illustration
Associate Clinical Professor
Dept of Dermatology
University of California, San Diego
San Diego, CA

Basil J Zitelli, MD
Editorial Board, Pediatrics Illustration
Professor of Pediatrics
University of Pittsburgh School of Medicine
Children's Hospital of Pittsburgh
Pittsburgh PA

Clinical Reviewers

Richard Averitte, MD
Dermatology
Chief Resident
Department of Dermatology
University Hospitals of Cleveland
Case Western Reserve University
Cleveland, OH

Elma D Baron, MD
Dermatology
Clinical Research Fellow
Department of Dermatology
University Hospitals of Cleveland
Case Western Reserve University School of
Medicine
Cleveland, OH

Thompson H Boyd, III, MD
Primary Care
Clinical Assistant Professor
Physician Liaison – Information Services
Department of Medicine
Hahnemann University Hospital
Philadelphia, PA

Rolland P Gyulai, MD, PhD
Dermatology
Research Fellow
Department of Dermatology
University Hospitals of Cleveland and Case
Western Reserve University
Cleveland, OH

Laurie G S Jacobson, MD
Dermatology
Dermatology Resident
Department of Dermatology
Case Western Reserve University
Cleveland, OH

Christine C Lin, MD
Dermatology
Chief Resident Physician
Department of Dermatology
University Hospitals of Cleveland
Cleveland, OH

Gregory J Raglow, MD, FAAFP
Internal Medicine
Primary Care Medical Director
Good Samaritan Family Practice Center
Phoenix, AZ

Douglas C Semler, MD
Dermatology
Chief Resident
Department of Dermatology
Case Western Reserve University and
Metrohealth Medical Center
Cleveland, OH

Andrea Trowers, MD
Dermatology
Department of Dermatology
University of Miami School of Medicine
Miami, FL

Editorial Faculty and Staff

Writers

Kim S Berman
Elly C Blake
Liza C Brettingham, MD, JCTGP
Patricia L Carroll, RN, CEN, RRT
Andrea L Clatworthy, PhD
Anne E Dyson, MB BS
Ewan M Gerard, MB ChB, MSc, MRCGP
Kelly D Karpa, RPh, PhD, BSPharm
Fiona McCrimmon, MBBS MRCGP

Shelley Minden
Beth E K Oliver, BSc Occupational Therapy
Elizabeth Robinson, MB ChB
Amber A Smith
Simon J Walker
Robert Whittle, MB BS (NSW)
Everetta M Woods
Tony M J Woolfson, MB BS, DM, MRCP

Staff

Management Team
Fiona Foley, Steven Merahn, MD, Daniel Pollock, Zak Knowles, Howard Croft, Tanya Thomas, Lucy Hamilton, Julie Volck, Bill Bruggemeyer, Andrea Ford

Editorial Team
Anne Dyson, Sadaf Hashmi, Debbie Goring, Louise Morrison, Ellen Haigh, Robert Whittle, Claire Champion, Caroline Barnett, Laurie Smith, Li Wan, Paul Mayhew, Carmen Jones, Fi Ward

Technical Team
Martin Miller, Narinder Chandi, Roy Patterson, Aaron McGrath, John Wylie, Sarah Craze, Cameron Sangster

We would also like to acknowledge the extraordinary contributions of the following individuals to the conceptualization and realization of PDxMD over the initial years of its growth and development:

Tim Hailstone, Jonathan Black, Alison Whitehouse, Jayne Harris, Angela Baggi, Sharon Bambaji, Sam Bedser, Layla van den Bergh, Stuart Boffey, Siobhan Egan, Helen Elder, Mark Mitchenall, Chris Moodie, Tony Pollard, Simon Seljeflot, Liz Southey, Tim Stentiford, Matthew Whyte

ACNE ROSACEA

DESCRIPTION

- Chronic facial skin disorder most commonly seen in individuals between the ages of 30 and 60 years
- More common in women than men, but often more severe in men
- Features include erythema, telangiectasia, papules, pustules and edema of midfacial skin
- Frequently causes significant psychologic distress
- Disease is progressive, commonly with periods of exacerbation and remission
- Originally termed 'acne rosacea' because of the similarity in appearance to acne vulgaris

ICD9 CODE
695.3 Rosacea

SYNONYMS
Rosacea.

CARDINAL FEATURES
- Characteristic pattern of facial involvement; rarely extrafacial
- Features include erythema, telangiectasia, papules, pustules, and edema of midfacial skin
- Eye involvement is common
- Disease is progressive, commonly with periods of exacerbation and remission
- Most commonly seen in individuals between the ages of 30 and 60; more common in women than men
- Often associated with easy flushing and blushing

CAUSES
Common causes
- Cause is largely unknown
- Theories suggest underlying vasomotor instability of the blood (circulatory system) or the skin mite *Demodex follicularum*, but there is little evidence for either

Contributory or predisposing factors
- Genetic predisposition: 40% of sufferers have a family member with the disease
- In sensitive individuals: sun exposure, stress, hot weather, alcohol, spicy foods, exercise, wind, hot baths, cold weather, hot drinks, skin care products, certain drugs
- Topical or oral steroid treatment

EPIDEMIOLOGY
Incidence and prevalence
FREQUENCY
- 50/1000
- Men: 20–30/1000; women: 60–80/1000

Demographics
AGE
- Peak age of onset: 30–45 years
- Rare in prepubescent children

GENDER
- Female:male approx. 3:1
- Women experience less severe disease than men

RACE
- Appears most often in individuals of northern and eastern European descent, such as Celtic or Scandinavian populations
- Occurs less often in individuals of Oriental, Polynesian or Hispanic origin
- Occurs rarely in African Americans

GENETICS
Family history predisposes to disease; 40% of sufferers have a family member with the disorder.

GEOGRAPHY
More common in areas where there are populations of individuals of northern and eastern European descent.

DIFFERENTIAL DIAGNOSIS

Acne vulgaris
Acne vulgaris is a chronic disease of the sebaceous follicle.

FEATURES
- Occurs most commonly in adolescents and young adults
- Scars, comedones, papules, pustules and nodules
- Back and chest involvement is common

Drug eruption
Reaction to drug, particularly bromides and iodides.

FEATURES
Flushing of face and body.

Dermatitis
Dermatitis is an inflammatory skin disorder, and may be seborrheic, contact, or perioral.

FEATURES
- Scaling
- Involvement of flexures

Systemic lupus erythematosus
Systemic lupus erythematosus (SLE) is a chronic multisystemic disease of autoimmune origin.

FEATURES
- Malar rash in midfacial region
- Rash on other light-exposed areas
- Systemic symptoms

Sarcoidosis
Sarcoidosis is a multisystem granulomatous disorder of unclear etiology characterized pathologically by the presence of noncaseating granulomas.

FEATURES
- Infiltrating plaques affecting the nose, cheeks or earlobes
- Systemic symptoms

Carcinoid syndrome
Carcinoid syndrome is a symptom complex characterized by paroxysmal vasomotor disturbances, diarrhea, bronchospasm, and cutaneous flushing.

FEATURES
- Telangiectasia, flushing attacks
- Hepatomegaly
- Systemic symptoms

SIGNS & SYMPTOMS
Signs
Early stage:

■ Transitory erythema of midfacial area (mainly cheeks and chin in women, includes nose in men)

Middle stage:

■ Episodic erythema of midfacial area (cheeks and chin only in women, includes nose in men)
■ Telangiectasia in affected areas
■ Papules and pustules
■ Mild conjunctivitis or blepharitis (can occur in up to 58% of patients)

Advanced stage:

■ Deep persistent erythema
■ Prominent and widespread facial telangiectasia
■ Papules and pustules
■ Increased skin and ocular inflammation
■ Persistent conjunctivitis or blepharitis
■ Edema in the skin, particularly above the nasolabial folds
■ Rhinophyma (usually in men, very rarely in women) caused by sebaceous gland hypertrophy

Symptoms
Early stage:

■ Episodic flushing triggered by local stimuli such as sunlight, hot drinks, alcohol, spicy foods and emotion
■ Redness (mainly cheeks and chin in women, includes nose in men)

Middle stage:

■ Persistent flushing sometimes accompanied by burning or stinging sensation
■ Numerous papules and pustules
■ Sensation of ocular grittiness

Advanced stage:

■ Permanent facial redness sometimes accompanied by burning or stinging sensation
■ Painful papules and pustules
■ Persistent eye irritation
■ Nasal swelling in men

ASSOCIATED DISORDERS
■ Conjunctivitis
■ Blepharitis

CONSIDER CONSULT
■ Refer if there is uncertainty regarding diagnosis

INVESTIGATION OF THE PATIENT
Direct questions to patient
Q Do you suffer from intense facial flushing triggered by any of the following: sun exposure, stress, hot weather, alcohol consumption, spicy foods, exercise, wind, hot baths, cold weather, hot drinks, skin care products? So-called flushers and blushers are signs of early-stage rosacea.

Q Do you suffer from episodic attacks of papules and/or pustules associated with the above triggers? Rosacea symptoms can be exacerbated by these triggers.

Q Are you taking any medication? Drug reaction can be confused with rosacea. Topical or oral steroid treatment can exacerbate symptoms of rosacea.

Family history

Q Do any family members have rosacea? 40% of sufferers have a family member with the disease.

Examination

- Is the patient well/unwell? If systemically unwell, suggests systemic lupus erythematosus, sarcoidosis or carcinoid syndrome
- Is the patient fair-skinned? Individuals of northern and eastern European descent with fair skin are most commonly affected

Examination of face:

- Rosacea is a centrofacial disease, principally localized on the nose, cheeks, chin, forehead, and glabella. It is very rarely found elsewhere
- Vivid red erythema and telangiectasias, papules (may be inflammatory or due to sebaceous gland hypertrophy), and pustules are hallmarks of rosacea
- Presence of comedones suggests acne vulgaris; rosacea by itself has no comedones
- Check for scaling. Alone it suggests seborrheic dermatitis. Perioral or flexure involvement suggests perioral or contact dermatitis
- Inspect eyes for signs of conjunctivitis or mild ocular involvement
- Check for edema in facial skin particularly above the nasolabial folds
- Check for rhinophyma in advanced-stage rosacea in men

Summary of investigative tests

- Rosacea is a clinical diagnosis as there is no specific laboratory test to confirm diagnosis
- Skin biopsy and histologic sections, which are normally performed by a specialist, can show a characteristic constellation of features, which may assist diagnosis in difficult cases

DIAGNOSTIC DECISION

- The diagnosis is based on clinical findings
- Episodic or persistent erythema of midfacial area (cheeks and chin only in women, includes nose in men), telangiectasia, papules and pustules, mild ocular involvement, sebaceous gland hypertrophy
- Absence of comedones or systemic symptoms
- Edema in the skin and rhinophyma (usually in men, very rarely in women) in advanced cases
- Suspect rosacea if patient presents with any of these clinical findings but no systemic symptoms or comedones. Take into account patient's race, sex and age

CLINICAL PEARLS

- Frequently mistaken for malar rash of systemic lupus erythematosus. One must look beyond red cheeks at finer points of differential diagnosis
- Presence of comedones suggests acne vulgaris rather than acne rosacea. Comedones need to be distinguished from follicular plugging of discoid lupus erythematosus

TREATMENT

CONSIDER CONSULT
- Consider referral to ophthalmologist in cases of severe ocular involvement
- Consider referral to plastic or dermatologic surgeon for treatment of rhinophyma

PATIENT AND CAREGIVER ISSUES
Patient or caregiver request
Patient may be aware of the enormous number of treatments for acne and rosacea and reported in the media and especially on the internet.

Health-seeking behavior
Has the patient been self-medicating? The patient may have been using OTC acne treatments, or steroid preparations, that can make the symptoms worse.

MANAGEMENT ISSUES
Goals
- Calm down any presenting flare-up
- Reduce frequency and intensity of further flare-ups
- Slow or halt progression of disease

Management in special circumstances
COEXISTING MEDICATION
- Topical or oral steroid treatment for a coexisting disease must be avoided and given only when condition is more serious than rosacea
- OTC acne treatments can exacerbate symptoms of rosacea

SPECIAL PATIENT GROUPS
- Suitable antibiotics can be given during pregnancy
- Never give isotretinoin or oral metronidazole during pregnancy or whilst breast-feeding

PATIENT SATISFACTION/LIFESTYLE PRIORITIES
- Conspicuous facial redness and blemishes of rosacea can have a deep impact on the life of an affected individual: 75% of sufferers feel low self-esteem; 56% feel they have been robbed of pleasure or happiness
- Treatment should be aggressive in patients who are sensitive to their appearance

SUMMARY OF THERAPEUTIC OPTIONS
Choices
- Advise patient on lifestyle recommendations, e.g. sunscreen which is just as important as drug therapy
- Oral broad-spectrum antibiotics are first-choice drug therapy: tetracycline, doxycycline, minocycline and erythromycin. In cases of intolerance or resistance to these, ampicillin and metronidazole can be used; these are all off-label indications
- Topical metronidazole can be used in addition to oral antibiotics or during and after withdrawal to prevent relapse
- Topical clindamycin is as effective as oral tetracycline for pustular lesions; this is an off-label indication
- Oral isotretinoin can be very effective in resistant rosacea, but requires extensive monitoring of side effects; this is an off-label indication
- Crotamiton may be helpful in resistant cases when *Demodex folliculorum* infestation is present
- Cryosurgery, laser therapy and electrosurgery for rhinophyma. These procedures are usually performed by a specialist

Clinical pearls
- Therapies are suppressive, not curative
- Patients often benefit from cool compresses after activity that induces flushing/blushing (e.g. exertion, stress, heat, sun)

Never
Never give topical or oral steroid treatments, except in cases where there is a more serious coexisting disease.

FOLLOW UP
Plan for review
- Patients must take oral antibiotics for at least 3 weeks before any improvement can be seen. Review and revise treatment if not effective after 6 weeks
- Patients taking isotretinoin must be extensively monitored for side effects during the 5-month course of therapy

Information for patient or caregiver
- Lifestyle adjustments are an important part of the treatment
- Improvement will be gradual and perseverance is required, especially when there is a history of topical steroid use

DRUGS AND OTHER THERAPIES: DETAILS
Drugs
TETRACYCLINE
First-line antibiotic for controlling symptoms of rosacea; this is an off-label indication.

Dose
- 500mg orally twice daily to bring rosacea under control (one month)
- Taper down to 200mg orally twice daily for a further 2 months

Efficacy
Visible improvement in 6 weeks in most cases.

Risks/benefits
Risks:
- Compliance can be a problem
- Use caution in patients with hepatic impairment
- Use caution with repeated or prolonged doses

Benefits:
- Low cost
- Improves symptoms/appearance

Side effects and adverse reactions
- Cardiovascular system: pericarditis
- Central nervous system: headache, paresthesia, fever
- Gastrointestinal: abdominal pain, diarrhea, heartburn, hepatotoxicity, vomiting, nausea, dental staining, anorexia
- Genitourinary: polyuria, polydipsia, azotemia
- Hematologic: blood cell dyscrasias
- Skin: pruritus, rash, photosensitivity, changes in pigmentation, angioedema, stinging

Interactions (other drugs)

■ Antacids ■ Atovaquone ■ Barbiturates ■ Bismuth subsalicyclate ■ Calcium, iron, magnesium, zinc ■ Cephalosporins ■ Cholesytramine, colestipol ■ Carbamazepine ■ Digoxin ■ Ethanol ■ Methoxyflurane ■ Oral contraceptives ■ Penicillins ■ Phenytoin ■ Quinapril ■ Sodium bicarbonate ■ Vitamin A ■ Warfarin

Contraindications

■ Pregnancy and breast-feeding ■ Children less than 8 years ■ Severe renal disease

Acceptability to patient
High.

Follow up plan
Ask patient to return for review in one month.

Patient and caregiver information
Patients should be warned not to expect any visible results for at least 3 weeks.

DOXYCYCLINE
Used to control symptoms of rosacea; this is an off-label indication.

Dose
■ 50mg orally twice daily to bring rosacea under control (one month)
■ Taper down to 25mg orally twice daily for a further 2 months

Efficacy
Visible improvement after 6 weeks in most cases.

Risks/benefits
Risks:
■ Compliance can be a problem
■ Use caution in hepatic impairment
■ Use caution with repeated or prolonged doses

Benefits:
■ Low cost
■ Widely available

Side effects and adverse reactions
■ Cardiovascular system: pericarditis, angioedema
■ Central nervous system: fever, headache
■ Gastrointestinal: abdominal pain, diarrhea, heartburn, nausea, hepatotoxicity, vomiting, pseudomembranous colitis
■ Hematologic: blood cell disorders
■ Skin: pruritus, rash, photosensitivity, exfoliative dermatitis

Interactions (other drugs)

■ Antacids (magnesium, calcium) ■ Anticonvulsants (barbiturates, carbamazepine, phenytoin) ■ Bismuth ■ Cholestyramine ■ Ethanol ■ Mineral supplements (iron, zinc) ■ Oral contraceptives ■ Penicillins ■ Warfarin

Contraindications

■ Pregnancy and breast-feeding ■ Children less than 8 years

Acceptability to patient
High.

Follow up plan
Ask patient to return in one month for review.

Patient and caregiver information
Patients should be warned not to expect any visible results for at least 3 weeks.

MINOCYCLINE
Used to control symptoms of rosacea; this is an off-label indication.

Dose
- 50mg orally twice daily to bring rosacea under control (one month)
- Taper down to 10mg orally twice daily for a further 2 months

Efficacy
Visible results after 6 weeks in most cases.

Risks/benefits
Risks:
- Use of this drug may result in overgrowth of nonsusceptible organisms, including fungi. If superinfection occurs, the antibiotic should be discontinued
- Risk of pseudotumor cerebri (benign intracranial hypertension) in adults
- Photosensitivity manifested by an exaggerated sunburn reaction has been observed

Benefit: Low cost

Side effects and adverse reactions
- Cardiovascular system: pericarditis
- Central nervous system: benign intracranial hypertension (pseudotumor cerebri) in adults, headache, anaphylaxis
- Gastrointestinal: anorexia, nausea, vomiting, diarrhea, glossitis, dysphagia, enterocolitis, esophagitis and esophageal ulcerations
- Metabolic: pancreatitis, inflammatory lesions (with candidal overgrowth) in the anogenital region, increases in liver enzymes, hepatitis and liver failure
- Musculoskeletal: polyarthralgia
- Skin: maculopapular erythematous rashes, exfoliative dermatitis, erythema multiforme, Stevens-Johnson syndrome, photosensitivity, pigmentation of the skin and mucous membranes, urticaria, angioneurotic edema, anaphylactoid purpura, exacerbation of systemic lupus erythematosus, pulmonary infiltrates with eosinophilia
- Hematologic: hemolytic anemia, thrombocytopenia, neutropenia, and eosinophilia have been reported
- Other: with prolonged treatment, brown-black microscopic discoloration of the thyroid glands

Interactions (other drugs)
- Methoxyflurane (has been reported to result in fatal renal toxicity)
- Anticoagulants (may depress plasma prothrombin activity) ■ Penicillin (bactericidal action may be reduced) ■ Oral contraceptives (may reduce effectiveness of contraceptives) ■ Antacids containing aluminum, calcium, or magnesium, and iron-containing preparations (may impair absorption of minocycline)

Contraindications
- Children under 8 years of age
- Pregnancy and lactation
- Hypersensitivity to any of the tetracyclines

Acceptability to patient
High.

Follow up plan
Ask patient to return in one month for review.

Patient and caregiver information
Patients should be warned not to expect any visible results for at least 3 weeks.

ERYTHROMYCIN
Used to control symptoms of rosacea; this is an off-label indication.

Dose
- 500mg orally twice daily to bring rosacea under control (one month)
- Taper down to 100mg orally twice daily for a further 2 months

Efficacy
Visible results after 6 weeks in most cases.

Risks/benefits
Risks:
- Caution in hepatic and renal impairment, porphyria
- Avoid concomitant administration with terfenadine, astemizole and cisapride (these drugs have been discontinued).
- Use caution with repeated or prolonged therapy
- Potential risk of superinfection with resistant bacteria

Side effects and adverse reactions
- Cardiovascular system: dysrhythmias (uncommon)
- Eyes, ears, nose, and throat: deafness, tinnitus
- Gastrointestinal: anorexia, nausea, diarrhea, abdominal pain, vomiting, heartburn, hepatitis
- Genitourinary: candidiasis, vaginitis
- Skin: rashes, pruritus

Interactions (other drugs)
- Alfentanil
- Antiarrhythmic drugs (digoxin, disopyramide)
- Antihistamines (terfenadine, astemizole)
- Anticonvulsants (carbamazepine, valproic acid)
- Antiviral agents
- Benzodiazepines
- Bromocriptine
- Buspirone
- Cisapride
- Clozapine
- Colchicine
- Cyclosporine, tacrolimus
- Ergotamine
- Ethanol
- Felodipine
- Itraconazole
- Methylprednisolone
- Penicillin
- Quinidine
- Sildenafil
- Statins
- Theophylline
- Warfarin
- Zopiclone

Contraindications
- Liver disease
- Various infections (vaccinia, varicella, mycobacterial, fungal, viral)

Acceptability to patient
High.

Follow up plan
Ask patient to return in one month for review.

Patient and caregiver information
Patients should be warned not to expect any visible results for at least 3 weeks.

AMPICILLIN
Used to control symptoms of rosacea; this is an off-label indication.

Dose
- 250mg orally four times daily to bring rosacea under control (one month)
- Taper down to 100mg orally four times daily for further 2 months

Efficacy
Visible results after 6 weeks in most cases.

Risks/benefits
Risks:
- Use caution in renal disease, mononucleosis, and hypersensitivity to cephalosporins
- Use caution in neonates or the elderly
- Use caution in prolonged or repeated treatment
- Requires dosing four times daily; compliance can be difficult

Benefits:
- Low cost
- Useful when tetracyclines are not tolerated or are contraindicated
- Long duration of treatment

Side effects and adverse reactions
- Central nervous system: seizures, hallucinations, coma, anxiety
- Gastrointestinal: nausea, diarrhea, vomiting, altered liver function tests, pseudomembranous colitis
- Genitourinary: urinary problems, renal damage, candidiasis, vaginitis
- Hematologic: bleeding disorders, bone marrow depression
- Hypersensitivity reactions

Interactions (other drugs)
- Allopurinol (may increase incidence of rash) ■ Atenolol ■ Chloramphenicol (inhibits effect of ampicillin) ■ Macrolide and tetracycline antibiotics (inhibit effect of ampicillin) ■ Methotrexate ■ Oral contraceptives ■ Phenindione ■ Probenecid (decreases renal tubular secretion of ampicillin) ■ Warfarin

Contraindications
- Hypersensitivity to penicillins

Acceptability to patient
High.

Follow up plan
Ask patient to return in one month for review.

Patient and caregiver information
Patients should be warned not to expect any visible results for at least 3 weeks.

METRONIDAZOLE
Used to control symptoms of rosacea; this is an off-label indication.

Dose
250mg orally twice daily until symptoms subside (not to be taken for more than one month due to possible side effects).

Efficacy
Visible results after one month in most cases.

Risks/benefits
Risks:
- Nausea and vomiting likely if alcohol is taken
- Use caution in hepatic and renal impairment, central nervous system disease, or history of seizures

Benefit: Useful when standard antibiotic treatments are not effective

Side effects and adverse reactions
- Central nervous system: dizziness, headache, seizures, ataxia, peripheral neuropathy
- Gastrointestinal: nausea, vomiting, taste disturbance, diarrhea, abdominal pain, dry mouth, anorexia, constipation
- Genitourinary: urination difficulties, cystitis, vaginal dryness
- Hematologic: blood cell disorders
- Skin: rashes, itching, flushing

Interactions (other drugs)
- Alcohol ■ Antiepileptics ■ Anticoagulants ■ Barbiturates ■ Carbamazepine ■ Cholestyramine ■ Cimetidine ■ Colestipol ■ Disulfiram ■ Fluorouracil ■ Lithium

Contraindications
- Pregnancy and breast-feeding ■ Blood dyscrasias

Acceptability to patient
Moderate due to possible side effects.

Follow up plan
Ask patient to return in one month for review.

Patient and caregiver information
Patients should be warned not to expect any visible results for at least 2 weeks.

METRONIDAZOLE GEL
Used to control symptoms of rosacea.

Dose
- 0.75% gel, topical application: twice daily, after washing, for 2 months
- 1% solution, topical application: once daily for 2 months

Efficacy
Visible results after 3 weeks in most cases.

Risks/benefits
Risks:
- Avoid contact with the eyes
- Blood dyscrasia (either past or present)

Benefit: Low toxicity compared with oral administration

Side effects and adverse reactions
- Skin: burning, irritation, dryness, redness (transient)
- Central nervous system: numbness or tingling of the extremities
- Gastrointestinal: nausea, metallic taste in the mouth

Interactions (other drugs)
- **Oral anticoagulants**

Contraindications
- **Hypersensitivity to metronidazole or any constituents of the gel** ■ **Pregnancy and breast-feeding**

Acceptability to patient
High.

Follow up plan
Ask patient to return in one month for review.

Patient and caregiver information
- Patients should be warned not to expect any visible results for at least 3 weeks
- Patients should be warned to avoid contact between the gel and their eyes

CLINDAMYCIN TOPICAL
Available as lotion, solution, gel, or solution pledgets; this is an off-label indication.

Dose
- Apply topically to affected area twice daily
- Can be used chronically or as needed for flare-ups

Efficacy
As effective as 12-week course of oral tetracycline.

Risks/benefits
Risks:
- Hypersensitivity to clindamycin or lincomycin
- Use caution in pregnancy and lactation
- May irritate the eyes; avoid contact with the eyes
- May cause an unpleasant taste if contacts the mouth; caution required when administered near the mouth

Benefit: Effective as topical agent with minimal systemic absorption

Side effects and adverse reactions
- Skin: burning, itching, dryness, redness, oiliness, peeling, Gram-negative folliculitis
- Gastrointestinal: abdominal pain, diarrhea (sometimes bloody), colitis

Interactions (other drugs)
- None listed

Contraindications
- Hypersensitivity to clindamycin or lincomycin ▪ Regional enteritis (past or present) ▪ Ulcerative colitis (past or present) ▪ History of antibiotic-induced colitis

Acceptability to patient
Burning, itching, and dryness that can occur may be unacceptable to some patients. They may decrease applications to avoid this, resulting in decreased effectiveness of treatment.

Follow up plan
Ask patient to return in one month for review.

Patient and caregiver information
- Patients should be warned not to expect any visible results for at least 2–4 weeks
- Irritating symptoms will probably occur before there is evidence of clinical improvement
- Patients should understand that this is a chronic disorder that will wax and wane, and that preventive measures need to be continued even if medication is effective

ISOTRETINOIN

Used to control symptoms of rosacea and usually only given by a dermatologist; this is an off-label indication.

Dose
- 500mcg/kg/day orally with food for one month
- If good response, continue for further 3 months
- If little response, up to 1mg/kg/day for 3 months
- If intolerant, reduce dose to 200mcg/kg/day

Efficacy
Most patients see dramatic improvement and control of all symptoms except ocular involvement.

Risks/benefits
Risks:
- Can aggravate any ocular involvement
- Risk of mucocutaneous irritation, musculoskeletal symptoms, hyperlipidemia
- Risk of pseudotumor cerebri, diminished night vision

Benefit: Useful in severe cases and when standard antibiotic treatments are not effective

Side effects and adverse reactions
- Eyes, ears, nose, and throat: conjuctivitis
- Gastrointestinal: abdominal pain
- Hematologic: hematuria, increase in serum lipids
- Musculoskeletal: arthralgias/myalgias
- Skin: dryness of skin, epidermal fragility, may exacerbate ocular involvement at higher doses, cheilitis/drying of mucosal membranes

Interactions (other drugs)
- Vitamin A (enhances toxic effects) ▪ Tetracyline, minocycline (associated with pseudotumor cerebri or papilledema)

Contraindications
■ Pregnancy and breast-feeding ■ Renal or hepatic impairment ■ Hypervitaminosis A ■ Hyperlipidemia

Acceptability to patient
■ Pregnancy must be excluded before starting therapy. During therapy two different methods of contraception must be used and continued for two menstrual cycles following cessation of therapy
■ Wide range of significant side effects
■ Extensive monitoring required

Follow up plan
■ Patient requires extensive monitoring
■ Initially review at one-month and then 3-month intervals
■ Monitor: hepatic function and plasma lipids, blood glucose in diabetic patients, signs of keratitis, any significant side effects

Patient and caregiver information
■ Patients should be warned not to expect any visible results for at least 3 weeks
■ Patients should note any side effects

CROTAMITON LOTION
Dose
Apply topically for 12h once daily.

Efficacy
Effective in eliminating *Demodex folliculorum* infestation, a probable contributor to rosacea.

Risks/benefits
Risks:
■ Use caution with children and infants
■ Use caution in pregnancy and nursing mothers
■ Avoid use near eyes or on broken skin

Benefits:
■ Topical application with no systemic toxicity
■ Well tolerated, with minimal incidence of side effects such as rash, burning, itching
■ May be helpful in rosacea patients who have not responded to topical or systemic antibiotic therapy

Side effects and adverse reactions
Skin: irritation, rashes, contact dermatitis.

Interactions (other drugs)
■ None listed

Contraindications
■ Inflammation and abrasions in skin or mucous membranes

Acceptability to patient
Rarely a problem with a single application and limited incidence of side effects.

Follow up plan
Ask patient to return in one month for review.

Patient and caregiver information
Patients should be warned not to expect any visible results for at least 2–4 weeks.

Other therapies
SUNSCREEN
Efficacy
- Can be very effective in preventing flare-ups and in managing acute episodes
- Patient must use a sunscreen that does not cause irritation
- Alcohol-based sunscreens are more expensive but are less likely to exacerbate pustule formation

Acceptability to patient
High when benefits have been explained.

LIFESTYLE
- Avoidance of a variety of factors that can precipitate a flare-up of the flushing and skin changes (listed in order of occurrence): sun exposure, stress, hot weather, alcohol consumption, spicy foods, exercise, wind, hot baths, cold weather, hot drinks, skin-care products, certain drugs
- Education about these triggers can help patients to gain control over rosacea and this is an important part of therapy

RISKS/BENEFITS
Benefit: can be very effective in preventing flare-ups and in managing acute episodes of rosacea.

ACCEPTABILITY TO PATIENT
High when benefits have been explained.

FOLLOW UP PLAN
Patients should note factors that they believe may be triggers for review at each visit.

PATIENT AND CAREGIVER INFORMATION
Avoidance of triggers must be consistent.

EFFICACY OF THERAPIES
- Most cases respond well to oral antibiotics
- In difficult cases, oral metronidazole can be tried
- In all cases improvement will be gradual, with results seen in one month and courses of therapy lasting 5 months or more

Review period
One-month intervals.

PROGNOSIS
- Untreated, rosacea tends to be a persistent disease with periods of relapse and remission
- Combinations of antibiotic treatment, topical treatments and lifestyle recommendations will slow or halt chronic course of the disease in most cases and individuals can experience remission for many years
- A small number of individuals are resistant to therapy and will go on to develop advanced-stage disease
- Prognosis for eye involvement is excellent except in cases of ocular keratitis

Clinical pearls
- Careful attention to reducing triggers and calming flushing/blushing with cool compresses can be quite helpful. The motivated patient can learn a variety of tricks, which are useful in subsets of patients, from on-line resources
- Using alcohol-based sunscreens may prevent the exacerbation of pustules by oil-based products
- Patients need to understand that, just because they may be protected from the sun, they still need to stay cool

Therapeutic failure
- Failure to respond to antibiotic and topical therapy is rare: refer to dermatologist for possible isotretinoin treatment
- In cases where ocular involvement fails to respond to treatment, refer to ophthalmologist

Recurrence
- Periods of relapse and remission are a common feature of rosacea
- Consider referral to dermatologist if relapse is refractory to antibiotic and topical treatment

Deterioration
- Consider referral to dermatologist if skin changes deteriorate
- Consider referral to ophthalmologist if eye involvement deteriorates

COMPLICATIONS
- Mild eye involvement: conjunctivitis, blepharitis, irritation
- Serious eye involvement: keratitis
- Persistent edema leading to coarsening of skin and features
- Rhinophyma (usually only in men)
- Rosacea fulminans (pyoderma faciale): sudden onset of coalescing nodules, abscesses and sinuses which occurs very rarely. Consider referral to dermatologist
- Lupoid rosacea: clusters of large, dull red papules which are resistant to standard treatment. Consider referral to dermatologist
- Steroid rosacea: extremely severe symptoms following erroneous treatment of rosacea with topical steroids

CONSIDER CONSULT

- Consider referral to dermatologist: when symptoms do not improve with antibiotic and topical treatment, when rosacea fulminans is suspected, when lupoid rosacea is suspected
- Consider referral to ophthalmologist in cases of deteriorating ocular involvement

RISK FACTORS

- Fair-skinned 'flusher and blusher': associated with high risk of developing rosacea
- Patient has been taking a topical or oral steroid treatment: steroid treatments can precipitate first flare-up of rosacea in susceptible patients or can exacerbate symptoms in existing disease

MODIFY RISK FACTORS
Lifestyle and wellness
ALCOHOL AND DRUGS
Alcohol should be avoided if it precipitates symptoms.

DIET
Hot drinks and spicy food should be avoided if they precipitate symptoms.

ENVIRONMENT
Exposure to cold, heat or wind may precipitate symptoms and should be avoided where possible.

FAMILY HISTORY
40% of sufferers have a family member with the disease; where there is a family history, lifestyle recommendations should be followed where possible.

DRUG HISTORY
OTC acne treatments and treatments containing steroids can precipitate first flare-up of rosacea in susceptible patients or can exacerbate symptoms in existing disease.

PREVENT RECURRENCE

- Most patients at some point have a relapse of symptoms following a period of treatment, and lifestyle-induced remission
- Following the lifestyle recommendations is the most effective way of preventing relapse

Reassess coexisting disease
Consider withdrawal of steroid treatments for any less serious coexisting disease.

ASSOCIATIONS

National Rosacea Society
800 South Northwest Highway
Suite 200
Barrington, IL 60010
Tel: 1-888-NO-BLUSH
www.rosacea.org

Rosacea Awareness Program
368 Notre Dame Street West
Montreal (Quebec)
Canada, H2Y 1T9
Tel: 1-888-767-2232
www.rosaceainfo.com

KEY REFERENCES

- Rook A, Wilkinson DS, Ebling FJG. Textbook of dermatology. Malden (MA): Blackwell Science, 1986
- Habif. Clinical dermatology. Philadelphia: Mosby, 2002
- Freedberg I, Eisen, Wolff, et al. Fitzpatrick's dermatology in general medicine. New York: McGraw-Hill, 2000
- Sams WM, Lynch PJ. Principles and practice of dermatology. New York: Churchill Livingstone, 1990
- Millikan L. Recognizing rosacea. Postgrad Med 1999;105(2):149–50,153–8
- Zuber TJ. Rosacea. Primare Care 2000;27(2);309–18
- Thiboutot DM. Acne and rosacea. New and emerging therapies. Dermatol Clin 2000;18(1):63–71

FAQS
Question 1
What are the key distinguishing features of acne vulgaris and acne rosacea?

ANSWER 1
Acne vulgaris usually features comedones and rosacea does not. Acne rosacea usually features some degree of sebaceous hypertrophy and telangiectasia and acne vulgaris does not.

Question 2
My patient has erythema of the central face that is worsened by sunlight suggesting rosacea, yet has comedones in the ear, suggesting acne vulgaris. How do I reconcile these findings?

ANSWER 2
While concomitant acne vulgaris and rosacea can occur, one should seek a diagnosis that explains both findings. One should consider the possibility that the facial lesion represents a butterfly rash and the ear lesion is a discoid lesion with follicular plugging, suggesting a diagnosis of lupus erythematosus.

Question 3
My young adult patient has a parent with rosacea and easily flushes. What is the likelihood that she will develop rosacea?

ANSWER 3
While precise estimates are not available, your patient is demonstrating the flusher/blusher phenotype of an early rosacea patient. In the context of a positive family history, your patient has a high likelihood of progressive rosacea.

CONTRIBUTORS
Russell C Jones, MD, MPH
Seth R Stevens, MD
Richard Averitte, MD

ACNE VULGARIS

DESCRIPTION

- Acne vulgaris is the most common skin disorder
- Chronic disease of sebaceous follicle, primarily affecting face, chest, and back
- Onset typically occurs at puberty because of increased sebum production triggered by increased androgen levels
- Inflammation is due in part to over-proliferation of *Propionibacterium acnes*, an anaerobic Gram-positive organism that resides in follicles
- Classified on basis of type of lesions (comedonal noninflammatory vs inflammatory) and number of lesions present

URGENT ACTION

Although rare, a deterioration in acne accompanied by a high fever and myalgias may indicate acne fulminans, an acute ulcerative acne with systemic symptoms which is usually treated with oral corticosteroids.

KEY! DON'T MISS!

Severe acne accompanied by fever and musculoskeletal symptoms may indicate acne fulminans.

ICD9 CODE
706.1 Other acne

SYNONYMS
Acne.

CARDINAL FEATURES
- Chronic disease of sebaceous follicle, primarily affecting face, chest, and back
- Onset typically occurs at puberty because of increased sebum production triggered by increased androgen levels. Virtually all adolescents will be affected to varying degrees
- Follicular disruption of the comedo
- Comedonal lesions precede inflammatory lesions (papules, pustules)
- Scarring may result
- Treatment is based on type of lesions and number of lesions present

CAUSES
Common causes
- Increased androgen production
- Overactivity/hyperresponsiveness of sebaceous glands in response to androgens
- Colonization of *Propionibacterium acnes*, which metabolizes sebum to free fatty acid, leading to inflammatory lesions

Rare causes
Industrial exposure to halogenated hydrocarbons.

Serious causes
- Adrenal hyperplasia
- Polycystic ovarian syndrome

Contributory or predisposing factors
- Hot, humid climates
- Adolescence
- Hair greases or oil-based cosmetics
- Sports equipment rubbing and occluding skin
- Medications with iodine (found in some cough medicines)
- Some prescription drugs: lithium, isoniazid, phenytoin, corticosteroids, anabolic steroids, and oral contraceptives with high androgenic activity

EPIDEMIOLOGY
Incidence and prevalence
Nearly 100% of adolescents are affected; only 15% seek medical advice.

INCIDENCE
150/1000 adolescents.

PREVALENCE
- 1000/1000 at age 16 years
- 80/1000 ages 25–34 years
- 30/1000 ages 35–44 years

Demographics

AGE

- Triggered at adolescence
- Most severe between 16 and 18 years of age

GENDER

Equally common in males and females; tends to be more severe in males, but more persistent (into mid-20s or even later) in females.

RACE

Nodulocystic acne is more common in European-Americans than African-Americans.

GENETICS

50% of patients have a family history of acne.

DIFFERENTIAL DIAGNOSIS
Acne rosacea
Acne rosacea is a chronic facial skin disorder most commonly seen in individuals between the ages of 30 and 60 years.

FEATURES
- No comedonal stage
- Diffuse inflammation in center of face with seborrhea, telangiectasia, and erythematous papules, sebaceous hyperplasia and/or pustules
- Unlike acne vulgaris, acne rosacea rarely occurs on the chest, back, shoulders, or scalp

Folliculitis
Folliculitis is inflammation of hair follicles resulting from injury, infection, or irritation.

FEATURES
- Painful yellow pustules surrounded by erythema
- A central hair is present in pustules
- May increase in size if located in an area that is shaved
- May be associated with poorly chlorinated hot tubs (*Pseudomonas* folliculitis)

SIGNS & SYMPTOMS
Signs
- Open comedones (blackheads)
- Closed comedones (whiteheads)
- Papules/pustules
- Nodules/cysts
- Scarring
- Hypertrophy of sebaceous glands
- Oily skin

Symptoms
Numerous, sometimes painful, pus-filled lesions.

ASSOCIATED DISORDERS
- Acne mechanica: caused by mechanical pressure from sports or occupational equipment
- Acne fulminans: acute, febrile, ulcerative acne with inflamed and tender lesions on back and chest that heal by scarring; primarily occurs in males, and may be associated with bone lesions and musculoskeletal syndromes
- Acne conglobata: large abscesses with scarring occurring mostly in young males. Associated with dissecting cellulitis of the scalp (also known as perifolliculitis capitis abscedens et suffodiens of the scalp) and hidradenitis suppurativa
- Hidradenitis suppurativa: chronic, pus-filled lesions of axilla, groin, and perianal area occurring mostly in females. Can progress to disfiguring sinus tracts and malodorous discharge
- Acne excoriee des jeunes filles: mild acne accompanied by extensive excoriation and linear scarring, caused by patients picking lesions
- Infantile acne: begins at 3–6 months of age; may be associated with increased risk of acne vulgaris later in life

KEY! DON'T MISS!
Severe acne accompanied by fever and musculoskeletal symptoms may indicate acne fulminans.

CONSIDER CONSULT

- Acne excoriee des jeunes filles may require referral for psychiatric evaluation
- Severe acne accompanied by musculoskeletal symptoms may need to be referred to an oncologist to rule out malignant bone lesions
- If accompanied by hirsutism and irregular menses, then referral for evaluation of androgen excess/polycystic ovary disease may be indicated

INVESTIGATION OF THE PATIENT
Direct questions to patient

Q For how long has acne been a problem for you/how frequently is acne a problem for you? May identify premenstrual flares.

Q Are you using any other medications? Corticosteroids, anabolic steroids, isoniazid, phenytoin, and oral contraceptives with high androgenic activity may worsen acne.

Q Are you experiencing any other symptoms? If patient is generally well, acne fulminans is unlikely even if acne is severe.

Q Do you have a history of oligomenorrhea or hirsutism? If present, these hormonal abnormalities may suggest acne caused by hyperandrogenism. Polycystic ovarian syndrome and adrenal hyperplasia should be considered.

Q Do you use hormonal contraception? Some hormonal contraceptives worsen acne whereas others (low androgens) have been shown to be beneficial.

Contributory or predisposing factors

Q What recreational sports do you play? Shoulder pads, helmets, and chinstraps may exacerbate acne.

Q What are your dress code requirements at work? Helmets/hard hats may exacerbate acne.

Q What type of cosmetics/hair products do you use? Oil-based cosmetics and greasy hair products may contribute to acne.

Family history

Q Do other members of your family have acne? 50% of patients have a positive family history.

Examination

- Examine the affected areas of skin, noting the type of lesions and how many lesions are present. Treatment depends on acne classification
- Perform a general examination and measure the patient's temperature in order to determine whether the patient is generally well. Acute onset/worsening of acne coupled with fever and musculoskeletal symptoms may indicate acne fulminans

Summary of investigative tests

- Laboratory work is not routinely needed for most patients with acne
- Testosterone and metabolites, as well as luteinizing hormone (LH) and follicle-stimulating hormone (FSH) ratio, are particularly useful in identifying hyperandrogenism as a cause of acne in women with treatment-resistant, late-onset, or persistent lesions

DIAGNOSTIC DECISION

Diagnosis is based on the clinical features:
- Mild acne: few to several papules/pustules and no nodules
- Moderate acne: several to many papules/pustules and few to several nodules
- Severe acne: numerous or extensive papules/pustules and many nodules

Guidelines
- The American Academy of Dermatology. Guidelines for care of acne vulgaris. [1]
- Pochi PE, Shalita AR, Strauss JS, et al. Report of the Consensus Conference on Acne Classification. Washington, D.C., March 24 and 25, 1990. [2]

CLINICAL PEARLS
Usually the diagnosis of acne vulgaris is not difficult. Distinction from acne rosacea can normally be made based on younger patient age, presence of comedones, and absence of sebaceous hyperplasia. Chest and back are frequently involved in acne vulgaris and rarely in rosacea.

THE TESTS
Body fluids
TESTOSTERONE AND METABOLITES
Description
Blood sample.

Advantages/Disadvantages
Advantages:
- Simple test
- May identify androgen excess as a contributing cause of acne

Normal
Testosterone:
- Males: 280–1100ng/dL (9.72–38.17nmol/L)
- Females: 15–70ng/dL (0.52–2.43nmol/L)

Dehydroepiandrosterone sulfate (DHEAS):
- Males: 1.7–6.7mcg/mL (4.6–18.2mcmol/L)
- Females: premenopausal 0.5–5.4mcg/mL (1.4–14.7mcmol/L); postmenopausal 0.3–2.6mcg/mL (0.8–7.1mcmol/L)

Abnormal
- Values elevated above normal
- Keep in mind the possibility of a false-positive result

DHEAS:
- 4000–8000ng/mL: associated with congenital adrenal hyperplasia
- >8000ng/mL: rule out adrenal tumor

Cause of abnormal result
- Ovarian tumor
- Adrenal tumor
- Dehydroepiandrosterone supplements

Drugs, disorders and other factors that may alter results
Athletes taking dehydroepiandrosterone supplements.

LUTEINIZING HORMONE (LH) AND FOLLICLE-STIMULATING HORMONE (FSH) RATIO
Description
Blood sample.

Advantages/Disadvantages
Advantages:
- Simple test
- May identify androgen excess as a contributing cause of acne

Normal
LH/FSH ratio <2.

Abnormal
Values elevated above normal.

Cause of abnormal result
- Polycystic ovary disease
- Ovarian tumor

CONSIDER CONSULT
- Recalcitrant nodular or cystic acne or acne that leaves deep facial scars may require referral to a dermatologist

PATIENT AND CAREGIVER ISSUES
Patient or caregiver request
- **I heard that sexual activity/masturbation causes acne. Is this true?** Acne occurs due to overactive and plugged oil glands
- **Does having acne mean that I do not wash frequently enough or scrub hard enough?** Acne is caused by plugged oil glands. Washing gently with a mild soap twice daily is sufficient. Avoid scrubbing as this only irritates the oil glands and may contribute to inflammation
- **Do I need to avoid chocolate or fried foods?** Acne is not caused by chocolate or fried foods. No dietary restrictions exist when treating acne
- **Can I 'pop' the lesions?** It is best not to squeeze the lesions because of risk of infection and potential scarring
- **How long will it take to see a response from medication?** This will depend on the drug used. Typically effects may be observed after 4 weeks, but 8–12 weeks are usually required for maximal response

Health-seeking behavior
- **Have you tried any other medications, and what results have you had?** Provides insight into products that cause excessive irritation or allergic reactions. May assist in determining whether treatment failures were due to insufficient compliance or duration of use
- **Are you currently using any medications to treat acne?** Many nonprescription acne medications are irritating and may limit patient tolerability of more effective therapies

MANAGEMENT ISSUES
Goals
- Lessen physical discomfort from inflamed lesions
- Improve patient's appearance
- Avoid adverse psychologic impact
- Prevent or minimize scarring

Management in special circumstances
- Females of child-bearing potential present some unique circumstances
- Antibiotic therapy, frequently used to treat inflammatory acne, may reduce the effectiveness of oral contraceptives
- All females should have a negative serum pregnancy test and be using effective contraception before receiving isotretinoin
- Tetracyclines have adverse effects on bone and teeth development in utero, and should be avoided during pregnancy or in children

COEXISTING MEDICATION
Advise women relying on hormonal therapy for contraceptive purposes that a backup method of birth control should be considered while using antibiotics concomitantly.

SPECIAL PATIENT GROUPS
Avoid isotretinoin in females who are pregnant or possibly could become pregnant, because this drug may result in teratogenic effects.

Most patients report an improvement in acne following several months of therapy. Most side effects are associated with skin irritation.

SUMMARY OF THERAPEUTIC OPTIONS
Choices
The appropriate choice of drug depends upon the type of acne (comedonal, inflammatory) and its severity (mild, moderate, severe).

Topical – nonantibiotics:
- Salicylic acid is a comedolytic and may be used for noninflammatory acne
- Benzoyl peroxide is an effective antimicrobial and comedolytic for treating inflammatory and noninflammatory acne
- Tazarotene possesses comedolytic properties, making it a choice for mild-to-moderate facial acne. However, it is expensive
- Azelaic acid is effective for mild-to-moderate inflammatory acne because of its antimicrobial and comedolytic properties. It is also useful for noninflammatory acne. It may be less irritating than other preparations
- Adapalene is as efficacious as tretinoin for mild-to-moderate noninflammatory acne, with greater tolerability
- Tretinoin is the drug of choice for treating moderate-to-severe noninflammatory comedonal acne. Tretinoin prevents new comedones from forming and eliminates those that are already present

Antibiotics - topical and systemic:
- Antibiotics may be used in the treatment of inflammatory acne. They improve acne by inhibiting the growth of *Propionibacterium acnes*, thus decreasing the concentration of free fatty acids and the resultant inflammatory lesions. Tetracyclines in particular have some anti-inflammatory properties as well. Oral and topical preparations may be used
- Some of the choices include tetracycline and its derivatives minocycline and doxycycline (first-line oral agents), erythromycin (oral agent of choice for pregnant women, young children, and those unable to tolerate tetracycline derivatives), topical benzoyl peroxide/erythromycin (where the combination of drugs has a synergistic effect and reduces risk of resistance to erythromycin)
- Clindamycin is a second-choice antibiotic because of its potential for pseudomembranous colitis
- Metronidazole is a topical antibiotic that is useful for mild inflammatory acne
- Trimethoprim/sulfamethoxazole is useful for treating resistant pustular acne or for acne lesions that contain Gram-negative organisms, which sometimes occur following the eradication of *P. acnes*
- Ampicillin is useful for mild-to-moderate inflammatory acne that is not responsive to tetracycline and for treating cysts/pustules caused by Gram-negative organisms following long-term use of oral antibiotics
- Cephalexin is useful for treating antibiotic-resistant pustular acne caused by *P. acnes*

Systemic – nonantibiotics:
- Ethinyl estradiol/norgestimate and other oral contraceptives with no or minimal androgenic effects are an effective treatment for moderate inflammatory acne caused by excessive androgen secretion in females
- Spironolactone functions as an androgen receptor blocker and inhibitor of 5-alpha reductase, and may be an effective treatment for acne that is unresponsive to first-line agents

- Oral corticosteroids in high doses are restricted to recalcitrant severe acne for limited periods of time because of the potential side effects. Low dosages are indicated in those with demonstrated androgen excess or in those with elevated dehydroepiandrosterone sulfate (DHEAS) associated with an 11- or 21-hydroxylase deficiency
- Isotretinoin is used for severe, nodulocystic acne or moderate noncystic inflammatory acne with the potential for scarring. It may induce a prolonged remission

Intralesional:
- Intralesional corticosteroids such as triamcinolone acetonide are effective for treating individual nodulocystic lesions

Alternative treatments:
- As a rich source of chromium, brewer's yeast may be a natural alternative for treatment of acne

Nondrug treatments:
- Lesion extraction or drainage may be necessary to remove open comedones and speed healing of pustules/cysts
- When excessive scarring is present, cryotherapy, dermabrasion, laser resurfacing, chemical peels, punch grafting, and collagen injections may be performed

Guidelines
- The American Academy of Dermatology. Guidelines for care of acne vulgaris. [1]

The American Academy of Family Physicians has produced the following:
- Johnson BA, Nunley JR. Use of systematic agents in the treatment of acne vulgaris. [3]
- Russell JJ. Topical therapy for acne. [4]

Clinical pearls
- Patients should be off isotretinoin therapy for at least 6 months before undergoing a resurfacing procedure (e.g. dermabrasion) because of poor wound healing
- Some dermatologists rotate minocycline (in summer) and doxycycline (in winter) to reduce risk of adverse effects (lupus-like syndrome and photosensitivity, respectively)
- Lack of compliance and follow up can be significant barriers to successful treatment in adolescents. In particular, if parents have insisted that the adolescent patient seek treatment, then he/she may perceive this long-term treatment as being imposed on them. It is important to address these issues early

Never
Never prescribe isotretinoin to females without first obtaining a negative serum pregnancy result and establishing that reliable contraceptive methods are used.

FOLLOW UP
Initially, patients should be followed biweekly or monthly for assessment of acne and adverse effects from medication.

Plan for review
If improvements are not observed after adequate trials on a given medication and the patient has been compliant, then additional pharmacologic agents may be added or substituted, or a consult with a dermatologist may be indicated.

Information for patient or caregiver

- Acne exacerbations may occur initially after drug therapies are initiated
- Skin irritation commonly occurs, but usually resolves with continued medication use
- Compliance and follow up are important to assess success
- Long-term treatment may be necessary

DRUGS AND OTHER THERAPIES: DETAILS
Drugs
BENZOYL PEROXIDE

- Liquid (2.5–10%)
- Bar (5–10%)
- Mask (5%)
- Lotion (5–10%)
- Cream (5–10%)
- Gel (2.5–20%)
- Cleanser (10%)

Dose

- Cleanser: wash once or twice daily
- Other dosage forms: initially apply topically once daily; increase frequency to two or three times daily as tolerated/indicated

Efficacy

- Effective as an antibacterial agent with mild comedolytic properties
- Used for mild-to-moderate inflammatory or noninflammatory acne

Risks/benefits
Risks:

- Skin irritation: scaling, erythema, edema
- Bleaching of hair and colored fabrics

Benefits:

- May improve acne
- Kills bacteria through direct effects

Side effects and adverse reactions

- Skin irritation: peeling, erythema, edema
- Contact dermatitis

Interactions (other drugs)

- Tretinoin: increased skin irritation

Contraindications

- Known sensitivity to benzoyl peroxide or any of its components

Evidence
An RCT compared isotretinoin gel, its vehicle base, and benzoyl peroxide in patients with mild-to-moderate acne vulgaris. Benzoyl peroxide significantly reduced inflamed and noninflamed lesions at 4, 8, and 12 weeks. Isotretinoin also significantly reduced inflamed and noninflamed lesions, but was not as rapid in effect for inflamed lesions as benzoyl peroxide. Acne grade improved significantly by 4 weeks in the benzoyl peroxide-treated patients, and by 8 weeks in the isotretinoin-treated patients [5] *Level P*

Acceptability to patient
Excessive skin irritation may necessitate discontinuation of medication.

Follow up plan
- Evaluate patient at 4- to 5-week intervals
- Substitute a topical or oral antibiotic or consider alternative treatment if no response is observed following several weeks of therapy

Patient and caregiver information
- May cause transitory warmth or stinging sensation on skin
- Patient should expect drying and peeling
- Avoid contact with hair and fabrics
- Avoid other sources of skin irritation (sunlamps/sunlight, other topical acne medications)
- PABA (para-aminobenzoic acid)-containing sunscreens may cause transient skin irritation

TRETINOIN
- Cream (0.025–0.1%)
- Gel (0.025–0.1%)
- Liquid (0.05%) – most irritating

Dose
- Initiate therapy with lowest dose cream
- Apply topically once daily at bedtime
- Consider every other day application for sensitive or fair skin

Efficacy
Drug of choice for treating moderate-to-severe noninflammatory comedonal acne.

Risks/benefits
Risks:
- Severe local irritation
- Photosensitivity

Benefits:
- May improve acne
- May improve associated dyspigmentation, particularly in medium to darkly pigmented patients

Side effects and adverse reactions
Skin irritation: redness, edema, blistering, or crusting of sensitive skin, photosensitivity.

Interactions (other drugs)
- Tretinoin is photolabile (therefore, apply at bedtime) and demonstrates chemical instability in the presence of benzoyl peroxide (therefore, avoid applying benzoyl peroxide and tretinoin at the same time of the day) - Sulfur, resorcinol, benzoyl peroxide, salicylic acid: concomitant use may result in significant skin irritation

Contraindications
- Known or suspected pregnancy - Breast-feeding - Sunburn, eczema, or other chronic skin conditions of the face - Sensitivity to sunlight - Concurrent use of photosensitizers (e.g. thiazides, tetracyclines, fluoroquinolones, phenothiazines, sulfonamides) because of the possibility of augmented phototoxicity

Evidence
In a 12-week RCT, tretinoin 0.025% creams were found to be significantly superior to placebo in patients with mild-to-moderate acne [6] *Level P*

Acceptability to patient
Excessive skin irritation may necessitate discontinuation.

Follow up plan
Alternative treatment should be selected if adaptation to irritating effects has not occurred after 6 weeks or if improvements are not evident following 12 weeks of therapy.

Patient and caregiver information
- May cause acne flare-ups initially during first 2–4 weeks of treatment
- To be applied at bedtime, 30min after washing
- Patient should avoid excessive exposure to sunlight/sunlamps
- Transitory warmth or stinging sensation on skin may be experienced
- Redness and peeling are likely. Patient should discontinue use if discomfort is excessive

ADAPALENE
- Gel (0.1%)
- Cream (0.1%)

Dose
Apply a thin film topically once daily, usually at bedtime.

Efficacy
As efficacious as tretinoin for mild-to-moderate noninflammatory acne, with greater tolerability.

Risks/benefits
Risk: skin irritation
Benefit: may improve acne with less irritation and in a quicker manner than tretinoin

Side effects and adverse reactions
Skin irritation: burning, itching, drying, erythema, peeling.

Interactions (other drugs)
- Adapalene is photostable and demonstrates chemical stability in the presence of benzoyl peroxide

Contraindications
- Adapalene cream and gel should not be administered to individuals who are hypersensitive to adapalene or any of the components in the cream vehicle or gel

Evidence
A multicenter RCT compared adapalene 0.1% solution with tretinoin 0.025% gel over 12 weeks in patients with acne vulgaris. Both treatments were found to be clinically and statistically effective in reducing inflammatory and noninflammatory lesions compared with baseline [7] *Level P*

Acceptability to patient
Well tolerated by patients.

Follow up plan
Consider alternative treatment if results are not evident after 8–12 weeks of therapy.

Patient and caregiver information
- To be applied at bedtime after washing
- Exacerbation may occur initially
- Local skin irritation, including burning and itching are common after application

TAZAROTENE
Gel (0.05–0.1%).

Dose
Cleanse the face gently. After the skin is dry, apply a thin film of tazarotene ($2mg/cm^2$) once a day, in the evening, to the skin where acne lesions appear. Use enough to cover the entire affected area. Tazarotene was investigated for up to 12 weeks during clinical trials for acne.

Efficacy
- Effective for mild-to-moderate comedonal acne
- Offers no apparent advantage over tretinoin or adapalene

Risks/benefits
Risks:
- Skin irritation
- Very expensive

Benefit: May improve acne

Side effects and adverse reactions
Skin irritation: desquamation, pruritis, burning, stinging, dryness, discoloration.

Interactions (other drugs)
- Tazarotene appears to be photostable ■ Tetracyclines and sulfonamides: concomitant administration may increase risk of photosensitization

Contraindications
- Pregnancy category X

Evidence
An RCT compared topical tazarotene gel vs vehicle gel in patients with mild-to-moderate facial acne vulgaris. Compared with its vehicle, treatment with tazarotene gel resulted in significantly greater reductions in noninflammatory and total lesion counts at all follow up visits, and inflammatory lesion counts after 12 weeks [8] *Level P*

Acceptability to patient
Skin irritation may necessitate discontinuation of treatment.

Follow up plan
Consider alternative therapy if improvement is not evident following 12 weeks of treatment.

Patient and caregiver information
- Application may cause transitory burning or stinging
- Excessive exposure to sunlight/sunlamps should be avoided
- Not to be used on sunburned skin until fully recovered
- Patient should discontinue if itching, burning, redness, or peeling is excessive

AZELAIC ACID
Cream (20%).

Dose
After the skin is thoroughly washed and patted dry, a thin film of azelaic acid cream 20% should be gently but thoroughly massaged into the affected areas twice daily, in the morning and evening. The hands should be washed following application. The duration of use of azelaic acid cream 20% can vary from person to person and depends on the severity of the acne. Improvement of the condition occurs in the majority of patients with inflammatory lesions within 4 weeks.

Efficacy
- Effective for mild-to-moderate inflammatory acne because of its antimicrobial and comedolytic properties
- As effective as topical tretinoin, benzoyl peroxide, or erythromycin

Risks/benefits
Risks:
- Skin irritation
- Hypopigmentation with darker skin types

Benefits:
- May improve acne
- Reduces postinflammatory hyperpigmentation caused by inflammatory acne
- No photosensitization
- Appropriate therapeutic choice for patients unwilling or unable to avoid the sun

Side effects and adverse reactions
- Skin irritation: pruritus, burning, stinging, erythema, dryness, peeling, rash
- Depigmentation

Interactions (other drugs)
- Tretinoin: beneficial synergistic effects

Contraindications
- Azelaic acid cream 20% is contraindicated in individuals who have shown hypersensitivity to any of its components

Evidence
Azelaic acid 20% cream was compared with its vehicle in a 3-month, double-blind study of patients with moderate inflammatory acne, and was compared with 0.05% tretinoin cream in a 6-month single-blind study of patients with comedonal acne. In both studies, azelaic acid significantly reduced the number of acne lesions, and resulted in clinically relevant improvements. Azelaic acid was significantly more effective than its vehicle, and was as effective as tretinoin in reducing the number of comedones [9] *Level P*

Acceptability to patient
Reported side effects are usually mild and transient, which increases patient compliance and acceptability.

Follow up plan
Consider alternative therapy if improvements are not observed following 12 weeks of treatment.

Patient and caregiver information
- Patient should report abnormal changes in skin color to physician
- Temporary skin irritation may occur if applied to broken or inflamed skin, but this commonly subsides. If irritation persists, patient should apply only once daily or discontinue use until effects have subsided

ERYTHROMYCIN
- Oral solution (1.5–2.0%)
- Gel (2%)
- Ointment (2%)
- Pledget (2%)

Dose
- Oral: 250–500mg twice daily; dosage or frequency of administration may be decreased after control is attained
- Topical pledget: 2% pad should be rubbed over the affected area twice daily after skin is thoroughly washed with warm water and soap and patted dry. Acne lesions on the face, neck, shoulder, chest, and back may be treated in this manner. Additional pledgets may be used, if needed. Each pledget should be used once and discarded
- Topical ointment: apply to the affected area twice daily after the skin is thoroughly washed with warm water and soap and patted dry

Efficacy
- Effective for mild-to-moderate inflammatory acne
- Improves acne by inhibiting growth and activity of *Propionibacterium acnes*, and therefore decreases inflammation

Risks/benefits
Risk: May contribute to the development of antibiotic-resistant micro-organisms

Benefits:
- May improve acne
- Does not cause photosensitivity
- Safe for use during pregnancy, lactation, and in children under 8 years of age

Side effects and adverse reactions
- Oral: gastrointestinal upset
- Genitourinary: *Candida* vaginitis
- Topical: local irritation

Interactions (other drugs)
- Oral contraceptives: antibiotics may decrease contraceptive efficacy

Contraindications
- Hypersensitivity to macrolide antibiotics ■ Epithelial herpes simplex keratitis ■ Fungal infections of the eye, mycobacterial infections of the eye, viral infections (vaccinia, varicella)
- Erythromycin is contraindicated in patients with known hypersensitivity to this antibiotic

Evidence
- Erythromycin 2% gel was compared with its vehicle in a double-blind, controlled trial of patients with mild-to-moderate acne vulgaris. Erythromycin was significantly more effective than its vehicle in reducing the number of inflammatory and noninflammatory lesions [10] *Level P*
- A double-blind study compared systemic erythromycin with doxycycline in patients with facial acne vulgaris. Both antibiotics produced a significant improvement in acne, without any difference between the two therapies [11] *Level P*

Acceptability to patient
Generally well tolerated.

Follow up plan
Consider isotretinoin or referral to a dermatologist if oral antibiotic therapy fails to improve inflammatory acne following 12 weeks of treatment.

Patient and caregiver information
- To be taken with food if stomach upset occurs with oral erythromycin
- Patient should notify physician if any of the following occur with oral erythromycin: nausea, vomiting, diarrhea, stomach cramps, abdominal pain, yellowing of skin or eyes, darkened urine, pale stools, or unusual tiredness

ERYTHROMYCIN/BENZOYL PEROXIDE
Erythromycin (3%)/benzoyl peroxide (5%) gel.

Dose
Apply topically twice daily, morning and evening, or as directed by physician, to affected areas after the skin is thoroughly washed, rinsed with warm water, and gently patted dry.

Efficacy
Synergistic antimicrobial effects treat mild-to-moderate inflammatory acne.

Risks/benefits
Risks:
- Skin irritation
- Photosensitivity

Benefit: The combination of drugs reduces development of *Propionibacterium acnes* resistance to erythromycin

Side effects and adverse reactions
Skin: dryness, erythema, pruritus.

Interactions (other drugs)
- Benzoyl peroxide (increased skin irritation may occur)

Contraindications
- Benzoyl peroxide and erythromycin topical gel is contraindicated in those patients with a history of hypersensitivity to erythromycin, benzoyl peroxide, or any of the other listed ingredients ■ Not for ophthalmic use. Avoid contact with eyes and mucous membranes ■ The use of antibiotic agents may be associated with the overgrowth of antibiotic-resistant organisms ■ Pregnancy category C ■ Breast-feeding ■ Safety and effectiveness in children below the age of 12 have not been established

Evidence
An RCT compared the efficacy of benzoyl peroxide/erythromycin gel with erythromycin/zinc in patients with acne vulgaris. Benzoyl peroxide/erythromycin resulted in significantly fewer inflammatory lesions and fewer comedones [12] *Level P*

Acceptability to patient
Excessive irritation may limit use of medication.

Follow up plan
Consider oral antibiotics if improvements have not been observed after 12 weeks of therapy.

Patient and caregiver information
- May cause transitory warmth or stinging of skin
- Expect dryness and peeling
- Avoid contact with hair and fabrics
- Avoid other sources of skin irritation (sunlight/sunlamps, or other topical medications)
- PABA-containing sunscreens may cause transient skin irritation
- Store in refrigerator; expiration date of 3 months

TETRACYCLINE
- Oral
- Topical solution (2.2mg/mL)
- Topical ointment (3%)

Dose
Oral: 250–500mg twice daily on an empty stomach; dosage or frequency of administration may be decreased after control is attained.

Efficacy
- Effective treatment for mild-to-moderate inflammatory acne by preventing growth and activity of *Propionibacterium acnes*, thereby decreasing inflammation
- Most frequently used oral antibiotic for acne treatment

Risks/benefits
Risks
Oral:
- Compliance can be a problem
- Use caution in patients with hepatic impairment
- Use caution with repeated or prolonged doses

Topical:
- Contains sodium bisulfite, a sulfite that may cause allergic-type reactions including anaphylactic symptoms and life-threatening or less severe asthmatic episodes in certain susceptible people
- For external use only and care should be taken to keep it out of the eyes, nose, and mouth
- Use caution during pregnancy and breast-feeding

Benefit: May improve acne

Side effects and adverse reactions
Oral:

- Cardiovascular system: pericarditis
- Central nervous system: headache, paresthesia, fever
- Gastrointestinal: abdominal pain, diarrhea, heartburn, hepatotoxicity, vomiting, nausea, dental staining, anorexia
- Genitourinary: polyuria, polydipsia, azotemia, *Candida* vaginitis
- Hematologic: blood cell dyscrasias
- Skin: pruritus, rash, photosensitivity, changes in pigmentation, angioedema, stinging
- Other: discoloration of teeth

Topical:

- Skin: severe dermatitis, stinging, burning sensation

Interactions (other drugs)
Oral:

- Antacids ■ Atovaquone ■ Barbiturates ■ Bismuth subsalicyclate ■ Calcium, iron, magnesium, zinc ■ Cephalosporins ■ Cholesytramine, colestipol ■ Carbamazepine ■ Digoxin ■ Ethanol ■ Methoxyflurane ■ Oral contraceptives ■ Penicillins ■ Phenytoin ■ Quinapril ■ Sodium bicarbonate ■ Vitamin A ■ Warfarin

Topical:

- None listed

Contraindications
Oral:

- Pregnancy and breast-feeding ■ Severe renal disease

Topical:

- Safety and effectiveness in children below the age of 11 has not yet been established

Evidence
An RCT compared topical tetracycline, 5% benzoyl peroxide gel, and oral oxytetrocycline in patients with mild-to-moderate acne. Facial acne improved significantly in all three treatment groups [13] *Level P*

Acceptability to patient
Generally well tolerated.

Follow up plan
Consider isotretinoin or referral to a dermatologist if oral antibiotic therapy fails to improve inflammatory acne following 12 weeks of treatment.

Patient and caregiver information

- Patient should avoid excessive sunlight/sunlamps
- Oral: to be taken on an empty stomach; coadministration with milk, antacids, or iron-containing products should be avoided
- Topical: yellowing of skin may occur, which may be minimized by washing
- The use of tetracycline or doxycycline during summer periods can be associated with photosensitivity. All patients should be instructed to cover up and use a sunscreen if they are out in the sun. For patients who feel they cannot comply because of work or lifestyle, another first-line treatment is probably indicated

MINOCYCLINE

Dose

The usual dosage of pellet-filled capsules is 100mg every 12h. Alternatively, if more frequent doses are preferred, two or four 50mg pellet-filled capsules may be given initially followed by one 50mg capsule four times daily.

Efficacy
- Effectively treats mild-to-moderate acne by inhibiting growth of *Propionibacterium acnes*
- Equally efficacious as doxycycline

Risks/benefits

Risks:
- Use of this drug may result in overgrowth of nonsusceptible organisms, including fungi. If superinfection occurs, the antibiotic should be discontinued
- Use caution with renal impairment
- Risk of pseudotumor cerebri (benign intracranial hypertension) in adults
- Photosensitivity manifested by an exaggerated sunburn reaction has been observed
- Central nervous system effects may make driving or operation of machinery hazardous
- Possible risk of neoplasia

Benefits:
- May improve acne
- Absorption is less affected by milk and food than tetracycline

Side effects and adverse reactions
- Cardiovascular system: pericarditis
- Central nervous system: bulging fontanelles in infants and benign intracranial hypertension (pseudotumor cerebri) in adults, headache, light-headedness, dizziness, vertigo
- Gastrointestinal: anorexia, nausea, vomiting, diarrhea, glossitis, dysphagia, enterocolitis, esophagitis and esophageal ulcerations
- Metabolic: pancreatitis, inflammatory lesions (with monilial overgrowth) in the anogenital region, increases in liver enzymes, hepatitis and liver failure
- Musculoskeletal: polyarthralgia
- Hypersensitivity and skin reactions: anaphylaxis, maculopapular erythematous rashes, exfoliative dermatitis, erythema multiforme, Stevens-Johnson syndrome, photosensitivity, pigmentation of the skin and mucous membranes, urticaria, angioneurotic edema, anaphylactoid purpura, exacerbation of systemic lupus erythematosus, pulmonary infiltrates with eosinophilia, transient lupus-like syndrome has also been reported with the capsules
- Hematologic: hemolytic anemia, thrombocytopenia, neutropenia and eosinophilia have been reported
- Renal toxicity: dose-related elevations in blood urea nitrogen (BUN) have been reported
- Other: with prolonged treatment, brown-black microscopic discoloration of the thyroid glands, tooth discoloration and enamel hypoplasia during tooth development

Interactions (other drugs)

Methoxyflurane (has been reported to result in fatal renal toxicity) **Anticoagulants (may depress plasma prothrombin activity)** **Penicillin (bactericidal action may be reduced)** **Oral contraceptives (may reduce effectiveness of contraceptives)** **Antacids containing aluminum, calcium, or magnesium, and iron-containing preparations (may impair absorption of minocycline)**

Contraindications
- **Pregnancy and lactation** **Hypersensitivity to any of the tetracyclines**

Evidence

- A systematic review found that minocycline is likely to be an effective treatment for moderate acne vulgaris; however, the review found no reliable evidence to justify the use of this drug as first-line therapy [14] *Level M*
- A double-blind study compared topical clindamycin with oral minocycline in patients with moderate-to-severe facial acne. Both treatments significantly improved acne grade and inflamed lesion counts from baseline. There was no significant difference between the treatment groups [15] *Level P*

Acceptability to patient
Generally well tolerated.

Follow up plan
Consider isotretinoin or referral to a dermatologist if oral antibiotic therapy fails to improve inflammatory acne following 12 weeks of treatment.

Patient and caregiver information

- Patients should avoid excessive sunlight/sunlamps
- The use of tetracycline or doxycycline during summer periods can be associated with photosensitivity. All patients should be instructed to cover up and use a sunscreen if they are out in the sun. For patients who feel they cannot comply because of work or lifestyle, another first-line treatment is probably indicated

DOXYCYCLINE
Dose
Orally, 100mg/day as a single dose or as 50mg every 12h.

Efficacy

- Effective treatment for mild-to-moderate inflammatory acne by eradication of *Propionibacterium acnes*
- As efficacious as minocycline

Risks/benefits
Risks:

- Compliance can be a problem
- Use caution in patients with hepatic impairment
- Use caution with repeated or prolonged doses

Benefits:

- May improve acne
- Usually less expensive than minocycline
- May be taken without regard to meals

Side effects and adverse reactions

- Cardiovascular system: pericarditis, angioedema
- Central nervous system: fever, headache
- Gastrointestinal: abdominal pain, diarrhea, heartburn, nausea, hepatotoxicity, vomiting, pseudomembranous colitis
- Hematologic: blood cell disorders
- Skin: pruritus, rash, photosensitivity, exfoliative dermatitis

Interactions (other drugs)
* Antacids (magnesium, calcium) * Anticonvulsants (barbiturates, carbamazepine, phenytoin) * Bismuth * Cholestyramine * Ethanol * Mineral supplements (iron, zinc) * Oral contraceptives * Penicillins * Warfarin

Contraindications
* Pregnancy and breast-feeding

Evidence
A double-blind study compared systemic erythromycin with doxycycline in patients with facial acne vulgaris. Both antibiotics produced a significant improvement in acne, without any difference between the two therapies [11] *Level P*

Acceptability to patient
Generally well tolerated.

Follow up plan
Consider isotretinoin therapy or referral to a dermatologist if oral antibiotic therapy fails to improve acne following 12 weeks of treatment.

Patient and caregiver information
* Patient should avoid excessive sunlight/sunlamps
* The use of tetracycline or doxycycline during summer periods can be associated with photosensitivity. All patients should be instructed to cover up and use a sunscreen if they are out in the sun. For patients who feel they cannot comply because of work or lifestyle, another first-line treatment is probably indicated
* May be taken with food or milk

CLINDAMYCIN
* Oral
* Topical solution, lotion, gel (1%)

Dose
* Oral: 75–300mg orally twice daily; may decrease dosage or frequency of administration once control is attained
* Topical: apply topically twice daily

Efficacy
Effective treatment for mild-to-moderate inflammatory acne by inhibiting growth and activity of *Propionibacterium acnes*. Most frequently used topical antibiotic for acne treatment.

Risks/benefits
Risks
Oral:
* Risk of pseudomembranous enterocolitis higher with clindamycin than with other antibiotics, patients developing diarrhea should be instructed to stop treatment immediately
* Use caution in hepatic or renal disease, or history of gastrointestinal disease, and tartrazine dye hypersensitivity
* Treatment failure can occur due to compliance problems

Topical:
- Hypersensitivity to clindamycin or lincomycin
- Caution in pregnancy and lactation
- May irritate the eyes; avoid contact with the eyes
- May cause an unpleasant taste if contacts the mouth; caution required when administered near the mouth

Side effects and adverse reactions
Oral:
- Central nervous system: headache, sleep disturbance, confusion, dizziness
- Gastrointestinal: pseudomembranous enterocolitis, abdominal pain, diarrhea, nausea, vomiting
- Genitourinary: vaginitis
- Hematologic: agranulocytosis
- General: hypersensitivity reactions (most commonly rashes)

Topical:
- Skin: burning, itching, dryness, redness, oiliness, peeling, Gram-negative folliculitis
- Gastrointestinal: abdominal pain, diarrhea (sometimes bloody), colitis

Interactions (other drugs)
Oral:
- **Aminoglycosides** ■ **Antacids** ■ **Loop diuretics** ■ **Probenecid**

Topical:
- **Neuromuscular blocking agents**

Contraindications
- **Hypersensitivity to clindamycin or lincomycin** ■ **Pregnancy category B** ■ **When clindamycin is administered to the pediatric population (birth to 16 years), appropriate monitoring of organ system functions is desirable**

Additional contraindications
Oral:
- **Enteritis**
- **Colitis**

Topical:
- **Regional enteritis (past or present)**
- **Ulcerative colitis (past or present)**
- **History of antibiotic-induced colitis**

Evidence
A double-blind study compared topical clindamycin with oral minocycline in patients with moderate-to-severe facial acne. Both treatments significantly improved acne grade and inflamed lesion counts from baseline. There was no significant difference between the treatment groups [15] *Level P*

Acceptability to patient
Generally well tolerated.

Follow up plan
Consider isotretinoin or referral to a dermatologist if oral antibiotic therapy fails to improve inflammatory acne following 12 weeks of treatment.

Patient and caregiver information
Patient should notify physician if diarrhea occurs.

TRIMETHOPRIM/SULFAMETHOXAZOLE
This is an off-label indication.

Dose
Trimethoprim (160mg)/sulfamethoxazole (800mg) orally twice daily.

Efficacy
Useful for treating resistant pustular acne or for lesions that contain Gram-negative organisms, which sometimes occur following the eradication of *Propionibaterium acnes.*

Risks/benefits
Risks:

- Use caution in renal and hepatic function impairment and G-6-PD deficiency
- Use caution in elderly patients receiving diuretics
- Risk of streptococcal pharyngitis

Benefit: May improve acne

Side effects and adverse reactions
- Central nervous system: seizures, anxiety, aseptic meningitis, ataxia, chills, depression, fatigue, headache, insomnia, vertigo
- Hematologic: agranulocytosis, aplastic anemia, thrombocytopenia, leukopenia, neutropenia, hemolytic anemia, megaloblastic anemia, hypoprothrombinemia, methemoglobinemia, eosinophilia
- Gastrointestinal: hepatitis (including cholestatic jaundice and hepatic necrosis), elevation of serum transaminase and bilirubin, pseudomembranous enterocolitis, pancreatitis, stomatitis, glossitis, nausea, emesis, abdominal pain, diarrhea, anorexia
- Genitourinary: renal failure, interstitial nephritis, BUN and serum creatinine elevation, toxic nephrosis with oliguria and anuria, and crystalluria
- Musculoskeletal: arthralgia, myalgia
- Respiratory: pulmonary infiltrates
- Skin: Stevens-Johnson syndrome, erythema multiforme, exfoliative dermatitis, generalized skin eruptions, photosensitivity, pruritus, urticaria, rash

Interactions (other drugs)
- Dapsone (may cause increased serum concentrations of both dapsone and trimethoprim-sulfamethoxazole) ▪ Disulfiram, metronidazole ▪ Methotrexate (increases methotrexate level) ▪ Oral anticoagulants (increases hypoprothrombinemic response) ▪ Oral hypoglycemics (may cause hypoglycemia) ▪ Phenytoin (may increase phenytoin concentration to toxic levels) ▪ Procainamide (increases procainamide level)

Contraindications
- Megaloblastic anemia secondary to folate deficiency ▪ Renal disease manifested by serum creatinine <15mL/min ▪ Should not be used in breast-feeding women or in pregnant women near term

Acceptability to patient
Generally well tolerated.

Follow up plan
Consider isotretinoin or referral to a dermatologist if oral antibiotics fail to improve inflammatory acne following 12 weeks of treatment.

Patient and caregiver information
- Take medication with a full glass of water
- Avoid excessive sunlight/sunlamps
- Notify physician if any of the following occur: blood in urine, rash, ringing in ears, difficult breathing, fever, sore throat, chills, and mouth sores

AMPICILLIN
This is an off-label indication.

Dose
500mg orally twice daily; dosage or frequency of administration may be decreased after control is attained.

Efficacy
Useful for mild-to-moderate inflammatory acne that is not responsive to tetracycline and for treating cysts/pustules caused by Gram-negative organisms following long-term use of oral antibiotics.

Risks/benefits
Risks:
- Use caution in renal disease, mononucleosis, and hypersensitivity to cephalosporins
- Use caution in prolonged or repeated treatment

Benefit: Safe for use during pregnancy

Side effects and adverse reactions
- Central nervous system: seizures, hallucinations, coma, anxiety
- Gastrointestinal: nausea, diarrhea, vomiting, altered liver function tests, pseudomembranous colitis
- Genitourinary: urinary problems, renal damage, candidiasis, vaginitis
- Hematologic: bleeding disorders, bone marrow depression
- Hypersensitivity reactions

Interactions (other drugs)
- Allopurinol (may increase incidence of rash) ▪ Atenolol ▪ Chloramphenicol (inhibit effect of ampicillin) ▪ Macrolide and tetracycline antibiotics (inhibit effect of ampicillin) ▪ Methotrexate ▪ Oral contraceptives

Contraindications
- Hypersensitivity to penicillins

Acceptability to patient
Generally well tolerated.

Follow up plan
Consider isotretinoin or referral to a dermatologist if oral antibiotic therapy fails to improve inflammatory acne after 12 weeks of therapy.

Patient and caregiver information
- Patient should take medication on an empty stomach
- Patient should notify physician if the following occur: skin rash, hives, diarrhea, breathing difficulties, black tongue, sore throat, nausea, vomiting, fever, swollen joints, unusual bleeding, or bruising

CEPHALEXIN
This is an off-label indication.

Dose
500mg orally twice daily; dosage or frequency of administration may be decreased once control is attained.

Efficacy
Useful for treating antibiotic-resistant pustular acne caused by *Propionibacterium acnes*.

Risks/benefits
Risks:
- Caution in patients with penicillin hypersensitivity
- Use caution in renal impairment and history of gastrointestinal disease
- Use caution in breast-feeding

Benefit: May improve acne

Side effects and adverse reactions
- Central nervous system: headache, sleep disturbance, confusion, dizziness
- Gastrointestinal: anorexia, nausea, diarrhea, abdominal pain
- Hematologic: pancytopenia
- Skin: rashes, erythema multiforme

Interactions (other drugs)
- Aminoglycosides ■ Loop diuretics ■ Probenecid ■ Polymixin B ■ Vancomycin ■ Penicillins ■ Warfarin

Contraindications
- Penicillin and cephalosporin hypersensitivity ■ True penicillin allergy (anaphylaxis, respiratory compromise) ■ True cephalosporin allergy

Acceptability to patient
Generally well tolerated.

Follow up plan
Consider isotretinoin or referral to a dermatologist if oral antibiotic therapy fails to improve acne following 12 weeks of treatment.

Patient and caregiver information
- To be taken with food or milk to minimize stomach upset
- Patient should notify physician if diarrhea occurs

ETHINYL ESTRADIOL/NORGESTIMATE
- Ethinyl estradiol (35mcg)/triphasic norgestimate (0.18mg, 0.215mg, 0.25mg)
- Other oral contraceptive combinations with low adrogenic activity may also be effective

Dose
One active tablet daily for 21 days followed by one placebo tablet for 7 days. After 28 tablets have been taken, a new course is started the next day.

Efficacy
Effective treatment for moderate inflammatory acne caused by excessive androgen secretion in females. Suppresses ovarian androgen levels.

Risks/benefits
Risks:
- Thromboembolic disorders
- Cardiovascular disorders

Benefit: May improve acne caused by androgen excess

Side effects and adverse reactions
- Central nervous system: migraine
- Gastrointestinal: gastrointestinal upset
- Genitourinary: breast tenderness, break-through bleeding during first few months of therapy

Interactions (other drugs)
- **Oral antibiotics: may decrease contraceptive efficacy**

Contraindications
- **Thromboembolic disorders** ▪ **Cardiovascular disorders** ▪ **Estrogen-dependent tumors** ▪ **Abnormal genital bleeding** ▪ **Jaundice/liver disease** ▪ **Pregnancy**

Evidence
An RCT compared norgestimate-ethinyl estradiol with placebo in the treatment of women with moderate acne vulgaris. There was significant improvement in inflammatory lesions, total lesions, and investigator's global assessment in patients receiving norgestimate-ethinyl estradiol compared with placebo [16] *Level P*

Acceptability to patient
Generally well tolerated.

Follow up plan
Consider isotretinoin or referral to a dermatologist if improvements are not seen following several months of treatment.

Patient and caregiver information
- If oral antibiotics are used concomitantly, patient should consider an alternative method of birth control
- May cause spotting during first few months of therapy
- To be taken with food or at bedtime if nausea is problematic

SPIRONOLACTONE
This is an off-label indication.

Dose
100–200mg/day orally.

Efficacy
Antiandrogenic properties suppress sebum production to reduce acne lesions in females; males do not tolerate endocrine side effects.

Risks/benefits
Risks:
- Spironolactone is a potassium-sparing diuretic; use caution with potassium supplements and hyponatremia
- Use caution in renal and hepatic impairment, diabetes, acidosis, and dehydration
- Use caution in pregnancy, menstrual problems, and gynecomastia

Benefit: May improve acne caused by hyperandrogen secretion

Side effects and adverse reactions
- Cardiovascular system: hypotension, bradycardia
- Central nervous system: headache, drowsiness
- Gastrointestinal: nausea, vomiting, diarrhea, bleeding, abdominal pain
- Genitourinary: menstrual irregularities, gynecomastia, hirsutism, impotence
- Metabolic: hyperkalemia, hyponatremia, acidosis
- Skin: rashes, pruritus

Interactions (other drugs)
- Angiotensin-converting enzyme (ACE) inhibitors ▪ Ammonium chloride ▪ Anticoagulants ▪ Angiotensin II receptor antagonists ▪ Cardiac glycosides ▪ Carbenoxolone ▪ Cyclosporine, tacrolimus ▪ Disopyramide ▪ Lithium ▪ Mitotane ▪ Potassium ▪ Salicylates

Contraindications
- Severe renal disease ▪ Anuria ▪ ACE inhibitors and angiotensin receptor antagonists in antikaliuretic therapy ▪ Hyperkalemia

Evidence
- A systematic review found no good-quality evidence on the treatment of acne vulgaris with spironolactone [17] *Level M*
- A crossover RCT compared spironolactone with placebo in women with acne vulgaris. Spironolactone was associated with significant improvement, as assessed by subjective benefit, number of inflamed lesions, and by an independently evaluated photographic method [18] *Level P*

Acceptability to patient
Generally well tolerated by women.

Follow up plan
Consider alternative therapy if acne lesions have not improved following 16 weeks of treatment.

Patient and caregiver information
- May cause drowsiness, lack of co-ordination, or mental confusion. Patient should use caution when performing tasks requiring alertness
- Patient should notify physician if the following occur: abdominal cramping, diarrhea, thirst, headache, rash, menstrual abnormalities, deepening of voice

ORAL CORTICOSTEROIDS
- Prednisone, dexamethasone
- This is an off-label indication

Dose
- Prednisone: 2.5–7.5mg at bedtime
- Dexamethasone: 0.125–0.5mg at bedtime

Efficacy
Useful in treating recalcitrant severe acne nonresponsive to oral contraceptives or spironolactone in patients with elevated dehydroepiandrosterone-sulfate levels.

Risks/benefits
Risks:
- False-negative skin allergy tests. Overwhelming septicemia if patient has an infection
- Loss of control of blood glucose in those with diabetes
- Use caution in elderly due to risk of diabetes and osteoporosis
- Use caution in patients with psychosis, seizure disorders, or myasthenia gravis
- Use caution in congestive heart failure, hypertension, ulcerative colitis, peptic ulcer, or esophagitis

Benefit: May improve acne

Side effects and adverse reactions
- Side effects are minimized by short duration of therapy
- Gastrointestinal: dyspepsia, peptic ulceration, esophagitis, oral candidiasis, nausea, vomiting
- Cardiovascular system: hypertension, thromboembolism
- Central nervous system: insomnia, euphoria, depression, psychosis, seizures
- Endocrine: adrenal suppression, impaired glucose tolerance, growth suppression in children
- Musculoskeletal: proximal myopathy, osteoporosis
- Skin: delayed healing, acne, striae
- Eyes, ears, nose, and throat: cataract, glaucoma, blurred vision

Interactions (other drugs)
- Adrenergic neurone blockers, alpha-blockers, beta-blockers, beta-2 agonists
- Aminoglutethimide - Anticonvulsants (carbamazepine, phenytoin, barbiturates) - Antidiabetics - Antidysrhythmics (calcium channel blockers, cardiac glycosides) - Antifungals (amphotericin, ketoconazole) - Antihypertensives (ACE inhibitors, diuretics: loop and thiazide, acetazolamide; angiotensin II receptor antagonists, clonidine, diazoxide, hydralazine, methyldopa, minoxidil) - Cyclosporine - Erythromycin - Methotrexate - Nonsteroidal anti-inflammatory drugs (NSAIDs) - Nitrates - Nitroprusside - Oral contraceptives - Rifampin - Ritonavir - Somatropin - Vaccines

Contraindications
- Systemic fungal infections - Administration of live virus vaccines

Acceptability to patient
Generally tolerated, although side effects may be limiting.

Follow up plan
Dosage should be increased if dehydroepiandrosterone sulfate levels have not lowered after 3–4 weeks of treatment. Patients should receive ACTH stimulation tests or have early morning cortisol levels drawn every few months to assess adrenal function. Therapy is usually continued for 6–12 months.

Patient and caregiver information
- Gastrointestinal upset may be minimized by taking medication with snacks or food
- Patient should notify physician if the following occur: unusual weight loss or gain, muscle weakness, swelling of face or ankles, tarry stools, vomiting blood, menstrual irregularities, fainting

ISOTRETINOIN
Dose
- 0.5–1.0mg/kg/day for 16–20 weeks
- 2.0mg/kg/day for 16–20 weeks may be used for recalcitrant cases or truncal acne

Efficacy
- Used for severe, nodulocystic acne or moderate noncystic inflammatory acne with the potential for scarring
- Isotretinoin is the only treatment that can produce prolonged remissions following a completed course of therapy

Risks/benefits
Risks:
- Can aggravate any ocular involvement
- Mucocutaneous irritation
- Pseudotumor cerebri
- Diminished night vision
- Musculoskeletal symptoms
- Hyperlipidemia

Benefit: Improvement in acne

Side effects and adverse reactions
- Eyes, ears, nose, and throat: conjuctivitis
- Gastrointestinal: abdominal pain
- Hematologic: hematuria, increase in serum lipids
- Musculoskeletal: arthralgias/myalgias
- Skin: dryness of skin, epidermal fragility, may exacerbate ocular involvement at higher doses, cheilitis/drying of mucosal membranes

Interactions (other drugs)
- **Vitamin A (enhances toxic effects)** ■ **Tetracyline, minocycline (associated with pseudotumor cerebri or papilledema)**

Contraindications
- **Pregnancy** ■ **Breast-feeding** ■ **Renal or hepatic impairment** ■ **Hypervitaminosis A** ■ **Hyperlipidemia**

Evidence
- Isotretinoin is only approved for the treatment of patients with severe, recalcitrant, cystic acne refractory to conventional anti-acne measures, including systemic antibiotics [1] *Level C*
- A prospective trial (no control group) found that response to isotretinoin was very good in 6.8% of patients, and good in 31.9% of patients. Scars were present in 89.4% of patients, with improvement occurring in 67.9% during treatment [19] *This study does not meet the criteria for level P*

Acceptability to patient
Adverse events are significant and may necessitate discontinuation of therapy.

Follow up plan
In females, pregnancy tests must be conducted before therapy and at monthly intervals. Serum lipids and liver enzymes should be monitored weekly or biweekly for the first month or until levels are stable; 16–20 weeks of therapy are needed for complete course.

Patient and caregiver information
- To be taken with meals
- Alcohol should be avoided
- Patient should not take vitamin A supplements
- Females must use two forms of contraception one month before, during treatment, and one month after treatment due to teratogenic potential
- Transient acne exacerbations may occur initially
- Emollients can be used to treat skin irritation caused by excessive dryness
- Sunlight/sunlamps should be avoided
- Patient should not donate blood for 30 days after discontinuing therapy
- Patient should not undergo wax depilation or laser resurfacing during and for 6 months after treatment because of risk for exuberant granulation reaction
- Patient should notify physician immediately if the following occur: visual disturbances, severe headache, abdominal pain, rectal bleeding or diarrhea, difficulty controlling blood sugar, and decreased tolerance of contact lenses

TRIAMCINOLONE ACETONIDE
- Triamcinolone acetonide injection
- This is an off-label indication

Dose
2.0–2.5mg/mL injected into acne lesions.

Efficacy
Intralesional corticosteroids are effective for treating nodulocystic lesions.

Risks/benefits
Risks:
- Risk of infection with intralesional injection
- Use caution with glomerulonephritis, ulcerative colitis, renal disease, AIDS, tuberculosis, ocular herpes simplex, live vaccines, viral and bacterial infections, diabetes mellitus, glaucoma, osteoporosis, hypertension, recent myocardial infarction
- Use caution in children and the elderly
- Use caution in psychosis
- Do not withdraw abruptly

Benefit: May improve acne

Side effects and adverse reactions
- Side effects are minimized by short duration of therapy
- Cardiovascular system: hypertension, thromboembolism
- Central nervous system: insomnia, euphoria, depression, psychosis, seizures
- Endocrine: adrenal suppression, impaired glucose tolerance, growth suppression in children
- Eyes, ears, nose and throat: cataract, glaucoma, blurred vision

- Gastrointestinal: dyspepsia, peptic ulceration, esophagitis, oral candidiasis, nausea, vomiting
- Musculoskeletal: proximal myopathy, osteoporosis
- Skin: delayed healing, acne, striae, transient atrophy at injection site

Interactions (other drugs)
- Aminoglutethimide ■ Antidiabetics ■ Barbiturates ■ Carbamazepine ■ Cholestyramine ■ Cholinesterase inhibitors ■ Cyclosporine ■ Diuretics ■ Estrogens ■ Isoniazid ■ Isoproterenol ■ NSAIDs ■ Phenytoin ■ Rifampin ■ Salicylates

Contraindications
- Local or systemic infection ■ Peptic ulcer ■ Pregnancy and breast-feeding

Acceptability to patient
Patients may be willing to tolerate intralesional injections if acne has been nonresponsive to more conventional therapies.

Follow up plan
Injections may be repeated after 3 weeks if necessary.

Patient and caregiver information
Skin changes (atrophy, hypopigmentation) are usually temporary and resolve in 4–6 months.

METRONIDAZOLE
- Metronidazole topical gel (0.75%)
- This is an off-label indication

Dose
Apply topically once or twice daily.

Efficacy
Beneficial for treatment of mild inflammatory acne.

Risks/benefits
Risks:
- Avoid contact with the eyes
- Blood dyscrasia (either past or present)

Benefit: May improve acne

Side effects and adverse reactions
- Skin: burning, irritation, dryness, redness (transient)
- Central nervous system: numbness or tingling of the extremities
- Gastrointestinal: nausea, metallic taste

Interactions (other drugs)
- Oral anticoagulants

Contraindications
- Hypersensitivity to metronidazole or any constituents of the gel ■ Pregnancy and lactation

Acceptability to patient
Generally well tolerated.

Follow up plan

Improvements are usually observed within 3 weeks. Consider alternative treatment if improvements are not observed following 8 weeks of therapy.

Patient and caregiver information
- Avoid contact with eyes
- Skin irritation is usually mild and transient

SALICYCLIC ACID
Salicylic acid, topical (0.5%–2.0%).

Dose

Apply thoroughly to the affected area and occlude the area at night. Preferably, the skin should be hydrated for at least 5min prior to application. The medication is washed off in the morning and if excessive drying and/or irritation is observed a bland cream or lotion may be applied.

Efficacy
- Keratolytic actions treat comedonal acne
- Less irritating than benzoyl peroxide and tretinoin, but not as effective
- Often used as an adjunct

Risks/benefits

Risks:
- Use caution in children
- Avoid contact with mucous membranes, eyes, and surrounding normal skin

Benefit: May improve noninflammatory acne

Side effects and adverse reactions
- Skin: irritation, sensitivity, dryness
- Systemic effects after long-term use (salicylism: dizziness, confusion, headache, tinnitus, hearing disturbances)

Interactions (other drugs)
- None listed

Contraindications
- Diabetes or other disorders with impaired blood circulation ■ Warts on mucous membranes, facial or genital areas ■ Warts with hairs growing from them ■ Moles, birthmarks ■ Infected or irritated skin

Acceptability to patient
Well tolerated.

Follow up plan
Consider alternative therapies if improvements are not observed following 4–6 weeks of treatment.

Patient and caregiver information
- For external use only
- May cause reddening or scaling of skin when used on open lesions

Surgical therapy
LESION EXTRACTION OR DRAINAGE
Extraction of comedones and drainage of pustules and cysts.

Efficacy
- Effective for removing comedones and draining pustules/cysts
- Speeds recovery of lesions, prevents subdermal rupture, and enhances cosmetic appearance

Risks/benefits
Benefits:
- Minimal risk of infection or scarring when performed correctly
- Improves appearance

Acceptability to patient
Generally well accepted.

Follow up plan
May need to be repeated every 3–4 weeks.

Patient and caregiver information
Patients should be discouraged from expressing contents of lesions themselves due to risk of infections and scarring.

Complementary therapy
BREWER'S YEAST
This is an alternative therapy.

Efficacy
- May be a natural, alternative, nonpharmacologic treatment to improve acne
- Brewer's yeast is a rich source of chromium, which is believed to improve acne

Risks/benefits
Risk: excessive flatulence
Benefit: may improve acne

Acceptability to patient
Well tolerated.

Follow up plan
Consider pharmacologic therapy if desired improvements are not observed.

Patient and caregiver information
- Should be avoided if there is a history of frequent yeast infections or osteoporosis
- Brewer's yeast is a nutritional supplement and differs from baker's yeast
- Patient should begin with one teaspoonful per day dissolved in water or juice and gradually increase the daily dose to 4 tablespoonfuls, in order to reduce the risk of flatulence

Other therapies
CRYOTHERAPY
Liquid nitrogen may produce superficial erythema and desquamation.

Efficacy
May be used if keloidal scar develops.

Risks/benefits
Risk: skin irritation
Benefit: may improve acne scarring

Evidence
In a double-blind study comparing intralesional triamcinolone with cryosurgery, the response to cryosurgery was better for the treatment early vascular lesions [20] *Level P*

Acceptability to patient
85% of patients show a moderate to good response in terms of keloid flattening.

Patient and caregiver information
Liquid nitrogen also reduces skin oiliness.

DERMABRASION

A high-speed motor-driven finely abrasive brush or wheel planes away the epidermis and upper dermis.

Efficacy
Extensive shallow pits, superficial scarring, or irregular skin contour may be smoothed with dermabrasion.

Risks/benefits
Risks:
- Infection
- Skin hypopigmentation, hyperpigmentation, and erythema
- May need to repeat procedure once or twice for optimal results

Benefits:
- May improve skin appearance, reducing scarring
- A major portion of face may be treated during a single session
- Relatively short healing time
- Predictable results in experienced hands

Acceptability to patient
Dyspigmentation and unpredictable results may be unacceptable.

Patient and caregiver information
- Dyspigmentation of the skin may occur
- Additional scarring may be created

LASER RESURFACING

Carbon dioxide laser or erbium:YAG laser destroys the epidermis and/or upper dermis.

Efficacy
- Erbium:YAG laser is used for more superficial scars
- Deeper scars may be smoothed with carbon dioxide laser

Risks/benefits
Risks:
- Infection
- Skin hypopigmentation, hyperpigmentation, and erythema
- Longer healing time and higher cost than dermabrasion
- May need to repeat procedure once or twice for optimal results

Benefits:
- May improve skin appearance, reducing scarring
- A major portion of face may be treated during a single session
- No bleeding, and no aerosolization of blood tissue and viral particles

Evidence
A systematic review found no good-quality evidence supporting the efficacy of laser therapy for treating atrophic or ice-pick acne scars [21] *Level M*

Acceptability to patient
Dyspigmentation and unpredictable results may be unacceptable.

Patient and caregiver information
- Dyspigmentation of the skin may occur
- Additional scarring may be created

CHEMICAL PEELS
Use 25% trichloracetic acid or phenol.

Efficacy
May be useful to treat extensive shallow pits, superficial scars, or irregular skin contours.

Risks/benefits
Risk: skin irritation
Benefit: may improve scarring

PUNCH EXCISION, ELEVATION, OR GRAFTING
Smoothing scarred skin contours by removal of deep scars, and/or replacement with full-thickness punch graft of normal postauricular skin.

Efficacy
- Useful methods to remove deep depressed scars
- Punch excision or grafting is effective for ice-pick scars
- Deep boxcar scars can be managed with punch excision or elevation

Risks/benefits
Risks:
- Irregular pigmenation, texture
- Pain
- Infection

Benefits:
- Removal of deep scars
- Autograft prevents rejection reactions

Acceptability to patient
Very well tolerated with acceptable results.

COLLAGEN INJECTIONS
Collagen suspensions are injected intradermally to correct scars.

Efficacy
Useful to smooth skin surface and to correct a small number of depressed acne scars.

Risks/benefits
Risks:
- Infection
- Effect only lasts 3–4 months
- Hypersensitivity reaction to bovine products

Benefit: Smoothes skin surface

Acceptability to patient
Well tolerated.

Patient and caregiver information
The duration of correction is not maintained permanently and may diminish over one year.

EFFICACY OF THERAPIES

In the normal course, pharmacologic treatments will result in improvement in acne within 2–4 months, depending on initial severity and drugs utilized.

Evidence

- Tretinoin creams have been found to be significantly superior to placebo in patients with mild-to-moderate acne [6] *Level P*
- Adapalene solution and tretinoin gel have been found to be clinically and statistically effective in reducing inflammatory and noninflammatory lesions compared with baseline [7] *Level P*
- Topical tazarotene gel has been shown to significantly reduce lesion counts (both inflammatory and noninflammatory) in patients with mild-to-moderate facial acne vulgaris [8] *Level P*
- Azelaic acid significantly reduced the number of acne lesions compared with its vehicle in a double-blind study of patients with moderate inflammatory acne [9] *Level P*
- Erythromycin was significantly more effective than its vehicle in reducing the number of inflammatory and noninflammatory lesions in patients with mild-to-moderate acne vulgaris [2] *Level P*
- An RCT compared the efficacy of benzoyl peroxide/erythromycin gel with erythromycin/zinc in patients with acne vulgaris. Benzoyl peroxide/erythromycin resulted in significantly fewer inflammatory lesions and fewer comedones [12] *Level P*
- Norgestimate-ethinyl estradiol significantly improved inflammatory lesions, total lesions, and investigator's global assessment compared with placebo in women with moderate acne vulgaris [16] *Level P*
- A systematic review found no good-quality evidence for the treatment of acne vulgaris with spironolactone [17] *Level M*
- A systematic review found that minocycline is likely to be an effective treatment for moderate acne vulgaris; however, the review found no reliable evidence to justify the use of this drug as first-line therapy [14] *Level M*
- A systematic review found no good-quality evidence supporting the efficacy of laser therapy for the treatment of atrophic or ice-pick acne scars [21] *Level M*
- Systemic erythromycin, doxycycline, topical tetracycline, benzoyl peroxide gel, oral oxytetracycline, topical clindamycin, and oral minocycline have been shown to produce a significant improvement from baseline in patients with facial acne vulgaris [13,14,15] *Level P*
- Benzoyl peroxide and isotretinoin gel significantly reduced inflamed and noninflamed lesions, and improved acne grade in patients with mild-to-moderate acne vulgaris [5] *Level P*

Review period

A minimum of 4 weeks may be sufficient for a trial of pharmacologic agents. However, 8–12 weeks may be required for maximal effects to be observed.

PROGNOSIS

There is no cure for acne, but it can be effectively managed. Spontaneous remission is usual.

Clinical pearls

- Patients whose parents had severe acne with residual scarring may have heightened fear of a similar result. This should be addressed by stating that newer medications (isotretinoin) will probably prevent that occurrence in them
- Psychologic distress in teenagers with acne should be assessed and managed as appropriate. Lack of compliance and follow up can be significant barriers to successful treatment in adolescents. In particular, if parents have insisted the adolescent patient seek treatment, he/she may perceive this long-term treatment as being imposed on them. It is important to address these issues early

Therapeutic failure

- When pharmacologic therapies fail, referral to a dermatologist may be indicated
- When facial scarring occurs following inflammatory acne treatment, referral to dermatologists or dermatologic surgeons may be necessary for dermabrasion, laser resurfacing, chemical peels, punch excision or grafting, or collagen injections

Recurrence

Acne recurrences are not uncommon, especially in adolescents. Long-term use of acne medications may be required even after patient's skin is clear. Alternatively, subsequent courses of isotretinoin treatment may be utilized.

Deterioration

Acute deterioration may require treatment with oral corticosteroids and may suggest acne fulminans.

COMPLICATIONS

- Acne fulminans: febrile acne accompanied by systemic symptoms
- Acne conglobata: large abscesses that heal by scarring
- Facial scarring: may be managed by dermatologist using dermabrasion, laser resurfacing, chemical peels, punch excision or grafting, or collagen injections
- Psychologic sequelae

CONSIDER CONSULT

- Referral is indicated if acne is unresponsive to oral antibiotics and topical therapies

PREVENTION

Washing twice daily and avoidance of oil-based cosmetics are good habits to follow.

RISK FACTORS

- **Family history:** in 50% there is a positive family history for acne and other sinus track diseases such as pilonidal sinus and hidradenitis suppurativa
- **Physical activity:** some sports equipment can aggravate acne
- **Medication history:** corticosteroids, anabolic steroids, oral contraceptives with high androgenic activity, isoniazid, phenytoin, and lithium may exacerbate acne

MODIFY RISK FACTORS

Presently, little is known about preventing the onset of acne. However, lifestyle and wellness modifications may have beneficial effects.

Lifestyle and wellness

DIET

There is no evidence to support exacerbation of acne by chocolate, shellfish, sweets, milk, and fatty foods.

PHYSICAL ACTIVITY

- Wash with a mild soap after exercise
- Avoid sports equipment that rubs or occludes skin whenever possible

FAMILY HISTORY

Begin pharmacologic treatment early when there is a positive family history.

DRUG HISTORY

If possible, avoid medications that are known to cause or aggravate acne, including oral contraceptives with high androgenic activity, corticosteroids, anabolic steroids, lithium, phenytoin, or isoniazid.

PREVENT RECURRENCE

Long-term therapy may be required to control acne, even after patient's skin has cleared. Isotretinoin is the only therapy demonstrated to induce prolonged remissions.

Reassess coexisting disease

Some medications tend to be comedogenic. If possible, the physician should avoid these medications when treating coexisting diseases, and the patient should also be informed of potential over-the-counter medications that may aggravate acne.

INTERACTION ALERT

The following may aggravate acne: lithium, phenytoin, corticosteroids/anabolic steroids, oral contraceptives with high androgenic activity, and iodides/bromides found in some cough medicines.

PATIENT SATISFACTION/LIFESTYLE PRIORITIES

Most patients experience improvements in acne following an appropriate course of therapy and experience minimal side effects, primarily involving skin irritation.

ASSOCIATIONS
American Academy of Dermatology
930 N. Meacham Rd
PO Box 4014
Schaumberg, IL 60168–4014
Tel: (708) 330–0230
www.aad.org

KEY REFERENCES

- Reisner RM. Management of acne. In: Goroll, ed. Primary care medicine, 3rd edn. Philadelphia: Lippincott-Raven Publishers, 1995
- Placzek M, Degitz K, Schmidt H, Plewig G. Acne fulminans in late-onset congenital adrenal hyperplasia. Lancet 1999;354:739–40
- Usatine RP, Quan MA. Pearls in the management of acne: an advanced approach. Primary Care 2000;27:289–308
- Fluhr JW, Gloor M, Merkel W, et al. Antibacterial and sebosuppressive efficacy of a combination of chloramphenicol and pale sulfonated shale oil. Multicentre, randomized, vehicle-controlled, double-blind study on 91 acne patients with acne papulopustulosa (Plewig and Kligman's grade II–III). Arzneimittelforschung 1998;48:188–96
- Acne, rosacea and related disorders. In: Habif, ed. Clinical dermatology, 3rd edn. St Louis, MO: Mosby-Year Book, 1996
- Pfenninger JL, Zuber TJ. Acne therapy. In: Pfenninger, ed. Procedures for primary care physicians. St Louis, MO: Mosby-Year Book, 1996
- White GM. The evolving role of retinoids in the management of cutaneous conditions: Recent findings in the epidemiologic evidence, classification, and subtypes of acne vulgaris. J Am Acad Dermatol 1998;39:S34–7
- Krowchuk DP. Managing acne in adolescents. Pediatr Clin North Am 2000; 47:841–57
- Hatwal A, Bhatt RP, Agrawal JK, et al. Spironolactone and cimetidine in the treatment of acne. Acta Derm Venereol 1988;68:84–7
- Schmidt JB. Other antiandrogens. Dermatology 1998;196:153–7

Evidence references and guidelines
1 The American Academy of Dermatology. Guidelines for care of acne vulgaris. J Am Acad Dermatol 1990;22:676–80
2 Pochi PE, Shalita AR, Strauss JS, et al. (1991) Report of the consensus conference on acne classification. Washington, D.C., March 24 and 25, 1990. J Am Acad Dermatol 24:495–500
3 Johnson BA, Nunley JR. Use of systematic agents in the treatment of acne vulgaris. Am Fam Physician 2000;62:1823–30, 1835–6
4 Russell JJ. Topical therapy for acne. Am Fam Physician 2000;61:357–66
5 Hughes BR, Norris JF, Cunliffe WJ. A double-blind evaluation of topical isotretinoin 0.05%, benzoyl peroxide 5% and placebo in patients with acne. Clin Exp Dermatol 1992;17:165–8. Medline
6 Lucky AW, Cullen SI, Funicella T, et al. Double-blind, vehicle controlled, multicenter comparison of two 0.025% tretinoin creams in patients with acne vulgaris. J Am Acad Dermatol 1998;38:S24–30. Medline
7 Ellis CN, Millikan LE, Smith EB, et al. Comparison of adapalene 0.1% solution and tretinoin 0.025% gel in the topical treatment of acne vulgaris. Br J Dermatol 1998;139(suppl 52):41–47. Medline
8 Shalita AR, Chalker DK, Griffith RF. Tazarotene gel is safe and effective in the treatment of acne vulgaris: a multicenter, double-blind, vehicle-controlled study. Cutis 1999;63:349–54. Medline
9 Katsambas A, Graupe K, Stratigos J. Clinical studies of 20% azelaic acid cream in the treatment of acne vulgaris. Comparison with vehicle and topical tretinoin. Acta Derm Venereol Suppl 1989;143:35–9. Medline
10 Pochi PE, Bagatell FK, Ellis CN, et al. Erythromycin 2 percent gel in the treatment of acne vulgaris. Cutis 1998;41:132–6. Medline
11 Bleeker J, Hellgren L, Vincent J. Effect of systemic erythromycin stearate on the inflammatory lesions and skin surface fatty acids in acne vulgaris. Dermatologica 1981;162:342–9. Medline
12 Chu A, Huber FJ, Plott RT. The comparative efficacy of benzoyl peroxide 5%/erythromycin 3% gel and erythromycin 4%/zinc 1.2% solution in the treatment of acne vulgaris. Br J Dermatol 1997;136:235–8. Medline

13 Norris JF, Hughes BR, Basey AJ, Cunliffe WJ. A comparison of the effectiveness of topical tetracycline, benzoyl-peroxide gel and oral oxytetracycline in the treatment of acne. Clin Exp Dermatol 1991;16:31–3. Medline

14 Garner SE, Eady EA, Popescu C, Newton J, Li Wan Po A. Minocycline for acne vulgaris: efficacy and safety (Cochrane Review). In: The Cochrane Library, 1, 2002. Oxford: Update Software

15 Sheehan-Dare RA, Papworth-Smith J, Cunliffe WJ. A double-blind comparison of topical clindamycin and oral minocycline in the treatment of acne vulgaris. Acta Derm Venereol 1990;70:534–7. Medline

16 Redmond GP, Olson WH, Lippman JS, et al. Norgestimate and ethinyl estradiol in the treatment of acne vulgaris: a randomized, placebo-controlled trial. Obstet Gynecol 1997; 89:615–22. Medline

17 Farquhar C, Lee O, Toomath R, Jepson R. Spironolactone versus placebo or in combination with steroids for hirsutism and/or acne (Cochrane Review). In: The Cochrane Library, 1, 2002. Oxford: Update Software

18 Muhlemann MF, Carter GD, Cream JJ, Wise P. Oral spironolactone: an effective treatment for acne vulgaris in women. Br J Dermatol 1986;115:227–32. Medline

19 Hermes B, Praetel C, Henz BM. Medium dose isotretinoin for the treatment of acne. J Eur Acad Dermatol Venereol 1998;11:117–21. Medline

20 Layton AM, Yip J, Cunliffe WJ. A comparison of intralesional triamcinolone and cryosurgery in the treatment of acne keloids. Br J Dermatol 1994;130:498–501. Medline

21 Jordan RE, Cummins CL, Burls AJE, Seukeran DC. Laser resurfacing for facial acne scars (Cochrane Review). In: The Cochrane Library, 1, 2002. Oxford: Update Software

FAQS
Question 1
What restrictions should be placed on diet?

ANSWER 1
None. No dietary component (greasy foods, chocolate, among other misconceptions) have been shown to worsen acne.

Question 2
Do blackheads indicate suboptimal hygiene?

ANSWER 2
No. Blackheads are not dirt, they are oxidized keratin. They are best removed by acne surgery or exfoliants.

Question 3
My 10-year-old patient has what appears to be acne. Is this possible?

ANSWER 3
Yes, and it should be taken seriously because early age of onset presages more severe acne later in life.

Question 4
My moderately pigmented patient has minimal acne but is distressed by marked hyperpigmented macules on the face. How do I approach such a patient?

ANSWER 4
Topical retinoids, such as tretinoin, are very useful in such cases because they should help not only with acne, but also with the postinflammatory hyperpigmentation. Often, in patients of African descent, the residua (dyspigmentation, keloidal scarring) are more bothersome than the otherwise minor primary acne lesions. Such patients need to be treated more aggressively because these residua can be as disturbing, if not more so, and last longer than the typical papules and pustules of acne.

CONTRIBUTORS
Russell C Jones, MD, MPH
Seth R Stevens, MD
Christine C Lin, MD

ALOPECIA

DESCRIPTION

- Loss of hair – may be scarring or nonscarring, localized or diffuse, reversible or permanent; may be confined to scalp or universal
- Inflammation, pruritis, and scaling may be present at site of hair loss
- Underlying causes are varied, including androgenic, infection, drug related, psychiatric, dermatologic, and systemic illness
- Treatment depends on underlying cause
- Psychologic impact of loss of hair in a culture in which hair has significant aesthetic value needs consideration

KEY! DON'T MISS!

- Cicatricial alopecia (scarring alopecia) and male-pattern androgenic alopecia with virilization or hirsutism in women, because early intervention may prevent further hair loss
- Hair loss due to metastatic carcinoma – biopsy is usually diagnostic

ICD9 CODE
- 704.00 Alopecia, unspecified
- 704.01 Alopecia areata
- 704.09 Other

SYNONYMS
- Androgenic alopecia
- Male-pattern baldness
- Female-pattern baldness
- Alopecia areata
- Cicatricial alopecia
- Telogen effluvium
- Allogen effluvium
- Traction alopecia
- Postpartum alopecia
- Hair loss

CARDINAL FEATURES
Androgenic alopecia (male-/female-pattern baldness):
- Localized and systemic hair loss
- Hair loss usually begins with the frontoparietal scalp and then the vertex
- Female-pattern baldness is similar but more diffuse, without complete baldness
- Male-pattern baldness in females is indicative of androgen excess and may be accompanied by hirsutism in mild cases and virilization in more serious ones

Alopecia areata:
- Second most common presentation of nonscarring alopecia
- Hair is rapidly lost in circular or oval patches

Telogen effluvium:
- Diffuse alopecia following a traumatic event
- Hair loss occurs approx. 3 months after the event
- Usually <50% of the scalp is affected
- Recovery is usually complete once triggering factor is resolved

Anagen effluvium:
- Diffuse hair loss occurring as a result of certain toxic exposures
- Following toxic exposure, hair growth is abruptly interrupted and anagen hair is shed after 1–4 weeks
- Rapidly affects 80–90% of the scalp
- Complete recovery can be expected once triggering factor is removed

Traction alopecia:
- Hair loss caused by direct insult to hair
- Usually caused by styling techniques such as hot rollers or braiding
- Pattern of hair loss relates directly to technique used
- If continued may progress to scarring

Trichotillomania (subtype of traction alopecia):
- Self-inflicted loss of hair, typically from frontoparietal region progressing backwards
- Regrowth of up to 1.5cm may also be visible before hair is long enough to pull again

Cicatricial alopecia (or scarring alopecia):
- Hair loss occurs with permanent destruction of hair follicles
- Often presents with inflammation arising from injury or disease
- Scalp lesions may also be present
- Initially localized, it may become diffuse in chronic presentations
- Scalp will gradually scar, becoming smooth without any evidence of hair follicles
- Once scarring is initiated, hair loss is permanent

Tinea capitis:
- Fungal infection causing hairs to break off close to the scalp leaving a 'black dot' effect
- Predominantly affects children

CAUSES
Common causes
Androgenic alopecia:
- Genetically determined
- Development is related to age and presence of androgenic hormones

Alopecia areata:
- Etiology is uncertain, but there is a genetic predisposition, and popular opinion favors an autoimmune response

Telogen effluvium:
- Normal hair cycle is interrupted so that anagen (growing) hairs are abruptly converted into telogen (resting) hairs which are subsequently shed after 2–4 months
- Hypothyroidism and hyperthyroidism

Tinea capitis:
- Ringworm of the scalp in which dermatophyte fungus invades the hair shaft. The most likely dermatophytes are *Microsporum* (from cats and dogs) and *Trichophyton* species

Rare causes
Androgenic alopecia:
- Drugs – testosterone, danazol, corticotropin, anabolic steroids, progesterone
- Adrenal tumor
- Pituitary tumor
- Carcinoid
- Male-pattern androgenic alopecia in a women may indicate an androgen excess due to: polycystic ovarian disease, hyperprolactinemia, ovarian tumor

Telogen effluvium:
- Childbirth (postpartum alopecia)
- Drugs (oral contraceptives, beta-blockers, anticoagulants, interferon, retinoids, lithium, nonsteroidal anti-inflammatories)
- Persistent high fever (as in typhoid, pneumonia)
- Severe illness (systemic lupus erythematosus, syphilis)
- Sudden starvation (e.g. crash diets) and inadequate diet (including iron and zinc deficiency)
- Psychologic stress
- Acute blood loss
- Major surgery

Anagen effluvium:
- Drugs: chemotherapeutic agents (most commonly methotrexate), allopurinol, bromocriptine, levodopa
- Poisons (arsenic, bismuth, borax, thallium, gold)
- Local X-ray and radiation therapy
- Mycosis fungoides

Metastatic carcinoma:
- Scalp is a relatively common site for cutaneous metastases. A patch of alopecia, particularly if there is any textural change in the scalp, may indicate such metastasis. This can occasionally be the initial presentation of a previously unidentified malignancy

Traction alopecia:
- Styling techniques (tightly wound hot rollers, tight braiding)
- Trichotillomania: conscious or subconscious habit (particularly in children), psychologic disturbance (more typically in adults)

Cicatricial alopecia:
- Physical trauma (burns, radiodermatitis)
- Infection (tuberculosis, syphilis)
- Congenital and developmental defects resulting in absent or incomplete hair follicles
- Lichen planus
- Discoid lupus erythematosus
- Cicatricial pemphigoid
- Sarcoidosis

Serious causes
Many serious illnesses can cause hair loss.

Contributory or predisposing factors
- Family history of baldness
- Old age
- Physical stress
- Psychologic stress
- Poor nutrition
- Pregnancy
- Regular use of aggressive hair styling techniques

EPIDEMIOLOGY
Incidence and prevalence

PREVALENCE
- 25% of men aged 25 years have some degree of clinically apparent androgenic alopecia
- 42% of men develop androgenic alopecia
- 0.1% of people develop alopecia areata

Demographics
GENDER
In trichotillomania the ratio of women to men is 2.5:1.

DIFFERENTIAL DIAGNOSIS
Polycystic ovarian disease
The key features of polycystic ovarian disease are as follows.

FEATURES
- Erratic menstrual periods or amenorrhea
- Excessive facial hair and other signs of hirsutism
- Tendency to weight gain
- Acne
- Decreased fertility

Cushing's syndrome
The key features of Cushing's syndrome are as follows.

FEATURES
- Facial adiposity (moon face)
- Increased adipose tissue in neck and trunk
- Weight gain
- Purple striae
- Hirsutism
- Emotional lability
- Hypertension
- Osteoporosis
- Loss of muscle mass

Hypothyroidism
The key features of hypothyroidism are as follows.

FEATURES
- Weight gain
- Feeling cold and sluggish
- Erratic menstrual periods in women

Hyperthyroidism
The key features of hyperthyroidism are as follows.

FEATURES
- Tremor
- Eye signs: erythema, lid retraction, stare
- Weight loss with increase in appetite
- Tachycardia
- Warm moist skin
- Fever
- Goiter

Systemic lupus erythematosus
Systemic lupus erythematosus may cause telogen effluvium during active phases of the disease; it is unlikely to cause scarring alopecia.

FEATURES
- Arthritis
- Fever and malaise
- Skin lesions
- Weight loss

Discoid lupus erythematosus
Commonly causes permanent hair loss; the itchy, erythematous, scaly areas that appear on the body can also affect the scalp, causing scarring alopecia.

FEATURES
- Skin lesions: dull red maculas with scales
- Lesions found on face, thorax, or upper extremities; rarely below waist
- Scarring alopecia with scalp lesions
- 'Carpet tack' appearance of skin when scale removed

Sarcoidosis
The key features of sarcoidosis are as follows.

FEATURES
- Skin lesions: plaques, papules, subcutaneous nodules
- Eye lesions
- Weight loss
- Fatigue
- Cough if pulmonary infiltration occurs
- Chest pain
- Breathlessness

Lichen planus
The key features of lichen planus are as follows.

FEATURES
- Skin lesions: small, flat, angular, violaceous; shiny papules
- Pruritus
- Mouth lesions: milky-white papules
- Scarring alopecia, which may result in total baldness

Seborrheic dermatitis
The key features of seborrheic dermatitis are as follows.

FEATURES
- Skin lesions: erythematous patches with yellow, greasy scales
- Lesions found bilaterally in hairy regions of the body, especially scalp, eyebrows, nasolabial folds, and sternum
- Red, smooth, glazed appearance in skin folds
- Chronic condition with remissions and exacerbations

Psoriasis
The key features of psoriasis are as follows.

FEATURES

- Skin lesions: erythematous patches with profuse proliferating white or silvery scales
- Lesions found on scalp (typically postauricular), trunk, limbs, face
- Nails may be pitted and/or thickened
- Chronic condition with remissions and exacerbations

Secondary syphilis

If the hair follicles are involved in secondary syphilis, then patchy alopecia will occur, giving a 'moth-eaten' look that may be confused with alopecia areata.

FEATURES

- Rash: maculas, papules and/or pustules
- Rash found initially on trunk spreading to whole body including palms and soles
- Lesions in mouth
- Adenopathy

SIGNS & SYMPTOMS
Signs

Androgenic alopecia:

- Pattern of terminal hair loss through a process referred to as 'miniaturization' initially from frontoparietal scalp, followed by vertex and occipital regions
- Female-pattern baldness is similar in pattern but more diffuse, with thinning throughout scalp and no complete hair loss; terminal hairs are replaced by fine vellus hairs
- Symmetric pattern of hair loss
- In female pattern baldness, frontal hairline is often spared
- Posterior and lateral margins are spared
- Male-pattern hair loss in a female: hirsutism may accompany scalp hair loss

Alopecia areata:

- Areas of round or oval hair loss
- Skin is smooth or may have short stubs of hair
- Hair is easily removed from edges of hairless patches when disease is active at that location
- Can progress to total baldness
- Tiny hairs with tapered tops ('exclamation mark hairs') may be seen within or around the edge of patches
- Eyebrows or lashes may be involved

Telogen effluvium:

- Diffuse hair loss of <50% of the scalp
- Frequently regrowth occurs in 4–6 months
- Evidence of systemic illness (systemic lupus erythematosus, hyperthyroidism, sarcoidosis)
- Loss of the lateral third of eyebrow in hypothyroidism

Anagen effluvium:

- Diffuse hair loss of 80–90% of the scalp
- Eyebrows and eyelashes are spared (they are not in active anagen phase)
- Under microscope hairs have a jagged or tapered end (pencil-point hairs)

Traction alopecia:

- Pattern of hair loss is dependant on injury to scalp
- Hair shaft fragments may be found in dermis and are surrounded by an inflammatory infiltrate
- Initially nonscarring if longstanding, then permanent damage to hair shaft may result

Trichotillomania (subtype of traction alopecia):
- Hair loss in typically frontoparietal area
- Affected area has irregular angulated border
- Presence of short, broken hairs randomly distributed in affected site; hair may regrow to 1.5cm before it can be pulled again
- In affected area no hair is released on gentle traction
- Eyebrows or lashes may be involved

Cicatricial alopecia:
- Typically hair loss is patchy and irregular
- Inflammation as a result of injury is often present
- Scarring and destruction of follicular units (sometimes only ascertained by biopsy)
- Erythema
- Scales
- Pustule formation
- Wood's light produces a fluorescent glow in area affected by fungal infection
- Evidence of systemic illness (lupus, sarcoidosis)
- Beau's lines on nails may suggest a systemic process affecting both nail and hair growth
- In congenital syndromes with structural defects of the hair shaft, hair may be sparse, fine, and wiry from early childhood
- Lichen planus: diffuse patchy scarring alopecia, additional lesions on skin, mucous membrane, and nails

Tinea capitis:
- Mild scaling
- Inflammation
- Erythema
- Pustules
- Broken hair shafts often leave residual black stumps (black dot ringworm)
- Wood's light produces a fluorescent glow
- Eventual scarring
- Positive culture

Symptoms
Androgenic alopecia:
- Gradual temporal hair recession (including midfrontal recession)
- Further gradual loss to frontal, vertex and occipital regions of scalp
- Female-pattern baldness is similar in pattern but more diffuse, with thinning throughout scalp and no complete hair loss

Alopecia areata:
- Sudden occurrence of one or more round or oval patches of hair loss, usually on scalp
- Regrowth begins in 1–3 months but may be followed by loss in the same or other areas
- Tends to involve pigmented hairs preferentially over nonpigmented hairs, causing hair to 'turn white'

Telogen effluvium:
- Diffuse loss of 30–40% of scalp hair
- Hair loss starts abruptly and continues for approx. 4 weeks

Anagen effluvium:
- Sudden and diffuse loss of 80–90% of scalp hair

Traction alopecia:
- Loss of hair

Trichotillomania:
- Loss of hair

Cicatricial alopecia:
- Patchy hair loss
- Itching and soreness

Tinea capitis:
- Patchy hair loss
- Pruritus

ASSOCIATED DISORDERS
Alopecia areata:
- Down syndrome
- Vitiligo
- Diabetes
- Autoimmune thyroid disease
- Pernicious anemia

KEY! DON'T MISS!
- Cicatricial alopecia (scarring alopecia) and male-pattern androgenic alopecia with virilization or hirsutism in women, because early intervention may prevent further hair loss
- Hair loss due to metastatic carcinoma – biopsy is usually diagnostic

CONSIDER CONSULT
- Male-pattern androgenic alopecia in women in conjunction with hirsutism or virilization should be referred to an endocrinologist for further investigation and treatment
- Severe alopecia areata may be referred to a dermatologist or trichologist
- Cicatricial alopecia may require referral to a dermatologist or rheumatologist to determine cause
- Metastatic carcinoma should prompt referral to an oncologist
- If a scalp biospy is considered appropriate, this should be performed by someone specifically trained in this procedure, as improper technique can reduce validity of test

INVESTIGATION OF THE PATIENT
Direct questions to patient
Q When did you last have a full head of hair? Telogen and anagen effluvium will usually present at <1 year; >1 year suggests a more insidious process. Male-pattern baldness starts after puberty; female-pattern baldness more typically presents or accelerates around time of menopause.
Q Has your hair loss been sudden or gradual? Telogen and anagen effluvium will present as sudden. Gradual hair loss in men is likely to be due to male-pattern baldness.

<1 year/sudden hair loss:
Q Have you gained or lost weight recently? Consider thyroid disorders.
Q Any recent pregnancy? Consider postpartum alopecia.
Q What medications have you been on in the last 6 months? Consider drug-related anagen or telogen effluvium.
Q Have you had an operation or general anesthetic in the last 6 months? Consider telogen effluvium.

Q Have you had any major psychologic stress in the past year such as death of a loved one or divorce? Consider telogen effluvium.

Q Have you been on a diet in the last 6 months? Consider telogen effluvium.

Q Have you been unwell recently? Consider an underlying disease. High fever can cause telogen effluvium as well as serious illness. It is rare for hair loss to be first or only presenting problem. In such cases appropriate examination usually reveals symptoms that were underappreciated.

>1 year/gradual hair loss:

Q Is there any pain, bleeding or itching from the scalp? Cicatricial alopecia may present with scalp discomfort.

Q Does your hair loss upset you? Treatment of alopecia may depend on the patient's perception of the loss.

Contributory or predisposing factors

Q Tell me what you would eat in a typical day. Poor nutrition, particularly iron or zinc deficiency, is a predisposing factor.

Q What sort of styling or dying do you use on your hair? Relaxers, perms, and bleaches can be damaging and result in hair fragility, so that hair breaks easily when brushed or washed. Many African-American women use a chemical treatment to straighten their hair. Overheating can cause a hair shaft abnormality known as 'bubble hair', which leads to fragility and hair breakage, e.g. if an overheating hair drying or styling tong is used.

Q Are you particularly stressed at the moment? Psychologic stress can be a contributing factor in trichotillomania, as well as a cause of telogen effluvium.

Family history

Q Do any other members of your family have a similar type of hair loss? Include maternal and paternal relatives, siblings, and children. Androgenic alopecia and some hair shaft abnormalities are heritable.

Examination

Pattern of hair loss:

▪ Is the hair loss localized, diffuse or patchy? Diffuse hair loss suggests effluvium

▪ What is the pattern of localized hair loss? Androgenic alopecia is symmetric; in male-pattern baldness hair loss typically begins with the frontoparietal scalp and then the vertex (Hamilton patterns). Female-pattern baldness is similar but more diffuse without complete baldness, and anterior hairline is spared (Ludwig pattern)

▪ What is the pattern of patchy hair loss? A moth-eaten pattern is indicative of syphilis and a serologic test should be ordered. Discrete round patches suggest alopecia areata. Trichotillomania typically progresses from frontoparietal region backwards; regrowth of up to 1.5cm may also be visible before hair is long enough to be pulled again. In traction alopecia, pattern of hair loss relates to technique used

Scalp:

▪ Is there any erythema? Erythema suggests a scalp biopsy may give helpful information as to nature of scalp disorder

▪ Scaling? Suggests seborrheic dermatitis, psoriasis, or tinea capitis. In the latter, Wood's light produces a fluorescent glow

▪ Pustules, crusts, and erosions? Suggest infection. Wood's light produces a fluorescent glow in area affected by fungal infection

▪ Scarring (loss of follicular units)? Altered scalp texture or nodularity may suggest infiltration by metastasis

Hair:
- **Exclamation mark hairs** (short hairs that taper as they approach scalp surface): characteristic of alopecia areata
- **Hair fragility:** determine by squeezing and rolling hair within a gauze pad. If hair is fragile, short fragments of hair remain on pad. This indicates traction alopecia or a hereditary hair shaft disorder
- **Pull test:** can assist in determining how much hair is being shed, and assess hair breakage. 20–40 hairs are firmly grasped and gentle traction applied. For normal hair loss one or two in 10 hairs should be extracted. In active androgenic alopecia and telogen effluvium, more than five in 10 will be extracted. Hairs should end with a visible depigmented bulb (telogen hairs). If there is no bulb suspect hair breakage. If regrowth hair is pulled from affected site and no hairs are extracted, suspect trichotillomania, because all hairs will be in the anagen (growing) phase
- **May be necessary to collect objective evidence of hair loss to differentiate perceived from genuine problems.** Patient combs hair first thing in the morning and collects hair lost daily in a clear plastic bag. Hair lost during washing should also be collected. Seven days should be sufficient. Patient counts hairs for each day and records the number on the bags. It is normal to lose 100 hairs a day plus 200–250 when washing (unless washing daily, when 100 would be normal)

Summary of investigative tests
- Venereal Disease Reference Laboratory (VDRL) test: serologic test for syphilis should be performed in all patients with unexplained hair loss
- Potassium hydroxide (KOH) preparation for fungal elements in patchy forms of alopecia associated with scaling or inflammation
- Wood's light examination and fungal culture if tinea capitis is suspected
- Complete blood count (CBC) to elicit anemia or lymphocytosis
- ESR to test for arthritic disease
- Thyroid-stimulating hormone assay to test for thyroid disease
- Pluck test to examine ratio of anagen to telogen hairs (trichogram), usually performed by a specialist
- Microscopic examination of hair shafts for hereditary hair-shaft disorders; normally performed by a specialist
- Scalp biopsy; usually performed by a specialist

DIAGNOSTIC DECISION
Androgenic alopecia (male-/female-pattern baldness):
- Patient and family history
- Examination of pattern of hair loss

Alopecia areata:
- Patient and family history
- Examination of pattern of hair loss, scalp, and hair
- If necessary, microscopic examination of hair and biopsy (usually performed by a specialist)

Telogen effluvium:
- Patient history
- Examination of pattern of hair loss, scalp, and hair, including pull test
- CBC to elicit anemia or lymphocytosis
- Serologic test may sometimes be performed to identify arthritic diseases

Anagen effluvium:
- Patient history
- Examination of pattern of hair loss

Trichotillomania:
- Patient history
- Examination including pull test

Cicatricial alopecia (or scarring alopecia):
- Patient and family history
- Examination of pattern of hair loss, scalp (including Wood's light) and hair
- KOH preparation for fungal elements in patchy forms of alopecia associated with scaling or inflammation

Tinea capitis:
- Patient history
- Examination of pattern of hair loss, scalp (including Wood's light), and hair
- Fungal culture

CLINICAL PEARLS
- Hair loss can be difficult to diagnose and emotionally difficult for patients. Referral to a dermatologist (one with particular expertise in hair loss, if available) can be very helpful for most patients without typical androgenic alopecia
- Examination of nails should be performed in all hair loss patients. If abnormalities are present, then suspicion for inflammatory disease, rather than androgenic alopecia, should be heightened

THE TESTS
Body fluids
VENEREAL DISEASE REFERENCE LABORATORY TEST
Description
- Blood test
- Performed as part of cerebrospinal fluid examination

Advantages/Disadvantages
Advantages:
- Inexpensive, fast, and convenient for screening large numbers of sera
- Results are quantitative and give an indication of disease activity

Disadvantages:
- Becomes positive 1–3 weeks after appearance of primary chancre, so can be negative in early syphilis
- In late syphilis, around 25% of untreated patients have a negative result

Normal
Nonreactive.

Abnormal
- Results are reported as borderline, weakly reactive or reactive; latter two are considered positive
- Quantitative reagin titers are reported for all positive results
- Keep in mind the possibility of a false-positive result

Cause of abnormal result
Presence of reagin antibodies in patient's serum as a result of infection with syphilis.

Drugs, disorders and other factors that may alter results
- False-positive results can occur in pneumonia, tuberculosis, chancroid, chicken pox, HIV infection, measles, malaria, pregnancy, intravenous drug use, history of multiple blood transfusions, autoimmune and connective tissue diseases, especially systemic lupus erythematosus
- A prozone reaction can occur – false-negative test due to high titer antibody; plasma should be diluted to assure 'negative' result is not due to prozone phenomenon

COMPLETE BLOOD COUNT
Description
Venous blood.

Advantages/Disadvantages
Advantage: inexpensive and readily available.

Normal
- Hemoglobin: women 12.0–16.0g/dL (120–160g/L); men 13.5–17.5g/dL (135–175g/L)
- Relative lymphocyte percentage: 15–40%
- Absolute lymphocyte count: 800–2200/mm^3

Abnormal
- Hemoglobin level: women <10g/dL (<100g/L); men <13.5g/dL (<135g/L)
- Lymphocyte count: >2200/mm^3
- Keep in mind the possibility of a falsely abnormal result

Cause of abnormal result
- Poor nutrition may result in anemia
- Rheumatologic disease may cause anemia and or leukocytosis

Drugs, disorders and other factors that may alter results
- Excessive fluid intake will decrease hemoglobin values
- Hemoglobin levels are normally decreased in pregnancy
- Many drugs are associated with anemia

ESR
Description
Blood sample.

Advantages/Disadvantages
Advantages:
- Simple, safe sample procedure that may be combined with other tests
- Elevated levels are observed in 90% of cases
- Indicates level of disease activity

Disadvantage: Sample needs to be sent away for analysis

Normal
Women 0–20mm/h; men 0–15mm/h (Westergren method).

Abnormal
- Women >30mm/h; men >20mm/h (Westergren method)
- Keep in mind the possibility of a false-positive result

Cause of abnormal result
Inflammatory disease activity.

Drugs, disorders and other factors that may alter results
Infections, myocardial infarction, neoplasms, hyperthyroidism, hypothyroidism.

THYROID-STIMULATING HORMONE ASSAY

Description
Venous blood sample.

Advantages/Disadvantages
Advantages:
■ Primary test used in diagnosis of hypothyroidism/hyperthyroidism
■ Relatively readily available
■ Assays are very sensitive to diagnose hypothyroidism and to monitor replacement therapy

Disadvantage: May be normal in suprathyroid hypothyroidism

Normal
2–11mcU/mL.

Abnormal
■ <2 or >11mcU/mL
■ Keep in mind the possibility of a falsely abnormal result

Cause of abnormal result
■ Raised thyroid-stimulating hormone (TSH) levels indicate hypothyroidism
■ Low TSH levels indicate hyperthyroidism
■ Normal or low TSH levels occur in suprathyroid hypothyroidism

Drugs, disorders and other factors that may alter results
Many factors can cause raised TSH levels, including:
■ Raised TSH, e.g. insufficient dose of euthyroid therapy; recovery from severe nonthyroid illness; Addison's disease; lithium, amiodarone, amphetamines; blood sample taken in the evening, the peak of the normal diurnal variation in TSH levels
■ Lowered TSH level, e.g. excessive hypothyroid therapy; severe nonthyroid illness; active thyroiditis; pituitary insufficiency, Cushing's syndrome

Biopsy
POTASSIUM HYDROXIDE PREPARATION
Description
For KOH wet mount of infected scales, material is scraped from an active area of the lesion and placed on a glass slide with 10–15% KOH with or without dimethyl sulfoxide (DMSO).

Advantages/Disadvantages
Advantages:
■ Can be performed quickly and easily in the clinic
■ Highly sensitive and specific for dermatophyte identification

Normal
No septate hyphae seen on microscope.

Abnormal
- Septate hyphae, pseudohyphae or yeast forms seen on microscope
- Keep in mind the possibility of a falsely abnormal result

Cause of abnormal result
- Hyphae: fungal infections
- Pseudohyphae or yeast forms: *Candida* or *Pityrosporum* infections

Special tests
TRICHOGRAM
Description
- Also known as 'pluck test'
- Around 50 hairs are grasped from affected area in a rubber-tipped hemostat 1cm from scalp. Hairs are extracted by pulling quickly and forcibly in direction of growth
- Hair roots are examined microscopically and a telogen count is determined

Advantages/Disadvantages
Advantage: inexpensive and easy to perform
Disadvantage: painful

Normal
10% telogen hairs.

Abnormal
- >50% telogen hairs
- Keep in mind the possibility of a falsely abnormal result

Cause of abnormal result
- >50% telogen hairs: telogen effluvium, syphilis, diffuse alopecia areata
- No telogen hairs: trichotillomania

Other tests
WOOD'S LIGHT EXAMINATION
Description
Scales scraped from infected area.

Advantages/Disadvantages
Advantage: easy to perform.

Normal
No fluorescence.

Abnormal
- Blue-green fluorescence: presence of *Microsporum audouinii* and *M. canis* (tinea capitis)
- Coral-red fluorescence: presence of *Corynebacterium minutissimum* (erythrasma)
- Pale yellow fluorescence: *Malassezia furfur* (pityriasis versicolor)

FUNGAL CULTURE
Description
Samples from infected area grown on Sabouraud's glucose agar (with an antibiotic such as chloramphenicol to inhibit bacterial overgrowth), or special media containing cycloheximide such as dermatophyte test medium (DTM), Mycosel, or Mycobiotic.

Advantages/Disadvantages
Advantage: Can distinguish causative organism

Disadvantages:
- Expensive and time consuming
- False-negative results can occur

Normal
No growth.

Abnormal
- Growth of dermatophytes
- Keep in mind the possibility of a falsely abnormal result

Cause of abnormal result
Presence of dermatophytes.

TREATMENT

CONSIDER CONSULT

- Cicatricial alopecia may require referral to a dermatologist or rheumatologist to initiate treatment
- Trichotillomania: patients with extensive involvement or those who persist in the habit should be referred for psychiatric evaluation

MANAGEMENT ISSUES
Goals

- To diagnose and treat underlying cause of alopecia to prevent further hair loss and/or scarring
- To reassure patient if hair loss is temporary
- To reduce hair loss where possible
- To assist patient in accepting the condition

Management in special circumstances

Alopecia is a common side effect of cancer chemotherapy. Use of 'cold caps' (a locally applied scalp-cooling system) has proved useful. Flexible, gel-filled caps are applied to the scalp before, during, and after administration of chemotherapy for intervals of 105–300min according to the chemotherapy regimen being administered.

PATIENT SATISFACTION/LIFESTYLE PRIORITIES

Hair loss may have a seriously detrimental effect on self-esteem of some patients; treatment of alopecia may depend on the patient's perception of the loss.

SUMMARY OF THERAPEUTIC OPTIONS
Choices

In addition to the following therapies, hair weaves and wigs can be considered in most cases of alopecia. Changes in hair care may help reduce rate of hair loss.

Androgenic alopecia (male-/female-pattern baldness):
- Treatment of choice for men is oral finasteride: this is not FDA approved for use in women because of possible effects on reproductive system of developing male fetus
- Alternatively, topical minoxidil is available over-the-counter and is approved for use in men and women
- Hair transplants can permanently restore hair, but many sessions are needed and cost is high
- Scalp reduction can provide an instant hair effect. An anteroposterior excision of bald vertex scalp with primary closure can be repeated every 4 weeks until hair margins converge or scalp tissue becomes too thin

Alopecia areata:
- Intralesional injections of corticosteroids is first-line therapy for adults; this treatment is normally managed by a dermatologist
- Minoxidil, as for androgenic alopecia, can be tried, but efficacy is not well established

Telogen and anagen effluvium, and cicatricial alopecia (scarring alopecia):
- Underlying cause should be treated

Traction alopecia:
- Patient education of cause of hair loss

Trichotillomania:
- Many cases resolve with discussion and understanding
- Parents can distract a child from hair pulling and avoid punitive measures

Tinea capitis:

- Griseofulvin: an oral antifungal agent is necessary as topical agents are not able to penetrate the hair follicle sufficiently

Clinical pearls

For most patients, 50% hair loss is required for it to be noticeable. Thus, significant loss usually has occurred with clinical presentation.

FOLLOW UP

Laboratory monitoring may be required if systemic medications are utilized to treat alopecia.

Plan for review

Follow up examinations for patients with severe disease.

Information for patient or caregiver

- Because of psychosocial impact of hair loss, it is important to explain diagnosis to patient and, where possible, to determine what they may expect in terms of continuing hair loss
- Patient should be informed that response to any therapy may be slow and may include hair regrowth and/or retardation of further thinning
- No medical treatment may be an appropriate option for certain patients
- Hair loss in traction alopecia may become permanent if styling technique is continued
- Wigs or hair weaves should be discussed if appropriate

DRUGS AND OTHER THERAPIES: DETAILS
Drugs
ORAL FINASTERIDE

- Treatment of choice for men in androgenic alopecia
- Not FDA approved for use in women because of possible effects on the reproductive system of the developing male fetus

Dose

- 1mg daily continued indefinitely
- Takes effect after a minimum of 3 months

Efficacy
70–80% of men will experience some hair regrowth.

Risks/benefits
Risks:

- Use caution in hepatic disease
- Use caution in obstructive uropathy
- Condoms should be used if partner is pregnant or likely to become pregnant (finasteride is excreted in semen)
- Women of child-bearing age should avoid handling crushed or broken tablets

Benefit: Hair regrowth is more immediate than with minoxidil

Side effects and adverse reactions

- Genitourinary: decreased libido, impotence, ejaculation disorders, breast tenderness and enlargement
- Hypersensitivity reactions

Interactions (other drugs)
- No known drug interactions

Contraindications
- Children - Women - Pregnancy

Acceptability to patient
Patient motivation is generally high.

Follow up plan
Follow up at patient's request.

Patient and caregiver information
Patients should be informed that discontinuation of treatment results in relapse; this medication must therefore be taken for life, or until hair loss is no longer important to patient.

MINOXIDIL
Topical minoxidil may be used in either androgenic alopecia or alopecia areata.

Dose
1mL of 2% or 5% solution applied to scalp twice daily.

Efficacy
- One-third of men who are under 30 years and have been losing hair for <5 years grow hair long enough to be cut or combed on the vertex
- Effect on frontoparietal area is not known

Risks/benefits
Risks:
- Use caution in pregnancy and breast-feeding
- Use caution in cardiac, cerebrovascular, and renal disease
- Use caution in angina, congestive heart failure, and pulmonary hypertension

Benefits:
- Some patients prefer a topical treatment over long-term oral drugs
- Approved for use in both men and women
- Available over-the-counter

Side effects and adverse reactions
- Gastrointestinal: nausea, vomiting
- Cardiovascular system: edema, hypotension, cardiac lesions, cardiac tamponade, pericardial effusion, reflux and sinus tachycardia, angina
- Genitourinary: sodium and water retention, mastalgia
- Central nervous system: headache
- Skin: hypertrichosis, rash, Stevens-Johnson syndrome

Interactions (other drugs)
- No known interactions with topical minoxidil

Contraindications
- Recent myocardial infarction
- Pheochromocytoma
- Dissecting aortic aneurysm

Acceptability to patient
Hair growth is only evident after 8–12 months; however, patient motivation is usually good.

Follow up plan
Follow up at patient's request.

Patient and caregiver information
- Should be applied to a dry scalp and hair should not be wet for 1h afterwards
- Spontaneous reversal to pretreatment state can be expected after 1–3 months if therapy is stopped

INTRALESIONAL INJECTIONS OF CORTICOSTEROIDS
Corticosteroid treatment is the treatment of choice in adult alopecia areata. Triamcinolone acetonide is the first-choice; alternatively, methylprednisolone. Treatment is usually initiated and managed by a dermatologist.

Dose
Triamcinolone acetonide:
- Intralesional injection with 5mg/mL to a maximum of 0.5mg/square inch of affected skin
- Multiple intradermal infections of 0.1mL per site, approx. 1cm apart
- Treatments repeated every 4–6 weeks
- Children under 10 years are not usually treated with intralesional steroids because of pain localized at injection sites

Efficacy
- Initial regrowth is often seen in 4–8 weeks
- Therapy in patients who do not respond after 6 months should be discontinued

Risks/benefits
Risks:
- Does not provide quick response; may take several hours for relief
- Use caution with glomerulonephritis, ulcerative colitis, renal disease
- Use caution with AIDS, tuberculosis, ocular herpes simplex, live vaccines, viral and bacterial infections
- Use caution in diabetes mellitus, glaucoma, osteoporosis, hypertension
- Use caution in children and the elderly
- Use caution in recent myocardial infarction
- Use caution in psychosis
- Do not withdraw abruptly

Side effects and adverse reactions
- Side effects are minimized by short duration of therapy
- Cardiovascular system: hypertension, thromboembolism
- Central nervous system: insomnia, euphoria, depression, psychosis, seizures
- Endocrine: adrenal suppression, impaired glucose tolerance, growth suppression in children
- Eyes, ears, nose, and throat: cataract, glaucoma, blurred vision
- Gastrointestinal: dyspepsia, peptic ulceration, esophagitis, oral candidiasis, nausea, vomiting
- Musculoskeletal: proximal myopathy, osteoporosis
- Skin: delayed healing, acne, striae, transient atrophy at injection site

Interactions (other drugs)
- Aminoglutethamide ■ Antidiabetics ■ Barbiturates ■ Carbamazepine ■ Cholestyramine ■ Cholinesterase inhibitors ■ Cyclosporine ■ Diuretics ■ Estrogens ■ Isoniazid ■ Isoproterenol ■ Nonsteroidal anti-inflammatory drugs ■ Phenytoin ■ Rifampin ■ Salicylates

Contraindications
- Local or systemic infection ▪ Peptic ulcer ▪ Pregnancy and breast-feeding

Acceptability to patient
Patients are often concerned about the long-term use of steroids, and treatment can be unpleasant. However, patient motivation is generally high.

Follow up plan
Follow up for success of therapy, further treatment, and side effects.

Patient and caregiver information
- Main side effect is transient atrophy at the injection sites
- If therapy is unsuccessful after 6 months it should be discontinued

GRISEOFULVIN
Treatment of choice in tinea capitis for over 40 years.

Dose
- Pediatric: approx. 5mg/lb of body weight/day for a minimum of 6 weeks
- Adult: 250mg twice daily for 6 weeks
- Medication is absorbed best with a fatty meal

Efficacy
Good efficacy, although drug resistance is an increasing concern.

Risks/benefits
Risks:
- Causes side effects in 20% of patients
- Use caution with known penicillin allergy

Side effects and adverse reactions
- Gastrointestinal: diarrhea, nausea, vomiting, gastrointestinal bleeding, hepatoxicity
- Hypersensitivity: rashes, photosensitivity
- Hematologic: leukopenia, agranulocytosis
- Central nervous system: headache, fatigue, insomnia, confusion, dizziness

Interactions (other drugs)
- Aspirin ▪ Cyclosporine ▪ Oral contraceptives ▪ Phenobarbital ▪ Tacrolimus ▪ Warfarin

Contraindications
- Lupus erythematosus ▪ Porphyria ▪ Pregnancy ▪ Severe liver disease

Acceptability to patient
Moderate as there is a high risk of side effects.

Follow up plan
Careful follow up for side effects, compliance, nonresponding lesions.

Patient and caregiver information
- Take with food
- Complete course of medication

Surgical therapy
HAIR TRANSPLANTS
- Consider in androgenic alopecia
- Androgen-independent hairs from lateral and posterior areas of scalp are removed in 4mm cylinders containing 8–15 hairs. 3.5mm cylinders of skin are removed from recipient sites and replaced with the 4mm grafts
- >300 grafts may be necessary, carried out over many sessions at least one month apart

Efficacy
If performed by a skilled surgeon, cosmetic results can be extremely effective.

Risks/benefits
Risk: surgical risks are present.

Acceptability to patient
- Time consuming
- Expensive

SCALP REDUCTION
- Consider in androgenic alopecia
- An anteroposterior elliptic excision of bald vertex scalp is carried out with primary closure
- Procedure can be repeated every 4 weeks until hair margins converge or scalp tissue becomes too thin

Risks/benefits
Benefit: instant hair effect can be achieved.

Other therapies
WIGS AND HAIR WEAVES
- Consider in most forms of alopecia
- Wigs are widely available
- Hair weave techniques have been refined: strands of human hair are applied to a thin nylon filament that is anchored to the scalp with the individual's own hair. Individual must return every 6 weeks for a haircut and tightening of the growing anchor hairs

Acceptability to patient
- Acceptability of wigs varies from individual to individual
- Hair weaves are generally successful but more expensive and time consuming

LIFESTYLE
Changes in hair care may help reduce rate of hair loss:
- Avoid alkaline pH shampoos
- Pat rather than rub hair dry with a towel
- Use a comb rather than a brush, and never brush hair when wet
- Use of a conditioner makes hair easier to comb
- Avoid bleaching, permanent waving, straightening, hot combs, overly hot dryers, and excessive sun exposure

RISKS/BENEFITS
Benefit: may help reduce unnecessary hair wastage.

ACCEPTABILITY TO PATIENT
Generally acceptable and easy to comply with, except where styling techniques are important to individual's self-image.

EFFICACY OF THERAPIES
Efficacy of treatments is highly variable.

PROGNOSIS
Androgenic alopecia (male-/female-pattern baldness):
- Depends on success of treatment

Alopecia areata:
- Regrowth of hair generally begins after 1–3 months but may be followed by cycles of loss and growth in same or other areas
- If involvement is limited, prognosis for permanent regrowth is excellent
- If involvement is extensive, as in alopecia totalis (where all scalp hair is lost) or alopecia universalis (where facial and body hair also is lost), cycles of growth and loss may occur but prognosis for longterm regrowth is poor

Telogen and anagen effluvium:
- Hair loss is rarely permanent

Traction alopecia:
- Unless scarring is initiated in severe cases, hair should regrow if the cause is removed

Trichotillomania:
- Good for psychologically stable patient; otherwise, prognosis depends on success of behavior modification treatment

Cicatricial alopecia:
- Once scarring is initiated, hair loss is permanent

Tinea capitis:
- Successful treatment results in full recovery, but reinfection is possible unless the source is traced and treated (e.g. family pet, school friends)

Clinical pearls
Occasionally, alopecia is associated with systemic disease. In other cases, it is a cosmetic problem, but one that may be very disturbing to the patient. Appropriate time must be made for these patients in order to allow for the additional counseling that is frequently required.

Deterioration
- Look for differential diagnosis
- Consider specialist referral

COMPLICATIONS
Hair loss may be severe and/or permanent and cause considerable emotional distress.

CONSIDER CONSULT
- Specialist referral is indicated for further treatment options even in cases of only moderate success in the office of the PCP

RISK FACTORS

- In androgenic alopecia, family history: the disorder is genetically determined
- In telogen effluvium, diet: crash dieting can precipitate hair loss
- In anagen effluvium, medication history: chemotherapy can cause hair loss

MODIFY RISK FACTORS

Cold caps can help prevent hair loss after chemotherapy.

ASSOCIATIONS

American Academy of Dermatology
Alopecia Areata Foundation
714 C St, Suite 202
San Rafael, CA 94901
Tel: (415) 456–4644
www.aad.org

KEY REFERENCES

- Shellow VR. Approach to the patient with hair loss. In: Goroll AH, Mulley AG Jr. Primary care medicine. 3rd edn. Philadelphia (PA): Lippincott-Raven Publishers, 1995
- Habif TP. Hair diseases. In: Habif TP. Clinical dermatology. St Louis (MO): Mosby-Year Book, 1996
- Rietschel RL. Clinical aspects of hair disorders. Dermatol Clin 1996;14:691–5
- Sperling LC, Mezebish DS. Office dermatology, part 1: hair diseases. Med Clin N Am 1998;82:1155–69
- Farrell A, Sinclair R, Dawber R. Disorders of the hair and scalp. Oxford: Health Press, 2000

FAQS
Question 1
What abnormalities of nails are associated with hair loss?

ANSWER 1
- Alopecia areata: pits
- Inflammatory dermatoses: psoriasis – oil spots, pits; lichen planus – pterygium; connective tissue disease (e.g. lupus erythematosus) – periungual telangiectasia

Question 2
How quickly does minoxidil work?

ANSWER 2
Frequently, it takes many months (6 or more). Patients must be motivated to use therapy for several months without improvement or they will be frustrated and quit before adequate trial.

Question 3
Does hair loss that is not cosmetically significant warrant investigation?

ANSWER 3
Yes, alopecia off the scalp is not androgenic, and thus may be a sign of systemic disease.

CONTRIBUTORS

Randolph L Pearson, MD
Seth R Stevens, MD
Richard Averitte, MD

BASAL CELL CARCINOMA

DESCRIPTION

- Most common malignant skin tumor arising from the basal cells of the epidermis
- Macroscopic appearance of the lesions is varied
- There are four main subtypes: nodular, superficial, pigmented, and aggressive growth type (morpheaform or infiltrative)
- Malignant nature of the tumor lies in its potential for local rather than metastatic growth
- Main causative factor is accumulative exposure to sunlight
- Most occur on the upper part of the face

KEY! DON'T MISS!

- Involvement of local structures or regional lymph nodes
- Possibility that lesion may be a melanoma (pigmented basal cell carcinomas have a similar appearance to melanoma, and amelanotic melanoma should be considered)

ICD9 CODE

- 173.9 Basal cell carcinoma, site unspecified
- 173.3 Basal cell carcinoma, face
- 173.4 Basal cell carcinoma, neck or scalp
- 173.5 Basal cell carcinoma of the trunk
- 173.6 Basal cell carcinoma, upper limb
- 173.7 Basal cell carcinoma, lower limb

SYNONYMS

- Rodent ulcer
- Basal cell epithelioma
- Basalioma

CARDINAL FEATURES

- Most common malignant skin tumor arising from the basal cells of the epidermis
- There are four main subtypes: nodular, superficial, pigmented, and aggressive growth type (morpheaform or infiltrative)
- These subtypes vary with respect to macroscopic appearance (and thus presentation), histology, and biologic aggressiveness
- Most common presentation is the nodular type, with a papule that has a pearly, shiny border, and surface telangiectasia. The lesion often ulcerates in the center, thus causing the characteristic bleeding and scabbing lesion that heals and recurs
- Morpheaform basal cell carcinoma is the most biologically aggressive
- They rarely metastasize: their malignant potential lies in their ability to invade and destroy local tissues, such as bone and brain
- Main causative factor is accumulative exposure to sunlight
- 85% occur on the face and neck, as these areas are most exposed to the sun
- Treatment depends on the site and size of the tumor, tumor margins, and histology

CAUSES

Common causes

- Exposure to sunlight, most importantly ultraviolet B (UVB) radiation
- Exposure to UVA and UVB radiation in tanning salons

Rare causes

- In some areas, exposure to inorganic arsenic from industrial sources or well water. Arsenic was historically used in some skin preparations
- *Calymmatobacterium granulomatis* and granuloma inguinale
- Basal cell nevus syndrome or nevoid basal cell carcinoma syndrome (gene defect: PTCH or patched gene)

Contributory or predisposing factors

- Fair skin and the propensity to freckle or burn rather than tan in the sun
- History of repeated sunburn or childhood exposure to the sun
- Outdoor occupation
- Immunosuppression from disease (HIV) or drugs
- Genetic disorders (e.g. xeroderma pigmentosum, nevoid basal cell carcinoma syndrome, albinism)
- Personal or family history of basal cell carcinoma
- History of radiation treatment

EPIDEMIOLOGY
Incidence and prevalence
Most common type of skin cancer.

INCIDENCE
- Average incidence in the US: 1.91 per 1000 Caucasians
- Incidence is increasing worldwide

FREQUENCY
900,000 cases are identified each year in the US.

Demographics
AGE
- Incidence increases with increasing age
- Most basal cell carcinomas are seen after the age of 40
- Those seen in patients <35 years are usually of the most aggressive type

GENDER
Males are more commonly affected than females, although female incidence is increasing.

RACE
Seen almost exclusively in Caucasians.

GENETICS
- Basal cell carcinoma nevus syndrome is a genetically linked autosomal dominant disorder characterized by multiple basal cell carcinomas as well as other features
- Xeroderma pigmentosum is a rare genetic disorder characterized by oversensitivity to UV radiation

GEOGRAPHY
Areas with warm/hot climates (tropical and subtropical regions), e.g. southern states of the US and Australia, where a significant proportion of the population is of Celtic origin.

SOCIOECONOMIC STATUS
- Outdoor workers have more sun exposure and, thus, higher risk for developing basal cell carcinoma
- Lack of education about sun protection is a risk factor

DIFFERENTIAL DIAGNOSIS
Differential diagnoses consist of other skin lesions, most of which are also related to repeated sun exposure.

Solar keratosis (actinic keratosis)
The key features of solar keratosis (actinic keratosis) are as follows.

FEATURES
- May be considered a premalignant skin lesion (may transform into squamous cell carcinoma)
- Caused by long-term sun exposure
- Most often seen on face, neck, hands, and arms
- Flat, brown, localized lesions
- Most common in older people with a long history of sun exposure

Seborrheic keratosis
Benign skin lesion.

FEATURES
- Common in elderly population
- Pigmented raised lesion, with a greasy surface

Squamous cell carcinoma
Squamous cell carcinoma is the second most common type of skin cancer.
FEATURES
- Usually occurs in sun-exposed areas of skin
- May arise from chronic ulcers or scars
- More likely to metastasize than basal cell carcinoma
- Typical presentation is an ulcerated nodule or a superficial plaque

Melanoma
Melanoma is a malignant and aggressive skin tumor.

FEATURES
- Usual presentation is a pigmented, irregular lesion, or a change in a pre-existing nevus
- Metastasis is common and the 5-year survival rate for patients with metastatic melanoma is low
- May be amelanotic or pigmented

Molluscum contagiosum
Molluscum contagiosum is a viral skin disorder.

FEATURES
- Skin papules that are pearly white or flesh-colored and have an umbilicated center
- No raised edge
- Lesions may be itchy or tender
- Seen on genitalia in adults, and face, trunk, and limbs in children

Nummular eczema (discoid eczema)
FEATURES
- Tends to be chronic, with periods of quiescence and exacerbation
- Discrete, coin-shaped patches of skin, most commonly on the arms, back, buttocks, and lower legs

- May be crusted, scaling, and extremely itchy
- More common during the winter months
- Cause is unknown

Scar

Scar formation is a naturally occurring phenomenon after deep injury to the skin, usually associated with connective tissue hyperplasia.

FEATURES

- Characteristic history (injury, surgery in the affected area)
- Epidermis is usually slightly hypotrophic and lacks skin appendages; underlying connective tissue is hypertrophic
- Requires no treatment unless hypertrophy is excessive

Bowen's disease

Squamous cell carcinoma *in situ*, with potential for significant lateral spread.

FEATURES

- Single lesion in two-thirds of cases
- Lesion up to several centimeters in diameter, with a sharply demarcated, irregular border
- Lesion is asymptomatic
- May occur on sun-exposed or covered skin (head and neck most commonly involved) and on mucous membranes

Morphea or localized scleroderma

Autoimmune disorder of unknown cause, which rarely develops into systemic disease, known as systemic sclerosis.

FEATURES

- Thickening and induration of the skin and subcutaneous tissue due to excessive collagen deposition
- Starts as patches of yellowish or ivory-colored rigid, dry skin. The lesions subsequently become hard, slightly depressed plaques which usually have a whitish or yellowish center surrounded by a purplish halo
- Single or multiple cutaneous lesion can develop
- Usually no internal involvement

SIGNS & SYMPTOMS
Signs

- Appearance of the lesion depends on the subtype
- Nodular lesions appear: raised pink or pearly white papules which may have a translucent, rolled, pearly edge, and surface telangiectasia. As they grow, central ulceration may be a feature, and a scab or crust may be seen
- Pigmented basal cell carcinomas: similar appearance to melanoma or seborrheic keratosis; the pearly raised border is seen
- Morpheaform lesions: usually flat and scaly, waxy and yellow-white with an indistinct border
- Superficial basal cell carcinomas: pearly white border surrounding a red scaling plaque; most often seen on the trunk and limbs
- Presence of other skin lesions related to sunlight exposure is common
- If the lesion has invaded the surrounding tissues, it may be fixated rather than freely movable over deep structures
- Lymphadenopathy is extremely rare

Symptoms

- Typical presenting complaint is an irritating skin lesion that has been bleeding or scabbing recurrently
- Itchy lesion
- Pain is rare
- Often asymptomatic

ASSOCIATED DISORDERS

Other disorders commonly caused by exposure to ultraviolet (UV) radiation:

- Squamous cell carcinoma
- Malignant melanoma
- Actinic keratosis

KEY! DON'T MISS!

- Involvement of local structures or regional lymph nodes
- Possibility that lesion may be a melanoma (pigmented basal cell carcinomas have a similar appearance to melanoma, and amelanotic melanoma should be considered)

CONSIDER CONSULT

Refer for biopsy of suspicious lesions and appropriate counseling regarding treatment options.

INVESTIGATION OF THE PATIENT
Direct questions to patient

Q **For how long have you noticed the lesion?** Due to the ulcerated area's intermittently scabbing, patients often assume their condition to be improving, thus delaying treatment.

Q **What is your occupation?** Outdoor occupations have more sun exposure.

Q **Have you ever been treated for or noticed other lesions?** A previous history of basal cell carcinoma is a risk factor for development of new lesions, including other photoinduced malignancies.

Q **Have you had skeletal abnormalities identified?** Odontogenic cysts and bifid ribs are part of the basal cell nevus syndrome.

Contributory or predisposing factors

Q **Have you had a lot of exposure to sunlight?** UV radiation is the main risk factor for skin cancers.

Q **Do you visit tanning salons?** Exposure to UVA and UVB radiation can occur with this type of tanning.

Q **Are you currently taking any medications?** Immune suppression is a risk factor for skin cancer.

Q **Have you ever received radiotherapy?** Radiotherapy is a risk factor for skin cancer.

Family history

Q **Has anyone in your family been treated for basal cell carcinoma?** Family history is a known risk factor for basal cell carcinoma.

Examination

- General examination will usually reveal fair skin and freckles
- Examine the lesion in bright white or natural light for specific features of basal cell carcinoma
- Examine for local invasion of surrounding and underlying tissues. Basal cell carcinomas can infiltrate local tissues if they are not treated promptly. In almost all cases, however, the clinically apparent lesion is much smaller than the actual extent of the tumor
- Examine the regional lymph nodes for any local spread
- Examine skin for other lesions, paying particular attention to the scalp, face, ears, medial canthus, and within the nasolabial folds. All of the skin should be examined

Summary of investigative tests
- Only investigation of use is a biopsy of the lesion
- Biopsy allows for confirmation of the diagnosis and, in some instances, concurrent treatment of the lesion by removing it completely
- Either a partial (punch or shave) or an excisional biopsy may performed
- Excisional biopsy is the 'gold standard' technique and is the method of choice if the diagnosis is in doubt (e.g. pigmented basal cell carcinoma may be similar in appearance to melanoma)

DIAGNOSTIC DECISION
Diagnosis is based on clinical features of the lesion and is confirmed by biopsy. Biopsy also gives information on histology and depth of invasion.

Guidelines
The American Academy of Dermatology. Guidelines of care for basal cell carcinoma.[1]

CLINICAL PEARLS
- The presence of basal cell carcinoma is an indication of the appropriate genetic background (e.g. pigmentation) and environmental exposure (e.g. UV radiation in sunlight) to warrant close inspection for squamous cell carcinoma as well as additional basal cell carcinomas
- Particularly in early disease, it can be difficult to distinguish basal cell carcinoma from other neoplastic lesions. In these instances, punch biopsy should be obtained to preclude missing the opportunity for important diagnostic and prognostic data regarding a melanoma. Alternatively, one does not want to subject a patient to definitive therapy for presumed cancer if the lesion is benign

THE TESTS
Biopsy
EXCISIONAL BIOPSY
Description
The 'gold standard' for biopsy techniques. The entire macroscopic lesion is removed for histologic examination.

Advantages/Disadvantages
Advantages:
- Allows simultaneous treatment of the lesion if the entire lesion is removed
- Full-thickness biopsy with margins is obtained

Disadvantages:
- Microscopic margins of the lesion cannot be assessed at the time of the procedure
- Requires appropriate training
- More time-consuming than other biopsy techniques

Normal
Normal skin histology.

Abnormal
- Histologic appearance consistent with basal cell carcinoma – nidus of basal cells extending into the dermis; neoplastic cells resemble normal basal cells with large basophilic oval nuclei; mitoses are rarely seen
- Keep in mind the possibility of a falsely abnormal result

PUNCH BIOPSY
Description

A method for obtaining a sample of the lesion with a disposable punch device.

Advantages/Disadvantages
Advantages:
- Simple procedure
- Provides a full-thickness skin biopsy
- Minimal skin damage and scarring

Disadvantage: Not suitable for malignant melanoma or pigmented basal cell carcinoma

Normal
Normal histology.

Abnormal
- Histology consistent with basal cell carcinoma – nidus of basal cells extending into the dermis; neoplastic cells resemble normal basal cells with large basophilic oval nuclei; mitoses are rarely seen
- Keep in mind the possibility of a falsely abnormal result

SHAVE BIOPSY
Description
A method for obtaining a sample of the lesion when a full-thickness sample is not required. A surgical blade is passed through the skin and underneath the lesion.

Advantages/Disadvantages
Advantages:
- Excellent cosmetic results
- Suitable for nodular, raised lesions

Disadvantage: Full-thickness sample is not obtained; if the lesion is in fact a melanoma, it does not provide critical prognostic information which is crucial to determine the utility of adjunctive therapy

Normal
Normal skin histology.
Abnormal
- Histology consistent with basal cell carcinoma – nidus of basal cells extending into the dermis; neoplastic cells resemble normal basal cells with large basophilic oval nuclei; mitoses are rarely seen
- Keep in mind the possibility of a falsely abnormal result

TREATMENT

CONSIDER CONSULT

- Refer if lesion has features consistent with an aggressive growth pattern
- Consider referral if lesion is on the nose or eyelid (an area that is prone to recurrence, and where excision or biopsy may be difficult)
- Refer if there is local tissue or lymph node involvement
- Refer for specialized treatment if the lesion is recurrent or in a high-risk area (ear, nose, nasolabial fold, periorbital area, and scalp)
- Refer if Mohs' micrographic surgery or radiation therapy will be the treatment of choice
- Refer if there is local invasion into nearby structures (thus requiring extensive surgery)
- Refer if the lesion is difficult to remove, or if the wound will require skin grafting

PATIENT AND CAREGIVER ISSUES
Patient or caregiver request

- **Is this type of cancer dangerous?** Basal cell carcinomas rarely metastasize, but they can destroy local tissues
- **Was the cancer caused by sunburn?** Exposure to sunlight is the most common causative factor for the development of basal cell carcinoma
- **Do I need chemotherapy?** Systemic chemotherapy is not indicated
- **Will I get any more cancers?** Patients who have had one basal cell carcinoma are at a higher risk for developing further lesions and should be followed-up regularly and long term

Health-seeking behavior

- **Have you delayed seeking treatment?** Patients often delay seeking treatment, as the lesions periodically scab and improve
- **Have you had lesions treated in the past?** Increased risk for further basal cell carcinoma is noted in these cases

MANAGEMENT ISSUES
Goals

- Removal of the entire lesion
- Preservation of the maximum amount of normal tissue
- Achievement of the optimal cosmetic result
- Prevention of local (and metastatic) spread
- Education on skin cancer prevention, including skin self-examination and sun protection

Management in special circumstances
COEXISTING DISEASE

- Radiotherapy is contraindicated in patients with xeroderma pigmentosum and nevoid basal cell carcinoma
- Patients who are immunocompromised or taking immunosuppressive therapy are more likely to have tumors with aggressive biologic behavior, and should be treated accordingly

COEXISTING MEDICATION
Corticosteroid use (long-term) affects wound healing and, thus, must be considered when deciding on therapy.

SPECIAL PATIENT GROUPS

- Radiation therapy or cryotherapy may be used for any patients who will not tolerate extensive surgery (e.g. elderly patients)
- Definitive treatment may not be required in terminally ill patients

PATIENT SATISFACTION/LIFESTYLE PRIORITIES
Some patients will be more concerned about a good cosmetic result than others.

SUMMARY OF THERAPEUTIC OPTIONS
Choices
General considerations:

- Guidelines for the management of basal cell carcinoma are complicated because there are several well accepted surgical and nonsurgical approaches. All methods may be curative for some lesions, but no single treatment method is applicable for all basal cell carcinomas
- The treatment choice for basal cell carcinoma is dependent on the lesion (site, size, histology, primary or recurrent lesion, growth rate, margins) and the patient (age, medical status, psychologic factors, medications)
- Recurrence rate should be the primary consideration in treatment choice, but must be balanced against other factors
- Small lesions in low-risk areas of the nodular, pigmented, or superficial type are effectively managed with most treatment choices
- Large, ulcerated, recurrent, or infiltrative morpheaform lesions may require a more aggressive approach to treatment

Forms of therapy:

- Curettage and electrosurgery is useful for small, nodular lesions (<6mm diameter) regardless of site; some larger lesions in low-risk sites (e.g. lower limbs, neck); and superficial primary lesions. It is not suitable for eyelid or lip lesions
- Cryotherapy is useful for small nodular and superficial primary lesions, when there are multiple lesions or when other forms of surgery are contraindicated
- Surgical excision is used for primary and recurrent lesions. This method is preferred for larger lesions (>2cm) on the cheek, forehead, trunk, and legs. This is the treatment of choice for nodular and superficial lesions when surgery is not contraindicated
- Mohs' micrographic surgery is performed by a subspecialist and is the preferred treatment for high-risk primary lesions (lesions on nose or eyelid or with an aggressive growth pattern or poorly defined clinical margins, and large tumors), and recurrent tumors. It is also indicated when maximum preservation of uninvolved surrounding tissue is desired (e.g. eyelid, nose)
- Radiation therapy is used for some primary tumors in patients who are not fit for surgery or for the palliation of inoperable tumors. It may also be used in areas where tumors are difficult to excise or where it is important to preserve surrounding tissue (e.g. lip). Its use is declining
- Laser surgery, phototherapy, and intralesional interferon therapy are examples of newer treatment methods. These therapies do not have proven efficacy, as they are still in the investigational phase, and are instituted by a specialist
- In addition to these therapeutic options, the patient should be advised to avoid excessive exposure to sunlight

Guidelines

- The American Academy of Dermatology. Guidelines of care for basal cell carcinoma. [1]
- The National Comprehensive Cancer Network (NCCN) guidelines of care for nonmelanoma skin cancers. [2]
- The American Academy of Family Physicians has published information on basal cell carcinoma. [3]

Clinical pearls

■ Basal cell carcinomas do not grow as discrete balls of cells. Rather, they usually grow with extensions that can be impossible to see. Therefore, treatment by curettage and electrodessication should be performed only by those with sufficient experience to be able to distinguish malignant from adjacent normal tissue. This tendency to track results in the desirability of Mohs' surgery for lesions in embryologic fusion planes
■ Basal cell carcinomas are slow growing and rarely metastasize. Risk-benefit analysis ratios should be considered in patients who are otherwise in poor health (i.e. with a short life expectancy) before embarking on costly treatments, or those that may require significant care at home

Never

Never treat a basal cell carcinoma with topical 5-fluorouracil, as it is associated with subdermal and clinically undetectable extension of the tumor under a healed epidermis.

FOLLOW UP
Plan for review

■ Long-term follow up is required due to the risk of recurrence and of further primary lesions developing
■ Early detection of new lesions allows for a simpler treatment approach with a higher cure rate and less morbidity
■ One suggested plan for follow up is: 3-monthly for 3 years, 6-monthly for 5 years, and yearly thereafter

Information for patient or caregiver

■ Patient must carefully and regularly self-examine their skin for early detection of new lesions
■ Patient must avoid further sun exposure to prevent the development of new lesions
■ Patient must be given advice regarding skin protection (such as sunscreen) when exposed to the sun

DRUGS AND OTHER THERAPIES: DETAILS
Surgical therapy
CURETTAGE AND ELECTROSURGERY

The lesion is alternately debrided with a curette, and then an extra margin of tissue can be destroyed by electrodessication, electrocoagulation, or electrocautery.

Efficacy

■ Effective for the treatment of small (<6mm) primary lesions that are well defined (nodular and superficial types)
■ When used appropriately, the 5-year cure rate is >90%
■ Not as effective in recurrent lesions that are in scar tissue
■ Not as effective for high-risk lesions

Risks/benefits
Risks:

■ Higher recurrence rate
■ Wound will take 4–6 weeks to heal
■ Leaves a hyper- or hypopigmented, atrophic or hypertrophic scar
■ A blind method of removal, thus provides no margins to ensure the lesion is completely removed

Benefits:
- Requires training and experience in the technique, but is easy to learn and perform
- Tissue should break down easily, thus confirming the clinical impression during the procedure
- Curette can be used in combination with cryotherapy or as a first-stage debulking procedure in combination with other therapies
- Inexpensive and time-efficient

Evidence
Curettage and electrosurgery is a useful treatment option for selected low-risk lesions (usually primary lesions) [1] *Level C*

Acceptability to patient
Patients who desire a good cosmetic result may find this treatment unacceptable.

Follow up plan
Wound can take up to 6 weeks to heal and should be monitored over this time period.

Patient and caregiver information
Patient should be told immediately to report any sign of wound infection or recurrence of tumor at the site of therapy.

SIMPLE EXCISION
- Surgical excision of the lesion with a margin of macroscopically normal tissue
- Simple surgical excision is the treatment of choice for small nodular or superficial tumors

Efficacy
- Useful for primary and recurrent tumors
- Recurrence depends on the initial size of the tumor and on the surgical margins achieved
- Effective for larger lesions (>2cm are most often excised)

Risks/benefits
Risks:
- Complete excision with wide tumor margins is not always achieved, as the procedure depends on clinical judgment
- Some normal tissue must be sacrificed
- Training for the procedure is required and it is time-consuming
- In the overwhelming majority of cases excisions are performed under local anesthetic on an outpatient basis; rarely, depending on the size of the lesion, it may need to be performed as an inpatient under general anesthetic

Benefits:
- Allows histologic examination of the tumor margins
- Can be used for large tumors with clearly defined borders
- Acceptable cosmetic result
- Faster healing than with other methods
- Better results for larger (>2cm) lesions

Evidence
- Surgical excision is effective for the treatment of primary and recurrent basal cell carcinomas [3] *Level C*
- A RCT compared surgery and radiotherapy for the treatment of primary basal cell carcinomas of the face (<4cm). Treatment failure rates at 4 years were lower for patients treated surgically, and cosmetic results were significantly better with surgery [4] *Level P*

Acceptability to patient
Generally well tolerated.

Follow up plan
Patients should be seen in the postoperative period for inspection of the wound and removal of sutures.

Patient and caregiver information
Patient should be told immediately to report any sign of infection or recurrence of tumor at the site of therapy.

MOHS' MICROGRAPHIC SURGERY
Microsurgically controlled removal of the lesion by a specialist.

Efficacy
- Effective for both primary and secondary lesions
- Lowest recurrence rate of all treatments at 5 years

Risks/benefits
Risks:
- Relatively expensive
- Time-consuming

Benefits:
- Useful for lesions in high-risk areas or lesions that are biologically aggressive
- Surgical margins are assessed during the procedure to ensure they are clear of tumor, while preserving the maximum amount of normal tissue
- Has the lowest recurrence rate at 5 years
- Excellent cosmetic results when combined with cosmetic repair. Usually, training in Mohs' surgery includes such repair techniques

Evidence
- Mohs' micrographic surgery is an effective treatment option for high-risk and recurrent lesions [3] *Level C*
- A systematic review of prospective trials found that recurrence rates after 5 years for tumors treated with Mohs' micrographic surgery were lower that those for surgical excision, cryosurgery, and curettage and electodessication [5] *Level P*

Acceptability to patient
Generally well accepted, as there is low recurrence and a good cosmetic result, although it is more expensive.

Follow up plan
Postoperative specialist follow up is required.

Patient and caregiver information
Patient should be told immediately to report any sign of wound infection or recurrence of tumor at the site of therapy.

Radiation therapy
RADIOTHERAPY
Radiation therapy may be used in patients who will not tolerate surgery, or for palliation of inoperable tumors. Its use for basal cell carcinoma is declining.

Efficacy
Radiation cure rates for small, nonaggressive tumors are close to 90%.

Risks/benefits
Risks:
- Poor cosmetic result (especially evident at 5 years postsurgery)
- Healing time may be longer
- Contraindicated for patients with xeroderma pigmentosum or nevoid basal cell carcinoma, as it may induce more tumors at the treatment site
- Local pain and inflammation are common side effects
- More expensive than surgical treatment
- Secondary malignancies may develop several years afterward as a result of the treatment
- Radiodermatitis may develop
- Treatment period is 3–4 weeks

Benefits:
- No anesthetic or surgical risk
- Can be useful in areas where preservation of surrounding tissues is important for cosmetic regions (e.g. eyelid, lips)

Evidence
- Radiation therapy is a useful treatment option for selected BCCs [1] *Level C*
- A RCT compared surgery and radiotherapy for the treatment of primary basal cell carcinomas of the face (<4cm). Treatment failure rates at 4 years were lower for patients treated surgically, and cosmetic results were significantly better with surgery [4] *Level P*

Acceptability to patient
Usually acceptable to patients in whom other therapies are contraindicated.

Follow up plan
Patient should be followed up during the course of the 4-week treatment.

Other therapies
CRYOTHERAPY
Cryotherapy destroys tissue by reducing the temperature of the lesion to tumoricidal levels. Liquid nitrogen is administered with a spray device or cryoprobe.

Efficacy
- Effective for small, well-defined primary tumors of the nodular and superficial histologic subtypes
- Cure rates are 98% in some series

Risks/benefits
Risks:
- Contraindicated in patients with cold intolerance, cryoglobulinemia, cryofibrinogenemia, or platelet deficiency
- Pigment loss over the scar, hypertrophic scarring, and neuropathies are possible complications
- May have severe postoperative pain and swelling, and blistering of the wound

Benefits:

- Useful when there are multiple lesions
- Useful in elderly or patients with coexisting disease where other forms of surgery may be contraindicated
- Anesthesia is not usually required for small lesions
- Inexpensive and time-efficient

Evidence

- Cryosurgery is useful for the treatment of primary basal cell carcinomas, and some recurrent lesions [1] *Level C*
- A systematic review of prospective trials found that cryotherapy is superior to curettage and electrodessication in terms of 5-year recurrence rate, but is less effective than surgery [4] *Level P*

Acceptability to patient
Patients who desire a good cosmetic result may find this treatment unacceptable.

Follow up plan
Patient should be followed up to ensure there is adequate analgesia and wound healing.

Patient and caregiver information

- Patients should be informed that a wound may appear a few days after treatment
- Wound should be washed daily with soap and water
- Patients should immediately report any sign of infection or recurrence of tumor at the site of therapy

LIFESTYLE
Avoid excessive exposure to the sun and employ methods to reduce harmful effects of ultraviolet (UV) radiation when in sun (e.g. wear a hat, long-sleeved shirt, sunscreen).

RISKS/BENEFITS
Benefit: reduces the risk of sun exposure-related skin disorders.

ACCEPTABILITY TO PATIENT
May be difficult if occupation is outdoors.

EFFICACY OF THERAPIES
- Cure rates vary with the size, location, and histology of the lesion
- Low-risk basal cell carcinoma may be successfully treated in >90% of cases
- Electrodessication and curettage gives 5-year cure rates of >90% for selected tumors (<2cm, nodular). It is less effective than other types of surgery and cryotherapy
- Cryosurgery cure rates for primary basal cell carcinoma have been reported to be as high as 98% with careful patient selection
- Excisional surgery cure rates as high as 98% have been reported. Simple excision is second only to Mohs' micrographic surgery in terms of recurrence rates
- Mohs' micrographic surgery has a cure rate of 99.8% for primary and recurrent basal cell carcinoma. It has the lowest 5-year recurrence rate of all therapies
- Radiation therapy cure rates for small, nonaggressive tumors are close to 90%

Evidence
- Treatment failure rates at 4 years for primary facial basal cell carcinomas (<4cm) have been found to be lower for patients treated surgically than with radiotherapy. Also, cosmetic results were significantly better with surgery in this RCT [4] *Level P*
- A systematic review of prospective trials found that recurrence rates after 5 years for tumors treated with Mohs' micrographic surgery were lower that those for surgical excision, cryosurgery, and curettage and electrodessication [5] *Level P*

Review period
Patients should be followed periodically for 5 years or more.

PROGNOSIS
Primary tumors of the ears, eyelids, scalp, and nose have the highest recurrence rates.

Clinical pearls
- The prognosis of individual lesions, even those that are recurrent, are quite good. Some patients, not uncommonly, will have several (to several dozen or even more) lesions over several decades due to the field effect of exposure to UV and the genetic predisposition. Regardless, life expectancy is not significantly reduced
- The danger from basal cell carcinomas arises from their ability to track along and invade vital structures, particularly given their predilection for the face and ears. At other sites they can become large fungating tumors with healing issues and risk of infection
- Photoprotection can reduce risk of new tumors

Therapeutic failure
- Therapeutic failure may occur if the margins of the tumor are not completely excised
- Inadequate treatment can transform lesions into more biologically aggressive tumors

Recurrence
- Tumors that recur are best treated by Mohs' micrographic surgery; 96% of recurrent tumors (which were previously treated with other methods) are cured when treated with Mohs' micrographic surgery
- Most recurrences occur in the first 5 years following treatment

Terminal illness
Palliation or observation may be considered in terminally ill patients.

COMPLICATIONS

- Disfigurement or poor cosmetic result after treatment
- Local recurrence and spread
- Invasion of adjacent structures (e.g. eye, brain) is possible, especially when tumors that originated on the nose or medial canthus are inadequately treated
- Death occurs very rarely if there is intracranial invasion or erosion of major blood vessels

CONSIDER CONSULT

- Virtually all lesions benefit from treatment by someone (usually a dermatologist) with special training in the treatment of basal cell carcinomas, in order to minimize the removal of normal tissue while maximizing the chance for cure
- Refer for specialist management if there is recurrence at the primary treatment site

PREVENTION

- Avoidance of sun exposure and protection from the sun
- Detection of early cancers prevents complications such as invasion and ulceration

MODIFY RISK FACTORS

Education regarding sun protection and avoidance is an important preventive measure for all skin cancers.

Lifestyle and wellness

ENVIRONMENT
- Patients should be advised to avoid direct exposure to the sun between the hours of 10 a.m. and 3 p.m.
- Patients should wear protective clothing, sunscreen, and hats while outdoors

FAMILY HISTORY
Patients with family members who have had basal cell carcinoma are at higher risk for developing the condition. They may benefit from counseling regarding sun protection and skin self-examination.

CHEMOPROPHYLAXIS
Treatment with retinoids is a possible medical prophylactic. This treatment is still in the investigative phase.

Cost/efficacy
Efficacy is unknown.

SCREENING

The effectiveness of screening for skin cancer is incompletely determined. There is some reasonably strong evidence that knowledge regarding skin cancer can be improved with promotional brochures and educational programs. The American Academy of Dermatology sponsors annual free skin cancer screenings in most US cities and large towns.

Guidelines
- The United States Preventive Services Task Force has developed guidelines. Screening for skin cancer: recommendations and rationale. [6]
- The American College of Preventive Medicine. Screening for skin cancer. [7]

SKIN EXAMINATION
- Clinicians may educate at-risk patients on the relevant signs and symptoms and the potential benefits of self-examination
- Clinicians should include skin examination as part of the routine examination
- There is insufficient evidence to recommend for or against counseling patients to perform periodic skin self-examination or for examination by the PCP

Cost/efficacy
- Effectiveness of screening for skin cancer has not been proven
- Screening involves a 3-min visual inspection of the entire skin surface, which is a fast, noninvasive, and sensitive screening method
- Screening is most cost-effective when directed at high-risk populations (personal or family history of skin cancer, outdoor occupation)

- Counseling on self-examination has little cost because education on how to perform the examination is all that is required
- Basal cell carcinoma has a better than 95% cure rate if detected and treated early
- Early treatment of basal cell carcinoma may decrease morbidity and improve the cosmetic result

PREVENT RECURRENCE

- Prevention of recurrence in a treated lesion is achieved by appropriate initial assessment and therapy
- Prevention of the development of further basal cell carcinoma is best achieved by avoidance of sun exposure and sun protection. Avoiding direct exposure to the sun between the hours of 10 a.m. and 3 p.m., and wearing protective clothing and hats are recommended. It is generally accepted that sunscreen does lower the risk of skin cancer, but there is no direct evidence to support this for basal cell carcinomas
- Skin self-examination is recommended, but there is no evidence to confirm that it improves outcome

ASSOCIATIONS

American Academy of Dermatology
930 N Meacham Road
PO Box 4014
Schaumburg, IL 60168–4014
Tel: (847) 330–0230
Fax: (847) 330–0050
http://www.aad.org/

American Cancer Society
Tel: (800) ACS–2345
http://www3.cancer.org/

Cancer Management Manual
BC Cancer Agency
600 West 10th Avenue
Vancouver, BC
Canada V5Z 4E6
http://www.bccancer.bc.ca/cmm/skin/02.shtml#1

KEY REFERENCES

- Garner KL, Rodney WM. Basal and squamous carcinoma. Primary care. Clin Office Pract 2000;27:447–58
- Basal cell carcinoma of the skin CancerNet (A Service of the National Cancer Institute)
- Ferrini R, Perlman M, Hill L. Screening for skin cancer American College of Preventive Medicine Practice policy statement. Am J Prev Med 1998;14:80–2 Available at the National Guideline Clearinghouse (http://www.guidelines.gov/FRAMESETS/guideline_fs.asp?guideline=000558&sSearch_st)
- Feightner JW. Prevention of skin cancer. In: Canadian Task Force on the Periodic Health Examination. Canadian guide to clinical preventive health care. Ottawa: Health Canada 1994: 850–9. Available at the National Guideline Clearinghouse
- Screening for skin cancer – including counseling to prevent skin cancer. Guide to clinical preventive services, 2nd edn. Baltimore: Williams and Wilkins; 1996, p141–52
- Rose LC. Recognizing neoplastic skin lesions: a photo guide. American Family Physician 1998;58:873–84, 887–8. Produced by the American Academy of Family Physicians

Evidence references and guidelines

1 The American Academy of Dermatology. Guidelines of care for basal cell carcinoma. The Committee on Guidelines of Care and the Task Force on Basal Cell Carcinoma. J Am Acad Dermatol 1992;26:117–20
2 The National Comprehensive Cancer Network (NCCN) guidelines of care for nonmelanoma skin cancers. Dermatol Surg 2000;26:289–92.
3 The American Academy of Family Physicians have published information on basal cell carcinoma. Jerant AF, Johnson JT, Sheridan CD, Caffrey TJ. Early detection and treatment of skin cancer. American Family Physician 2000;62:357–68, 375–6, 381–2
4 Avril MF, Auperin A, Margulis A, et al. Basal cell carcinoma of the face: surgery or radiotherapy? Results of a randomized study. Br J Cancer 1997;76:100–6. Medline
5 Thissen MR, Neumann MH, Schouten LJ. A systematic review of treatment modalities for primary basal cell carcinoma. Arch Dermatol 1999;135:1177–83. Medline
6 The United States Preventive Services Task Force have developed guidelines. Screening for skin cancer: recommendations and rationale. Am J Prev Med 2001;20(3 Suppl):44–6. Available at the National Guideline Clearinghouse
7 The American College of Preventive Medicine. Ferrini RL, Perlman M, Hill L. Screening for skin cancer. Practice Guidelines Committee. Am J Prev Med 1998;14:80–2. Available at the National Guideline Clearinghouse

FAQS
Question 1
Can basal cell carcinoma occur in darkly pigmented people?

ANSWER 1
While basal cell carcinoma is reported to occur rarely in darkly pigmented patients, it is not so rare that an otherwise suspicious lesion can be discounted. It should be approached in the same manner as if the lesion were arising in a lightly pigmented individual.

Question 2
What feature best distinguishes seborrheic keratosis from basal cell carcinoma?

ANSWER 2
Seborrheic keratoses frequently have a pitted surface, whereas basal cell carcinomas are usually smoother, resulting in a shinier surface.

CONTRIBUTORS
Gordon H Baustian, MD
Seth R Stevens, MD
Rolland P Gyulai, MD, PhD

CELLULITUS

DESCRIPTION

- A spreading, acute inflammation of the dermis and subcutaneous tissue, sometimes involving muscle. Hallmarks are erythema, edema, tenderness, warmth, and indistinct margins
- Most frequently occurs on the face, lower legs, or feet. Also found on the scalp, the perianal area, and the sites of traumatic wounds, burns, animal bites, and surgical incisions
- Patients most likely to develop cellulitis are those with diabetes, immunodeficiency diseases, previous cellulitis, venous, and/or lymphatic compromise

URGENT ACTION

Check for signs of necrotizing infection:

- Edema extending beyond area of erythema
- Bullae formation
- Skin anesthesia
- Crepitus
- Discoloration affecting an entire limb or at a distant site on the same limb
- Extremely toxic appearance of patient

Immediate hospitalization and aggressive surgical management is required for necrotizing infection. Rapid hospitalization is also required for deep and quickly spreading infections, particularly those on the face or hand.

KEY! DON'T MISS!

Signs of necrotizing infection: edema extending beyond the area of erythema, bullae formation (particularly if filled with clear, maroon, or violaceous fluid), skin anesthesia, crepitus, discoloration affecting an entire limb, pain in excess of apparent erythema, and/or extremely toxic appearance of patient. Immediate hospitalization and aggressive surgical management required.

ICD9 CODE
682.9 Cellulitis
376.01 Orbital cellulitis

CARDINAL FEATURES
- Acute, spreading inflammation of the dermis and subcutaneous tissues
- Muscle may also be affected
- Affected areas are warm, red, edematous, suppurative, and tender
- Borders are diffuse and not palpable
- Lymphatic streaking and lymphadenopathy may be present
- Most frequently occurs on the face, lower legs, feet, scalp, and perianal area
- Can affect traumatic wounds, burns, animal bites, and surgical incisions
- Patients most frequently affected are those with diabetes, immunodeficiency diseases, previous cellulitis, venous, and/or lymphatic compromise
- The infectious agent is most frequently group A streptococcus or *Staphylococcus aureus*
- In the past, the most common infectious agent among children was *Hemophilus influenzae*, but since the introduction of the Hib vaccine (*Hemophilus influenzae* type b), these infections are now rare

CAUSES
Common causes
- Group A beta-hemolytic streptococci (*Streptococcus pyogenes*)
- *Staphylococcus aureus*
- *Hemophilus influenzae*
- Group B, C, D, or G beta-hemolytic streptococci

Rare causes
- Aerobic Gram-negative bacilli, including *Escherichia coli* and *Pseudomonas aeruginosa* (may occur with granulocytopenia, diabetic foot ulcers, severe tissue ischemia, and institutionalized patients)
- *Streptococcus agalactiae* (patients with diabetes mellitis or peripheral vascular disease)
- *Helicobacter cinaedi* (patients with immune deficiency)
- *Pasteurella multocida* (cat and dog bites)
- *Staphylococcus intermedius* (dog bites)
- *Capnocytophaga canimorsus* (dog bites)
- *Eikenella corrodens* (animal bites)
- *Bacteroides* species (animal bites)
- *Aeromonas hydrophila* (injuries in freshwater lakes, rivers, and streams)
- *Vibrio vulnificus* (injuries in salt water)
- *Erysipelothrix rhusiopathiae* (injuries from saltwater fish; also transmitted by farm animals)
- *Pseudomonas aeruginosa* (usually contracted by stepping on a nail and called sweaty tennis shoe syndrome; also suspected in intravenous drug users)
- *Mycobacterium marinum* (injuries in aquariums or swimming pools)
- Mixed aerobic-anaerobic flora (suspected in synergetic necrotizing cellulitis)
- Enterobacteriaceae (suspected in intravenous drug users)
- Fungi, including mucormycosis and aspergillosis (suspected with immunocompromised hosts and intravenous drug users)
- Atypical mycobacterium (suspected with immunocompromised hosts)
- *Clostridium perfringens* (may cause gas-forming cellulitis)
- Tuberculosis
- Syphilitic gumma

Serious causes

- Group A streptococci (several strains may cause severe infections leading to shock, multisystem organ failure, and death)
- *Hemophilus influenzae* (may be associated with gas formation or purulent collections. In nonvaccinated children younger than 3 years who lack an obvious portal of entry, meningitis should be considered)
- *Clostridium perfringens* (may cause gas gangrene if infection spreads to muscle)

Contributory or predisposing factors

- Break in the skin due to trauma, puncture, laceration, animal bite, or sting
- Burns
- Skin lesions caused by furuncle, ulcer, or fungal infection
- Surgical procedure or incision, including lymphadenectomy, saphenous vein stripping, and mastectomy
- Previous cellulitis
- Diabetes mellitus
- Lymphatic stasis
- Peripheral vascular disease
- Chronic steroid use
- Intravenous drug addiction
- AIDS or other immunodeficiency disorder
- Liver disease
- Renal failure
- Occupational exposure: farm workers; gardeners; handlers of fish, shellfish, and aquariums

EPIDEMIOLOGY
Incidence and prevalence

FREQUENCY
Common in the US, but because it is a nonreportable infection, exact incidence is not known.

Demographics
AGE

- Facial cellulitis usually occurs in adults aged 50 or above, or children aged 6 months to 3 years
- Perianal cellulitis usually affects children

GENDER

- Perianal cellulitus is more common in males than females
- No gender difference for other types of cellulitis

GEOGRAPHY
Cellulitis caused by halophilic *Vibrio* species occurs in coastal areas (shellfish handlers).

SOCIOECONOMIC STATUS

- Immigrant populations who may not have been vaccinated against *Hemophilus influenzae* type b and tetanus are at increased risk of infection
- Overcrowded conditions may also exacerbate infection
- Farm, garden, fish, and shellfish workers at increased risk of infection by rare agents causing cellulitis

DIFFERENTIAL DIAGNOSIS
Thrombophlebitis
Thrombophlebitis is inflammation of a vein due to thrombus formation.

FEATURES
- Superficial thrombophlebitis causes the vein and surrounding area to be erythematous, warm, and painful. The vein is palpable and may appear as a red line
- Deep vein thrombophlebitis presents with pain, swelling, heat, and redness. If the lower extremity is affected, the patient may show a positive Homans' sign

Erysipelas
Intense inflammation of superficial skin layers with lymphatic involvement. Most commonly seen on the legs.

FEATURES
- Erythema
- Induration
- Sharply defined and elevated border

Peripheral vascular insufficiency
The main characteristics of peripheral vascular insufficiency are as follows:

FEATURES
- Pain
- Swelling and discoloration of skin
- Temperature changes
- Ischemic ulceration or gangrene
- Ischemia can be tested by applying finger pressure to induce blanching. A delayed return of normal color after release suggests reduced perfusion

Candida intertrigo
Superficial fungal infection found in skin folds or sites where clothing (commonly diaper) creates moist conditions.

FEATURES
- Erythema
- Moist lesions
- Ill-defined borders
- Rupturing of pustules causes erosion and peeling

Osteomyelitis
Osteomyelitis is an infection involving bone. Often chronic with sinus formation.

FEATURES
- Swelling
- Erythema
- Restricted movement
- In contiguous osteomyelitis, skin and soft tissue are chronically infected

Acute gout

Acute gout is an extremely painful arthritis typically affecting the first metatarsophalangeal joint. Caused by an inflammatory reaction associated with the deposition of urate crystals, and commonly associated with high alcohol consumption.

FEATURES
- Redness present in early stages of attack
- Exquisite pain
- Affected joints may be warm and swollen
- Skin deposits (tophi) may be present

Pseudogout

Arthritis due to deposition of calcium pyrophosphate dihydrate crystals in the cartilage of one or more joints.

FEATURES
- Periodic inflammation of joints
- Erythema, heat, and swelling
- Peak age 65–75 years, predominantly in females
- Knees, wrists, and shoulders are the most commonly affected joints, followed by ankles and elbows

Necrotizing fasciitis

Virulent infection primarily involving the deep layer of superficial fascia. May resemble cellulitis in early stages.

FEATURES
- Extremely toxic appearance of patient
- Diffuse swelling, bullae formation, crepitus, exudate with foul-smelling odor
- Shiny, tense skin in early stages; later turns dusky and then bronze
- *Streptococcus pyogenes* causes the most fulminant cases

Contact dermatitis

Distribution corresponds precisely to areas of exposure, often revealing the culpable irritant, e.g. sock lines, placement of jewelry

FEATURES
- Erythema with vesicles or pustules
- Patients report itching or stinging

SIGNS & SYMPTOMS
Signs

Localized signs:
- Spreading, acute inflammation of dermis and subcutaneous tissue
- Affected skin shows erythema, tenderness, and warmth
- Margins indistinct and not palpable
- Skin may have infiltrated surface resembling an orange peel (peau d'orange)
- Possible lymphangitis and regional lymphadenopathy

Systemic signs:
- Fever
- Chills
- Tachycardia
- Hypotension
- Delirium

Orbital cellulitis:
- Lid edema and redness
- Proptosis
- Tenderness
- Vision loss and afferent pupil defect
- Extraocular muscle restriction
- Systemic illness and fever

Preseptal cellulitis:
- Lid edema and redness
- Tenderness
- Absence of proptosis
- Absence of extraocular muscle restriction
- Absence of fever

Symptoms
- Redness
- Swelling
- Warmth
- Tenderness or pain
- Fever
- Chills or sweats
- Malaise
- Headache
- Enlarged lymph nodes near the inflamed area
- Orbital cellulitis: bulging eye, swollen eyelids, pain, changes in vision, inability to move the affected eye, headaches, and vomiting
- Preseptal cellulitis: eyelids are swollen, red, and painful. Vision and movement of the eye are not impaired, and fever is rare

KEY! DON'T MISS!
Signs of necrotizing infection: edema extending beyond the area of erythema, bullae formation (particularly if filled with clear, maroon, or violaceous fluid), skin anesthesia, crepitus, discoloration affecting an entire limb, pain in excess of apparent erythema, and/or extremely toxic appearance of patient. Immediate hospitalization and aggressive surgical management required.

CONSIDER CONSULT
- Suspected necrotizing infection, deep or quickly spreading infection (particularly on the face and hands), and orbital cellulitis require referral for further investigation and treatment
- If there is no response to empirical oral antibiotics, referral for further investigation is required

INVESTIGATION OF THE PATIENT
Direct questions to patient
Q Was this problem preceded by an injury? Answer may provide clues to the infectious organism, e.g. *Pasteurella multocida* likely in cellulitis following a dog bite.

Q What vaccinations have you received? Tetanus vaccine may be necessary. Previous Hib (*Haemophilus influenzae* type b) vaccination helps rule out *Hemophilus influenzae.*

Q Are you taking ibuprofen for fever? This may delay some symptoms of cellulitis, particularly that accompanied by varicella.

Contributory or predisposing factors
Q Do you have any other medical conditions? Several conditions predispose to severe forms of cellulitis. These include diabetes mellitus, lymphatic stasis, peripheral vascular disease, chickenpox, AIDS or other immunodeficiency disorder, liver disease, or renal failure.

Q Have you had any operations? Patients who are asplenic are at increased risk of infection.

Q Are you taking any drugs at the moment, prescribed or recreational? Intravenous drugs, immunosuppressive therapy, chemotherapy, or steroid therapy all predispose to severe cellulitis.

Q Have you had cellulitis before? Previous history of cellulitis increases the risk of a recurrent attack. Recurrent staphylococcal infections may be associated with nasal carriage: culture and, if positive, treatment is appropriate.

Q What is your occupation? Cellulitis is an occupational hazard for farm workers, gardeners, and those who handle fish, shellfish, and aquariums.

Examination

- Assess the patient's overall status. If systemically unwell, septicemia is likely and the patient will need hospital referral. Extremely toxic appearance may suggest necrotizing condition
- Look for source of infection. This can give clues as to the etiology of the infection
- Check the temperature. Pyrexia suggests systemic infection. Patients with low-grade fever may be treated as outpatients; high fever signals the need for hospitalization
- Examine the affected area. Redness, warmth, and orange peel appearances are suggestive of cellulitis
- Assess the area for tenderness. Cellulitis can be painful
- What are the margins of the affected area like? Cellulitic infections have indistinct margins, which are not palpable
- How deep does the infected area appear to be? Cellulitis only affects the dermis and subcutaneous tissues. If joints are involved or there are draining sinuses consider further diagnoses
- Note the extent of infection. This is crucial to the assessment of the patient's response to treatment. With mild cases, an aid is to draw the approximate margin of affected area on skin with a ball point pen
- Check for lymphangitis and lymphadenopathy. Both signal the spread of infection
- Check the heart rate. Tachycardia may be present with necrotizing or severe infection
- Check the blood pressure. Hypotension may accompany systemic illness
- With infections around the eye, distinguish between orbital cellulitis (a medical emergency) and preseptal cellulitis (generally not an emergency). Proptosis and extraocular muscle restriction are present in orbital cellulitis but not in preseptal infection
- Examine the contralateral lower extremity. If both legs are erythematous and tender, consider stasis dermatitis rather than bilateral cellulitis

Summary of investigative tests

- Complete blood count is important with any instance of cellulitis to indicate if there is systemic infection
- Blood culture may indicate bacteremia and associated infectious agent
- Swab of drainage material may indicate infectious agent
- X-rays may reveal gas formation in suspected necrotizing infection. Usually performed by a specialist
- Punch biopsy of skin may reveal infectious agent. Normally performed by a specialist if patient is refractory to first-line treatment. These can be sent for culture as well as histopathology
- Computed tomography or magnetic resonance imaging may confirm necrotizing infection. Computed tomography is also used with orbital cellulitis to reveal orbital abscesses and sinus involvement. This is normally performed by a specialist

DIAGNOSTIC DECISION

Diagnosis is usually based on clinical presentation rather than identification of etiologic agent because attempts at identification usually fail.

CLINICAL PEARLS

Early recognition of the disease and institution of proper antibiotic treatment, and/or referral to the appropriate specialist if needed, is key to the management of cellulitis. Laboratory tests only support the diagnosis and may help monitor response to treatment.

THE TESTS
Body fluids
COMPLETE BLOOD COUNT
Description
Venous blood sample.

Advantages/Disadvantages
Advantages:
■ Quick, easy, inexpensive
■ Can indicate systemic response to infection

Normal
■ Red blood cells: 4.2–6.1x10^6/mcL
■ White blood cells: 4800–10,800/mcL
■ Neutrophils: 3150–6200/mcL
■ Lymphocytes: 1500–3000/mcL
■ Monocytes: 300–500/mcL
■ Eosinophils: 50–250/mcL
■ Basophils: 15–50/mcL
■ Platelets: 150,000–450,000/mm^3

Abnormal
■ Any value above or below normal range
■ Keep in mind the possibility of a false-positive/negative result

Cause of abnormal result
■ High white blood cells: probable infection
■ Low white blood cells: possible overwhelming infection
■ High neutrophil count: probable bacterial infection
■ High monocyte count: probable infection
■ Immature white blood cells: probable bacterial infection

Drugs, disorders and other factors that may alter results
Many other medical conditions and medications can alter the patient's hematological profile. Results must be interpreted using the clinical picture and the patient's previous medical and drug history.

BLOOD CULTURE
Description
■ 10mL venous blood sample taken during fever spike >38°C (100°F)
■ Two samples taken for aerobes and anaerobes

Advantages/Disadvantages
Advantages:
■ Quick, easy, inexpensive
■ If taken prior to antibiotic administration, will accurately reflect the drug sensitivities of the infectious agent
■ May reveal life-threatening bacteremia

Disadvantages:
- Low yield and not cost-effective if performed on inappropriate patient group
- Must take sample during temperature spike to increase chance of finding bacteria
- May have false-negative or false-positive results

Normal
- No bacteria isolated
- Sterile sample

Abnormal
- Any bacteria present in the blood
- Keep in mind the possibility of a false-positive result

Cause of abnormal result
Bacteremia.

Drugs, disorders and other factors that may alter results
- Sample can become contaminated by poor technique
- Previous or concurrent antibiotic therapy can alter bacterial sensitivities

SWAB FROM AFFECTED AREA
Description
- Sterile swabs used to take a sample of any drainage material from the affected area
- Sample analyzed for Gram stain, microscopy, culture, and sensitivity

Advantages/Disadvantages
Advantages:
- Quick, easy, inexpensive
- May reveal infective pathogen
- Gram stain will give quick results

Disadvantages:
- Causative organism is likely to be skin commensal
- Some organisms are hard to grow on culture

Abnormal
- Evidence of overgrowth of a skin commensal
- Presence of any other bacteria that are not commensals

Cause of abnormal result
Infection of the dermis and subcutaneous tissues.

Drugs, disorders and other factors that may alter results
- Cellulitis associated with chronic wounds (i.e. ulcers) often grow atypical bacteria
- Cellulitis that has had previous antibiotic therapy or is hospital-acquired may grow resistant strains (i.e. MRSA)

CONSIDER CONSULT
- Evidence of sepsis requires referral
- Any immunocompromised patient requires referral
- Refer patients at the extremes of age
- Patients with alcoholism or intravenous drug addiction, poorly controlled diabetes, and lymphatic compromise require referral

PATIENT AND CAREGIVER ISSUES

Patient or caregiver request
'Flesh-eating bacteria' have been in the news. This might prompt patient anxiety. It also may help encourage patients to complete their prescribed regimen of antibiotics.

Health-seeking behavior
- **Have you applied any creams or lotions to the affected area?** Patients may try over-the-counter or herbal remedies to alleviate symptoms
- **Have you tried elevating your legs?** This action can greatly decrease swelling and discomfort in cellulitic peripheries
- **Have you taken any medication to control pain or fever?** NSAIDs can mask signs and symptoms of a septic patient

MANAGEMENT ISSUES
Goals
- Identify infection
- Accurate diagnosis and recognition of patients requiring referral
- Eradicate infection
- Avert complications
- Control any underlying disease
- Prevent recurrences

Management in special circumstances
COEXISTING DISEASE
- Many patients who present with cellulitis have underlying medical conditions. The nature of these conditions greatly affects the management and threshold for hospital referral
- Patients with immunocompromise, diabetes mellitus, peripheral vascular disease, or asplenia can become victims of overwhelming sepsis without early recognition of severe infection

COEXISTING MEDICATION
Chemotherapeutic drugs, immunosuppressant drugs, and steroid therapy are associated with greater severity of cellulitis.

SPECIAL PATIENT GROUPS
- Intensive management is needed for geriatric patients and young children
- Intensive management is needed for intravenous drug users
- Pregnant women will require antibiotics that are safe for the fetus
- Institutionalized patients may grow organisms with resistance to common antibiotics

PATIENT SATISFACTION/LIFESTYLE PRIORITIES
Cellulitis can be very painful and extremely debilitating in terms of mobility.

SUMMARY OF THERAPEUTIC OPTIONS
Choices
- First-choice preferred drug category: first-generation cephalosporins
- Second-choice preferred drug: cloxacillin
- Third-choice preferred drug: dicloxacillin
- Alternative drug category: macrolide antibiotics
- Alternative drugs: amoxicillin-clavulanate, cefpodoxime, or cefdinir
- The affected limb should be immobilized and elevated, to reduce pain and swelling

Mild cellulitis:
- If the suspected infecting organism is *Staphylococcus aureus*, dicloxacillin should be the first-line treatment
- If *Streptococcus pyogenes* is suspected, phenoxymethylpenicillin is the first choice
- For patients who are hypersensitive to penicillin (excluding immediate hypersensitivity), cephalexin is the alternative drug of choice

Severe cellulitis:
- For both *Streptococcus* and *Staphylococcus* spp., dicloxacillin is the first-line therapy
- A cephalosporin should be used for patients who are hypersensitive to penicillin (excluding immediate hypersensitivity)
- Patients with immediate hypersensitivity should be treated with clindamycin

Clinical pearls
- Response to antibiotic therapy should always be assessed in about 48h. If there is no response at all, or there is continued progression of the disease, referral to a specialist may be necessary
- Simultaneous, bilateral lower extremity involvement is relatively uncommon (although it can occur in compromised patients or sequentially), whereas bilateral stasis dermatitis is common. In the absence of signs and symptoms beyond erythema, consider alternative diagnoses

Never
Never attempt to treat cellulitis with simply a topical antibiotic preparation.

FOLLOW UP
- Outpatients with mild cellulitis should be re-examined 24–48h after initiation of antibiotic treatment
- Those with underlying illness or severe cellulitis should receive intensive management in a hospital setting

Plan for review
- For outpatients with mild cellulitis, skin should be re-examined 24–48h after initiation of antibiotic treatment
- Check that the cellulitis has not spread
- Ensure that the antibiotics are not causing intolerable side effects
- Reiterate the need for patient compliance

Information for patient or caregiver
- Cellulitis is an infection of the skin that sometimes affects underlying tissues. It often occurs after the skin has been broken by an injury such as an animal bite or a puncture wound. In people with diabetes mellitus or certain other disorders, cellulitis may occur without any injury to the skin

- Symptoms of cellulitis are skin that is red, tender, swollen, and warm. The person may also have a fever and swollen glands
- Most instances of cellulitis are treated with oral antibiotics. In some cases, infections are severe and require hospitalization and intravenous antibiotics. Rarely, cellulitis may worsen, even after a person has begun taking antibiotics. If this occurs, it is important to contact your doctor immediately. It is also important to take the complete course of antibiotics prescribed by your doctor. This will help ensure that the infecting bacteria cannot re-emerge to cause a more serious condition

DRUGS AND OTHER THERAPIES: DETAILS
Drugs
FIRST-GENERATION CEPHALOSPORINS
First-generation cephalosporins include cephalexin, cefadroxil, cefazolin.

Dose
- Cephalexin: 500mg orally every 6h
- Cefadroxil: 1–2g orally once or twice a day
- Cefazolin: 250–500mg intramuscularly every 8h

Efficacy
Covers Gram-positive cocci, including *Staphylococcus* species.

Risks/benefits
Risks:
- Caution in patients with penicillin hypersensitivity
- Use caution in renal impairment and in history of gastrointestinal disease
- Use caution in breast-feeding

Benefits:
- Usually well tolerated
- Covers the most common bacteria that cause cellulitis

Side effects and adverse reactions
- Central nervous system: headache, sleep disturbance, confusion, dizziness, fever
- Gastrointestinal: nausea, vomiting, diarrhea, abdominal pain, pseudomembranous colitis, anorexia
- Genitourinary: renal toxicity, proteinuria
- Hematologic: blood cell disorders, bone marrow depression, pancytopenia
- Respiratory: dyspnea
- Skin: rash, pruritis, urticaria, Stevens-Johnson syndrome

Interactions (other drugs)
- Aminoglycosides ■ Aztreonam ■ Carbapenems ■ Chloramphenicol ■ Loop diuretics
- Macrolides ■ Penicillins ■ Polymyxin B ■ Probenecid ■ Tetracyclines ■ Vancomycin

Contraindications
- Infants less than one month old ■ Breast-feeding ■ Colitis ■ Gastrointestinal disease
- Intramuscular injections ■ Penicillin and cephalosporin hypersensitivity

Acceptability to patient
Usually very well accepted by patient.

Follow up plan
Skin should be examined 24–48h after patient initiates therapy.

Patient and caregiver information
Patients should promptly report signs of worsening infection.

CLOXACILLIN
Dose
- Adult: 250–500mg orally every 6h
- Child (less than 20kg): 12.5–25mg/kg orally every 6h (max 4g/day)

Efficacy
Highly active against most penicillinase-producing staphylococci.

Risks/benefits
Risks:
- Use caution in penicillin hypersensitivity
- Do not administer for prolonged or repeated doses

Benefits:
- Usually well tolerated
- Easy to take
- Covers most penicillinase-producing staphylococci

Side effects and adverse reactions
- Central nervous system: headache, fever, depression, anxiety, seizures
- Gastrointestinal: nausea, vomiting, diarrhea, abdominal pain, colitis, gastritis, anorexia
- Genitourinary: impotence, proteinuria, hematuria, vaginitis
- Hematologic: bone marrow depression, hemolytic anemia
- Skin: rashes

Interactions (other drugs)
- Aminoglycosides ■ Anticoagulants ■ Chloramphenicol ■ Erythromycin ■ Heparin ■ Tetracyclines ■ Oral contraceptives ■ Probenecid

Contraindications
- Penicillin hypersensitivity

Acceptability to patient
Usually very acceptable to the patient.

Follow up plan
Skin should be examined 24–48h after patient initiates therapy.

Patient and caregiver information
Patients should report signs of worsening infection.

DICLOXACILLIN
Dose
- Adult: 125–500mg orally every 6h
- Child (less than 40kg): 12.5–25mg/kg orally every 6h (max 4g/day)

Efficacy
Strongly active against penicillinase-producing staphylococci. Not effective against methicillin-resistant staphylococci or Gram-negative bacteria.

Risks/benefits
Risks:
- Use caution in patients with a history of gastrointestinal disease, and in those with eczema or asthma
- Use caution in breast-feeding

Benefits:
- Usually well tolerated
- Easy to take
- Strongly active against penicillinase-producing staphylococci

Side effects and adverse reactions
- Central nervous system: seizures, anxiety, lethargy
- Gastrointestinal: nausea, vomiting, diarrhea, pseudomembranous colitis, abdominal discomfort, gastrointestinal bleeding, elevated hepatic enzymes
- Hematologic: thrombocytopenia, leukopenia, neutropenia
- Skin: purpura, rashes, vasculitis, exfoliative dermatitis, maculopapular rash, Stevens-Johnson syndrome

Interactions (other drugs)
- Aminoglycosides ■ Chloramphenicol ■ Macrolide antibiotics ■ Methotrexate
- Oral contraceptives ■ Probenecid ■ Tetracycline antibiotics ■ Warfarin

Contraindications
- Hypersensitivity to penicillins

Acceptability to patient
Usually very acceptable to the patient.

Follow up plan
Examine skin 24–48h after patient initiates therapy.

Patient and caregiver information
Patients should report any signs of worsening infection.

MACROLIDE ANTIBIOTICS
Macrolide antibiotics include erythromycin, dirithromycin, clarithromycin.

Dose
- Erythromycin: 250–500mg orally every 6–12h
- Dirithromycin: 500mg orally every day
- Clarithromycin: 250mg orally every 12h

Efficacy
Covers Gram-positive cocci, most anaerobic bacteria, and some Gram-positive bacilli.

Risks/benefits
Risks:
- Caution in hepatic and renal impairment, porphyria
- Prolongs QT interval
- Avoid concomitant administration with terfenadine, astemizole, and cisapride
- Use caution with repeated or prolonged therapy
- Use caution in pregnancy

Benefits:
- Usually well tolerated
- Can be used in patients with penicillin sensitivity
- Broad spectrum of antimicrobial coverage

Side effects and adverse reactions
- Gastrointestinal: anorexia, nausea, diarrhea, abdominal pain, vomiting, heartburn, hepatitis
- Cardiovascular system: dysrhythmias (uncommon)
- Central nervous system: headache
- Skin: rashes, pruritis, vaginal candidiasis, Stevens-Johnson syndrome
- Ears, eyes, nose, and throat: deafness, tinnitus

Interactions (other drugs)
- Alfentanil ▪ Antiarrhythmic drugs (digoxin, disopyramide)
- Antihistamines (terfenadine, astemizole) ▪ Anticonvulsants (carbamazepine, valproic acid)
- Antiviral agents ▪ Benzodiazepines ▪ Bromocriptine ▪ Buspirone ▪ Cisapride
- Clozapine ▪ Colchicine ▪ Cyclosporine, tacrolimus ▪ Ergotamine ▪ Ethanol
- Felodipine ▪ Itraconazole ▪ Methylprednisolone ▪ Penicillin ▪ Quinidine ▪ Sildenafil
- Statins ▪ Theophylline ▪ Warfarin ▪ Zopiclone

Contraindications
- Liver disease ▪ Various infections (vaccinia, varicella, mycobacterial, fungal, viral)

Acceptability to patient
Generally acceptable.

Follow up plan
Examine the skin 24–48h after patient initiates therapy.

Patient and caregiver information
Patient should report any signs of worsening infection or side effects such as diarrhea.

AMOXICILLIN-CLAVULANATE
Dose
- Adult: 250 or 500mg tablet orally (each with 125mg clavulanic acid) every 8–12h
- Child less than 40kg: 20–40mg/kg per day orally (based on amoxicillin component) divided every 8–12h
- Neonates/infants less than 3 months: 30 mg/kg per day orally (amoxicillin) divided every 12h

Efficacy
Active against Gram-positive bacteria, including *Staphylococcus aureus* and *Streptococcus pneumoniae*.

Risks/benefits
Risks.
- Use caution if history of hypersensitivity to cephalosporins
- Use caution in renal failure and hepatic impairment
- Avoid use in mononucleosis

Benefits:
- Easy to take
- Good spectrum of antimicrobial coverage

Side effects and adverse reactions
- Central nervous system: headache, nausea
- Eyes, ears, nose, and throat: black tongue, oral thrush
- Gastrointestinal: diarrhea, abdominal pain, psuedomembranous colitis
- Hematologic: bone marrow suppression
- Respiratory: anaphylaxis
- Skin: allergic rashes, erythema multiforme

Interactions (other drugs)
- Atenolol ■ Chloramphenicol ■ Macrolide antibiotics ■ Methotrexate ■ Oral contraceptives ■ Tetracyclines

Contraindications
- Hypersensitivity to penicillins

Acceptability to patient
Generally acceptable.

Follow up plan
Skin should be examined 24–48h after patient initiates therapy.

Patient and caregiver information
Patient should report any signs of worsening infection.

CEFPODOXIME

Dose
- Adult: 400mg orally every 12h for 10 days
- Child (5–12 years): 10mg/kg per day orally divided every 12h

Efficacy
Active against Gram-negative bacteria.

Risks/benefits
Risks:
- Use caution in gastrointestinal disease and renal disease
- Use caution in pregnancy and breast-feeding

Side effects and adverse reactions

- Central nervous system: headache, anxiety, dizziness, flushing, fatigue, insomnia, weakness
- Ears, eyes, nose, and throat: epistaxis, rhinitis, tinnitus, ocular irritation
- Skin: rashes, irritation, itching, dermatitis
- Gastrointestinal: nausea, vomiting, diarrhea, pseudomembranous colitis, abdominal pain, flatulence, candidiasis
- Genitourinary: candidiasis, vaginitis, nephrotoxicity
- Hematologic: blood cell disorders

Interactions (other drugs)

- Aminoglycosides ■ Antacids ■ Chloramphenicol ■ Didanosine ■ H2-blockers
- Loop diuretics ■ Probenecid ■ Proton pump blockers

Contraindications

- Penicillin and cephalosporin hypersensitivity ■ Neonates and children

Acceptability to patient
Generally acceptable.

Follow up plan
Skin should be examined 24–48h after patient begins therapy.

Patient and caregiver information
Patients should report any signs of worsening infection.

CEFDINIR

Dose

- Adult: 300mg orally every 12h for 10 days
- Child (6 months–12 years): 7mg/kg orally every 12h for 10 days

Efficacy
Covers a wide range of Gram-positive and Gram-negative bacteria.

Risks/benefits
Risks:

- Use caution in renal disease, gastrointestinal disease, and coagulation or bleeding disorders
- Use caution in pregnancy, children, and the elderly
- Cefdinir oral suspension should not be used in diabetics

Benefit: Broad range of antimicrobial action

Side effects and adverse reactions

- Central nervous system: headache, asthenia, dizziness, drowsiness, insomnia, seizures
- Gastrointestinal: nausea, vomiting, diarrhea, constipation, flatulence, dyspepsia, abdominal pain, anorexia
- Genitourinary: candidiasis, vaginitis
- Skin: rashes, hypersensitivity reaction

Interactions (other drugs)

- Antacids, aluminium, magnesium salts ■ Other cephalosporins ■ Chloramphenicol
- Iron supplements

Contraindications
- Hypersensitivity to cefdinir and other cephalosporins
- Infants

Acceptability to patient
Generally acceptable.

Follow up plan
Skin should be examined 24–48h after patient initiates therapy.

Patient and caregiver information
Patients should report any signs of worsening infection.

Other therapies

IMMOBILIZE AND ELEVATE AFFECTED LIMB
Efficacy
- Reduces swelling
- Speeds recovery of infections on lower legs

Risks/benefits
Risk: Immobility increases risk of deep vein thrombosis

Benefits:
- Simple treatment
- Decreases pain and swelling

Acceptability to patient
Usually highly acceptable to the patient as it decreases pain and discomfort.

Patient and caregiver information
- Patient should understand that this may speed healing
- Should be advised to wiggle toes or flex ankles to decrease risk of DVT

EFFICACY OF THERAPIES

Mild cases of cellulitis treated with oral antibiotics on an outpatient basis typically resolve in 7–10 days.

Evidence

■ Several small RCTs have looked at various antibiotic regimens for the management of cellulitis and found approximately 70% cure rates for all antibiotics studied. This indicates that from a 'cure' point of view, there is no clear 'best choice' among antibiotics [1]
■ There is little evidence on the treatment of cellulitis [1]
■ There is no good evidence on optimal treatment duration, oral versus intravenous medications or antibiotic combination therapy [1]

Review period

24–48h.

PROGNOSIS

In most instances, resolves within 7–10 days after antibiotic treatment begins.

Clinical pearls

Marking the area of erythema with an indelible marker is a convenient way to follow progression or regression of the disease.

Therapeutic failure

■ Hospitalization and intravenous antibiotics
■ Surgical debridement may be necessary

Recurrence

■ For recurrent cellulitis of the legs, treat tinea pedis with antifungal agent
■ Identify and control any underlying medical condition that predisposes to cellulitis
■ With other instances of recurrence, prophylactic treatment with penicillin G (250–500mg orally twice a day) may be required

COMPLICATIONS

■ Bacteremia
■ Necrotizing fasciitis
■ Progressive bacterial synergistic gangrene
■ Local abscess
■ Superinfection with Gram-negative micro-organisms
■ Thrombophlebitis of lower legs
■ Lymphangitis
■ Complications of orbital cellulitis: cavernous sinus thrombosis, meningitis, intracranial infection, and septicemia

CONSIDER CONSULT

■ Refer patients whose cellulitis has worsened in the 48–72h after initiation of oral antibiotics

Treat diabetes mellitus and potential portals of entry (e.g. ulcers, dermatophyte infection).

RISK FACTORS

- Intravenous drug use: increases incidence and severity of cellulitis
- Environment: skin should be protected in instances of exposure to potentially harmful bacteria, especially if there are any breaks in the skin
- Physical activities: skin should be protected when engaging in activities that might cause injuries, such as bicycling or skating
- Immunization: vaccination against *Hemophilus influenzae* type b (Hib vaccine) protects children from a major and potentially serious cause of cellulitis

MODIFY RISK FACTORS

- Protect skin from injuries, particularly in environments that might harbor harmful bacteria
- When injuries do occur, clean affected skin immediately, apply antibiotic ointment, and notify a doctor of any signs of inflammation

Lifestyle and wellness
ALCOHOL AND DRUGS
Intravenous drug users are at risk of developing cellulitis, and often have severe complications from cellulitis.

PHYSICAL ACTIVITY
Skin should be protected when engaging in activities that might cause injuries, such as bicycling or skating.

ENVIRONMENT
Skin should be protected from injury in environments containing potential bacterial hazards, particularly farms, gardens, and brackish water.

DRUG HISTORY
Chemotherapy, immunosuppressants and steroid therapy cause increased severity of cellulitis.

IMMUNIZATION
Immunization against *Hemophilus influenzae* type b (Hib vaccine) protects children from a major and potentially serious cause of cellulitis.

Cost/efficacy
Highly cost-effective.

PREVENT RECURRENCE
Treat nasal carriers of *Staphylococcus aureus*.

Reassess coexisting disease
As underlying diseases can increase the risk of developing cellulitis, it is important to optimize control of the predisposing condition, e.g. meticulous blood sugar control for diabetes.

ASSOCIATIONS

American Academy of Dermatology
930 N. Meacham Rd
Schaumburg, IL 60173
Tel: (888) 462–3376
http://www.aad.org

KEY REFERENCES

- Habif TP. Clinical dermatology. Philadelphia: Mosby, 1996
- Rhody C. Bacterial infections of the skin. Prim Care 2000;27:2;459–73
- Subcutaneous tissue infections. In: Behrman RE, Kliegman RM, Arvin AM (eds). Nelson textbook of pediatrics, 16th edn. Philadelphia: WB Saunders, 2000
- Holten KB, Onusko EM. Appropriate prescribing of oral beta lactam antibiotics. Am Fam Physician 2000;62:3:611–20
- Stevens DL. Skin and soft tissue infections. National Foundation for Infectious Diseases. Clinical Update 1996;3:2 http://www.nfid.org/publications/clinicalupdates/id/skininfect.html
- Buttaravoli, Stair. 11.11 Erysipelas cellulitis lymphangitis, Common simple emergencies. National centre for emergency medicine informatics. Available at: http://www.ncemi.org/cse/cse1111.htm
- Bacterial infections of the skin. In: Freke T. The Merck manual. New Jersey: Merck Publications, 1999
- Group A streptococcal infections, NIAID fact sheet. Bethesda, MD. Available at: http://www.niaid.nih.gov/factsheets/strep.htm
- Sowka JW, Gurwood AS, Kabat AG. Review of optometry online: Handbook of ocular disease management: Orbital cellulitis. New York: Jobson Publishing, 2000. Available at: http://www.revoptom.com/HANDBOOK/SECT7g.HTM
- Wilson BA, Shannon MT, Stang CL. Nurses' drug guide 2000. Appleton & Lange, 1999
- O'Dell ML. Skin and wound infections: An overview. Am Fam Physician 1998;15:57(10):2424–32

Evidence references

1   Morris A. Cellulitis and erysipelas: Skin disorders. In: Clinical Evidence 2001; 5:1146–1149. London: BMJ Publishing Group

FAQS
Question 1

My patient has bilateral leg cellulitis, a normal white blood cell count, and no fever. Does she need hospitalization?

ANSWER 1
While the scenario described may indicate aggressive disease in a host who is unable to mount an adequate response, consider the possibility of vascular stasis dermatitis, particularly if in the setting of proximal edema in areas that are not erythematous.

Question 2
Can I treat mild cellulitis with mupiricin?

ANSWER 2
No, unlike impetigo, cellulitis should be treated with systemic antibiotics.

Question 3
My patient initially responded to oral dicloxicillin in a few days, and then developed painful erythema, fever, and an elevated white count, should I increase the dose?

ANSWER 3

No, if the dicloxicillin is inadequate, then therapy with another agent is recommended. Information on local resistance patterns can be obtained from the laboratory. Also, consider the possibility that the patient is developing a drug eruption such as a hypersensitivity syndrome or if mucosal involvement is present, Stevens-Johnson syndrome or toxic epidermal necrolysis and if appropriate discontinue antibiotic therapy.

Question 4

My patient has several chronic medical problems and cellulitis. Her dermatologist recommends treating her tinea pedis, which is the least of her problems. Why the recommendation?

ANSWER 4

Tinea pedis is a frequent portal of entry for cellulitis. Its treatment, therefore, can much reduce the likelihood of recurrent cellulitis.

Question 5

My patient has eczema as his only other medical condition, yet has recurrent *Staphylococcus aureus* infections. Is this because of his use of topical steroids impairing local immunity?

ANSWER 5

Not likely. Rather, atopic dermatitis patients are commonly colonized with *Staphylococcus aureus*. Several studies reveal that treating the eczematous skin with topical steroids actually reduces bacterial load.

CONTRIBUTORS

Randolph L Pearson, MD
Seth R Stevens, MD
Elma D Baron, MD

ATOPIC DERMATITIS

DESCRIPTION

- Atopic dermatitis is an inflammatory skin disorder
- Characterized by erythema, edema, intense pruritus, exudation, crusting, xerosis and lichenification
- Many patients with atopic dermatitis have elevated serum IgE levels (5– 10 times normal value)
- Some patients have a family history of allergy; or a personal history of asthma, hay fever, or allergic rhinitis

URGENT ACTION

In patients with impaired T-cell function, atopic dermatitis can be associated with potentially life-threatening infections caused by disseminated herpes virus infections (eczema herpeticum).

ICD9 CODE
691.8 Atopic dermatitis

SYNONYMS

- Atopic eczema, eczema, and atopic dermatitis
- Eczema is the general term that includes a number of skin conditions including atopic dermatitis, seborrheic dermatitis, dyshidrotic eczema, irritant contact dermatitis, and allergic contact dermatitis

CARDINAL FEATURES

Major features:
- Pruritus
- Typical morphology and distribution: Flexural lichenification, and facial and extensor involvement in infants and young children
- Chronic relapsing dermatitis
- Familial or personal history of atopy

Other features:
- Xerosis (dry skin)
- Keratosis pilaris
- Ichthyosis
- Pityriasis alba
- Palmar or plantar hyper linearity
- Dennie-Morgan lines (infraorital fold)
- White dermatographism
- Hand or foot dermatitis
- Cheilitis
- Susceptibility to cutaneous infection, especially Staphylococcus, herpes simplex and other viral infections, warts, molluscum contagiosum, dermatophytes
- Erythroderma
- Early age of onset
- Impaired cell-mediated immunity
- Immediate type 1 skin test response

CAUSES

Common causes
- True origin of disease unknown. Hypothesized to be multifactorial, including genetic, environmental, and infectious conditions
- Currently thought that there is a defect of a bone marrow-derived cell that causes a variety of cutaneous and generalized immune abnormalities

Contributory or predisposing factors
- Family history of allergy in the parents or in a sibling
- B cell IgE overproduction is predisposing factor (allergy)
- Depressed cell-mediated immunity

EPIDEMIOLOGY

Incidence and prevalence
Atopic dermatitis affects over 15 million children and adults in the United States.

INCIDENCE
5– 25 cases per 1000 persons.

FREQUENCY
Up to 15% of the population may suffer from atopic dermatitis during childhood.

Demographics
AGE
Highest incidence is among children (5–15%); 60% of cases appear during the first 12 months of life, the next 30% is seen before the age of 5. Onset is rarely seen after the age of 50.

GENDER
Affects both sexes equally.

GENETICS
There appears to be a genetic predisposition to atopic dermatitis; family history of allergy is positive in more than two-thirds of cases.

DIFFERENTIAL DIAGNOSIS
Scabies
FEATURES
- Itchy papules often excoriated
- Most common sites: webbing of fingers, wrist, buttocks
- Rarely affects face except in immunocompromised patients

Psoriasis
FEATURES
- Well-demarcated erythematous plaques with silvery scales
- Most common sites: gluteal fold, elbows, knees and scalp

Dermatitis herpetiformis
FEATURES
- Rare relapsing condition associated with gluten enteropathy
- Vesicular symmetrical eruptions
- Intense burning and itching
- Most common sites: limbs, buttocks and scalp

Contact dermatitis
FEATURES
- Follows contact with irritant or allergen, often within a few hours
- Symptoms may build up over prolonged contact
- Erythema, itching, scaling and fissuring
- Hands most commonly affected

Seborrheic dermatitis
FEATURES
- Characterized by erythematous, eczematous patches with yellow, greasy scales
- Most common sites: face, scalp, flexures, upper chest and back
- Etiology unknown

Candidiasis
FEATURES
- Erythematous wet, sometimes scaly skin
- Satellite lesions invariably found
- Skin folds most commonly affected

Lichen simplex chronicus
FEATURES
- Secondary to continual rubbing and scratching by the patient
- Well defined, thickened skin with pronounced skin creases
- Intensely itchy

Impetigo
FEATURES
- Yellow crusting, weeping lesions
- Common on the face in children
- May spread rapidly to other parts of the body
- Causative agent: *Staphylococcus* spp. and/or *Streptococcus* spp.

Ectodermal dysplasias
FEATURES
- Usually related to an X-linked recessive trait, principally seen in male patients
- Characterized by excessive skin peeling in newborns, paucity of sebaceous glands
- Skin is dry, finely wrinkled, hypopigmented, with prominent venous patterning

SIGNS & SYMPTOMS
Signs
Lesion distribution:
- Infants – lesions seen on trunk, face, and extensor surfaces
- Children – lesions seen on extensor surfaces, and the antecubital and popliteal fossae
- Older children, adolescents, and adults – lesions seen on face, neck, flexors surfaces, hands and feet

Lesion morphology:
- Infants – papules and vesicles that may develop oozing, crusty vesicles
- Children – dry and papular with circumscribed scaly patches
- Adults – dry, thick lesions, confluent papules, and lichenified plaques
- Facial erythema (mild to moderate)
- Infraorbital fold (Dennie's sign/Morgan line)
- Increased palmar linear markings
- Pityriasis alba
- Keratosis pilaris

Symptoms
- Pruritus
- Intense scratching – occurs throughout the day and is more intense at night
- Sleep is frequently disturbed
- Dryness of the skin (xerosis)
- Flaky skin

ASSOCIATED DISORDERS
- Secondary skin infections may be present (*Staphylococcus aureus*, herpes simplex, dermatophytosis)
- Keratoconjunctivitises and stellate anterior subcapsular cataracts are associated with atopic dermatitis, especially in patients with extensive skin changes. Cataracts may occur at an early age (often by age 20) and develop rapidly

CONSIDER CONSULT
- Erythroderma or extensive exfoliation
- When identification of trigger factors or allergens is needed
- When diagnosis of atopic dermatitis is in doubt

INVESTIGATION OF THE PATIENT
Direct questions to patient
Q Do you suffer from asthma, allergic rhinitis, contact allergies, or food-related exacerbations? Patients with atopy may have a combination of asthma, dermatitis and rhinitis.
Q How long have you had these symptoms, have you had these symptoms before? Dermatitis tends to follow a relapsing and remitting course over many years.
Q What is your occupation? Hairdressers, mechanics, health care workers have increased exposure to irritants and trigger factors.

Contributory or predisposing factors

Q Has the patient been under emotional stress? Stress may contribute to severity of attacks.

Q Is the patient aware of any clothing or chemical sensitivities? Irritating clothing or exposure to certain chemicals may trigger increase in severity of pruritus.

Q Has the patient recently been exposed to extremely hot or cold climate or environment? Increased sweating or extremely low humidity may worsen the condition.

Q Does the patient suffer from food allergies? Some children who are exposed to certain foods (eggs, fish, peanuts, soy, wheat, and milk) may provoke exacerbation of condition.

Q Has the patient been exposed to the allergens? Topical or inhalant allergens such as dust mites, proteins or animal dander are common causes of atopic dermatitis.

Q Has the patient been exposed to irritant factors? Has the patient been washing hands excessively? Increased skin dryness may predispose to bacterial infection.

Family history

Q Is there a member of the immediate family who has asthma, allergic rhinitis, atopic dermatitis? Atopic dermatitis is associated with inherited tendency for respiratory allergic disease.

Examination

- Is the patient experiencing pruritus? This is a major indicator of atopic dermatitis
- Where on body is skin affected? Facial and extensor involvement will be seen in infants and children. Flexural lichenification will be seen in adults
- How does the affected skin appear? Ichthyosis, white dermatographism, and eczema-perifollicular accentuation are associated with atopic dermatitis
- Does patient have nipple or hand dermatitis orcheilitis? These are all associated with atopic dermatitis
- Has patient a history of recurrent conjunctivitis? This could be indicative of immune system disfunction
- Does the patient have any signs of skin infections?

Summary of investigative tests

Investigative tests are not normally required to establish a diagnosis. The following tests are neither sensitive nor specific to atopic dermatitis:

- IgE level – elevated IgE is seen in 80–90% of atopic dermatitis cases, and the IgE level declines as the disease becomes controlled
- Eosinophil count – blood eosinophilia is frequently found in atopic dermatitis

Allergy skin testing with relevant allergens may provide information pertaining to allergens that trigger or contribute to the skin manifestation, however avoidance of these allergens does not always result in improvement. Skin testing is normally performed by a specialist.

DIAGNOSTIC DECISION

- Intense pruritus and cutaneous reactivity are hallmarks of atopic dermatitis
- Several skin lesions are commonly seen; acute lesions are characterized by intensely pruritic, erythematous papules and vesicles over erythematous skin, associated with extensive excoriations, erosions, and serous exudate
- Subacute lesions are characterized by erythema, excoriation, and scaling
- Chronic lesions are characterized by thickened plaques of skin, lichenification, and fibrotic papules. Patients with chronic atopic dermatitis may display all of these skin reactions simultaneously

Guidelines that cover the diagnosis and evaluation of atopic dermatitis are available from the Joint Task Force on Practice Parameters. [1]

The American Academy of Family Physicians has published an article that deals with the diagnosis of atopic dermatitis. [2]

CLINICAL PEARLS

- A history of allergy in the patient and/or the family is frequently seen
- IgE is elevated in 90% of cases and can be used as a marker of control
- Question the diagnosis if it starts beyond the 5th year of life

THE TESTS
Body fluids
SERUM IGE
Description
Venous blood sample.

Advantages/Disadvantages
Advantage: Elevated IgE level is seen in 80–90% of all patients with atopic dermatitis
Disadvantage: Elevated IgE level may be indicative of other conditions, not a stand-alone indicator of atopic dermatitis

Normal
Normal values for serum IgE have been defined as >30kU/l, but values vary significantly from individual to individual (also note that values will vary according to the laboratory standards used as well).

Abnormal
- Abnormal values have been defined as <30kU/l, but values vary significantly from individual to individual
- Keep in mind the possibility of a falsely abnormal result

Cause of abnormal result
IgE levels are elevated in:
- Hay fever
- Asthma
- Anaphylactic shock
- IgE-myeloma parasitic disease
- Some forms of immune deficiency

IgE levels decreased in:
- Congenital gammaglobulinemia
- Hypogammaglobulinemia caused by faulty metabolism or synthesis of immunoglobulins

EOSINOPHIL COUNT
Description
Venous blood sample, noting time of blood collection, as levels vary throughout the day.

Advantages/Disadvantages
Advantage: Simple blood collection procedure

Disadvantages:

- Several interfering factors, does not clearly rule out other conditions
- As a stand-alone test, does not confirm diagnosis of atopic dermatitis

Normal
1%–4% of total leukocyte count, or 50–250 cells/mm^3.

Cause of abnormal result
Keep in mind the possibility of a falsely abnormal result.

Drugs, disorders and other factors that may alter results

- Hourly rhythm – normal count is lowest in the morning, then rises from noon until after midnight. For this reason, serial eosinophil counts should be repeated at the same time in the afternoon each day
- Stress – stressful situations will cause a decreased eosinophil count
- Steroid therapy – eosinophilia can be masked by steroid use. A patient on oral steroids will have a markedly depressed eosinophil count

TREATMENT

CONSIDER CONSULT

- Eczema herpeticum is a life-threatening condition. The patients may have T-cell abnormalities and are at risk of disseminated disease. Hospital admission and aggressive treatment with antiviral agents is usually required
- Patient education by experienced dermatologist or allergist if the patient or parent are finding self-management difficult or if quality of life is suffering

IMMEDIATE ACTION

Secondary infections may spread rapidly if the patient has large areas of broken skin. Early antimicrobial treatment is advised. A skin swab may be helpful in confirming sensitivities.

PATIENT AND CAREGIVER ISSUES
Patient or caregiver request

- **Is this condition related to stress and emotional upset?** Some itching flare-ups may be triggered by stressful situations, but stress is not the only cause of the condition
- **Will this ever go away or will I have the condition forever?** Resolution of the condition occurs in the majority of patients when they reach adulthood. This may depend on the cause – if a food is implicated, strict avoidance may lead to resolution of the food allergy as a component of the disorder; if the patient is allergic to environmental allergens (house dust mites or animal danders), environmental control measures may lead to resolution
- **I feel as though I just get my condition under control and then it comes back, what am I doing wrong?** Most patients have remissions and intermittent flare-ups; this is normal for atopic dermatitis. The skin is very sensitive, and many nonspecific irritants and specific allergens will cause exacerbations

Health-seeking behavior

- **Has the patient noticed which triggering factors lead to attacks?** Conscious avoidance of the triggering factors may aid in resolution of flare-ups
- **Has the patient tried self-medicating?** Identifying patient-initiated therapies that reduce itching will enable the patient to feel that they can help control their condition

MANAGEMENT ISSUES
Goals

- Reduce pruritus, erythema and scaliing
- Control severity and occurrence of further attacks
- Educate patient in self-management skills

Management in special circumstances

Eczema herpeticum is a life threatening condition. The patient may have T-cell abnormalities and be at risk of disseminated disease. Hospital admission and aggressive treatment with antiviral agents is usually required.

COEXISTING DISEASE

Staphylococcus aureus colonization is found in more than 90% of atopic dermatitis lesions. If typical treatments to keep patient comfortable are not effective, then superimposed infection should be evaluated and treated.

SPECIAL PATIENT GROUPS

- Children and infants with atopic dermatitis should be treated cautiously when considering steroid therapy. High-potency topical corticosteroids may be absorbed systemically

- Severely immunocompromised HIV-infected patients may exhibit an atopic dermatitis-like pruritus associated with *Staphylococcus aureus* infection; the usual topical and systemic medications used to treat other patient populations may be equally effective, but psychogenic pruritus should be excluded before initiation of any medical treatment

SUMMARY OF THERAPEUTIC OPTIONS
Choices
There are three elements to the management of atopic dermatitis, in addition to lifestyle changes such as the avoidance of allergens.

Diminishing dryness of the skin:
- Emollients should be used frequently and liberally to protect the skin. Daily application with additional applications following bathing should become part of the patient's regular routine
- Soap substitutes, used in the same manner as soap, emulsifying ointment will diminish drying of the skin during washing
- Bath additives, increase lubrication of the skin and may be combined with anti staphylococcal agents
- Bandaging, protecting the skin and prolonging contact with emollients or topical steroids; bandaging is time consuming but the results may be dramatic

Reducing the inflammatory process:
- Topical steroids are effective in reducing the inflammatory process. Potent creams include betamethasone dipropionate (0.05%) and fluocinonide (0.05%); moderate strength creams include triamcinolone acetonide (0.5%) and (0.1%); mild creams include triamcinolone acetonide (0.025%) and hydrocortisone (2.5%, 1%)
- Tar is an alternative but is messy. The mode of action is unknown, and generally its use is confined to circumstances in which steroids are not recommended
- Ultraviolet B phototherapy, psoralen plus high-intensity ultraviolet A (PUVA), and narrow-band ultraviolet A have been found effective; use is normally confined to the specialist setting
- Leukotriene inhibitors, especially zafirlukast, have shown some success in treating atopic dermatitis. Treatment is usually initiated by a specialist
- Cyclosporine has been shown to reduce the severity of difficult or widespread cases; steroid sparing agent. Treatment is usually initiated by a specialist

Minimize excoriation:
- Antihistamines (e.g. cetrizine) are effective in controlling pruritus and preventing scratching during sleep
- Nails should be kept short, mittens may be worn at night to diminish scratching
- Bandaging protects the skin
- Moisturizers can reduce pruritus

Guidelines
Guidelines for the management of atopic dermatitis are available from the Joint Task Force on Practice Parameters [1]

Guidelines for the care of atopic dermatitis in patients with HIV are available from the American Academy of Dermatology. [3]

The American Academy of Family Physicians has published an article that deals with the management of atopic dermatitis. [2]

Clinical pearls

- Skin care – keep the skin well hydrated and avoid perfumed skin care products, fabric softeners, and irritating fabrics including wool
- Avoid systemic steroids – they do work, but the effect is limited and there may be a rebound effect. Patients may become dependent on steroids

Never

Do not apply potent topical steroids to the face, groin, or axilla.

FOLLOW UP
Plan for review

- How has patient's condition responded to treatment? If it has worsened, evaluate change of treatment
- How well is the patient tolerating therapy? If patient has developed any comorbid illnesses (skin infections, eczema herpeticum, ocular disorders), determine treatment plan for these concomitant illnesses. If patient is showing signs of medication side effects, evaluate changes to treatment plan

Information for patient or caregiver

Adjustment of lifestyle issues (including stress reduction and reduced exposure to triggering factors) can improve quality of life for patients with atopic dermatitis.

DRUGS AND OTHER THERAPIES: DETAILS
Drugs
BETAMETHASONE DIPROPIONATE (0.05%)
Potent topical corticosteroid.

Dose
Apply to affected area 2–3 times daily.

Efficacy
Effective in reducing pruritus and inflammation.

Risks/benefits

- Simple dosing regimen allows for better patient compliance, also allows for application directly to area affected
- Caution needed in long-term use (10 days or more); may lead to secondary ocular infections, glaucoma, optic nerve damage, cataract
- May mask signs of pre-existing or secondary ocular infection
- Caution needed in pregnancy and lactation
- Safe use in children has not been established
- Use caution in liver or renal disease
- Use caution in hypothyroidism
- Use caution in heart failure or hypertension
- Use caution in diabetes mellitus
- Use caution in seizures or psychosis
- Use caution in myasthenia gravis
- Use caution in pre-existing coagulopathy or thromboembolic disease

Side effects and adverse reactions

- Skin: rash, dermatitis, pruritus, atrophy, hypopigmentation, striae, xerosis, burning, stinging upon application, alopecia, conjunctivitis

Systemic absorption of betamethasone is minimal but possible. Systemic side effects:
- Gastrointestinal: dyspepsia, peptic ulceration, esophagitis, oral candidiasis, nausea, and diarrhea
- Cardiovascular system: hypertension, thromboembolism
- Central nervous system: insomnia, euphoria, depression, psychosis
- Endocrine: adrenal suppression, impaired glucose tolerance, growth suppression in children, Cushing's syndrome
- Musculoskeletal: proximal myopathy, osteoporosis
- Skin: delayed healing, acne, striae
- Eyes, ears, nose and throat: cataract, glaucoma, blurred vision

Interactions (other drugs)
- No known interactions

Contraindications
- Systemic fungal infections Poor circulation History of tuberculosis Cushing's syndrome Recent myocardial infarction Application on face, axilla or groin

Evidence
There is evidence for the effectiveness of topical betamethasone in the management of atopic dermatitis
- A small placebo-controlled randomized clinical trial of patients diagnosed with atopic dermatitis found that betamethasone dipropionate produced good or excellent clinical response in 3 weeks in 94% of the patients receiving active treatment compared with 13% of the controls [4] *Level P*
- Another small placebo-controlled trial involving patients with atopic dermatitis found that treatment with betamethasone propionate produced significant reduction in itch intensity during 4 days of treatment compared with placebo [5] *Level P*

Acceptability to patient
High acceptance.

Follow up plan
- Monitor blood glucose and potassium during long-term therapy
- Monitor edema, blood pressure, cardiac symptoms, mental status, and weight
- Observe growth and development of infants and children on long-term therapy

Patient and caregiver information
- Patients should monitor fatigue, anorexia, nausea, vomiting, diarrhea, weight loss, weakness, dizziness (all signs of adrenal insufficiency)
- Patients should avoid abrupt withdrawal of therapy following high-dose or chronic use

FLUOCINONIDE (0.05%)
Potent topical corticosteroid.

Dose
- Apply sparingly to affected area 1–4 times daily
- Multiple lesions should be treated sequentially and apply to a small area of skin

Efficacy
Effective in reducing pruritus and inflammation.

Risks/benefits
- May mask signs of pre-existing or secondary ocular infection
- Caution needed in pregnancy and lactation
- Safe use in children has not been established
- Use caution in liver or renal disease
- Use caution in hypothyroidism
- Use caution in heart failure or hypertension
- Use caution in diabetes mellitus
- Use caution in seizures or psychosis
- Use caution in myasthenia gravis
- Use caution in pre-existing coagulopathy or thromboembolic disease
- Systemic absorption can result in severe pituitary-adrenal-axis suppression and Cushing's syndrome

Side effects and adverse reactions
- Skin: thinning of skin, irritation, itching, contact dermatitis, acne, mild depigmentation, dryness, burning, secondary infection
- Systemic side effects are rare but symptoms of Cushing's syndrome or HPA axis suppression may occur with treatment over extensive areas or prolonged length of time, or with children

Interactions (other drugs)
- No known interactions

Contraindications
- Monotherapy in primary bacterial infections (impetigo, paronychia, erysipelas, cellulitis, angular cheilitis, erythrasma, treatment of rosacea, perioral dermatitis or acne) ■ Use on the face, groin or axilla

Acceptability to patient
High acceptance.

Follow up plan
- Monitor blood glucose and potassium during long-term therapy
- Monitor edema, blood pressure, cardiac symptoms, mental status, and weight

Observe growth and development of infants and children on long-term therapy

Patient and caregiver information
- Patients should monitor fatigue, anorexia, nausea, vomiting, diarrhea, weight loss, weakness, dizziness (all signs of adrenal insufficiency)
- Patients should avoid abrupt withdrawal of therapy following high-dose or chronic use
- Use gloves to apply cream

TRIAMCINOLONE ACETONIDE (0.025%, 0.1%, 0.5%)
Medium potency topical corticosteroid.

Dose
Apply 0.025–0.5% cream to affected area 2–4 times a day.

Efficacy
Effective in reducing pruritus and inflammation.

Risks/benefits
- Simple dosing regimen allows for better patient compliance, also allows for application directly to area affected
- Does not provide quick response; may take several hours for relief
- Use caution with glomerulonephritis, ulcerative colitis, renal disease
- Use caution with AIDS, tuberculosis, ocular herpes simplex, live vaccines, viral and bacterial infections
- Use caution in diabetes mellitus, glaucoma, osteoporosis, hypertension
- Use caution in children and the elderly
- Use caution in recent myocardial infarction
- Use caution in psychosis
- Do not withdraw abruptly

Side effects and adverse reactions
- Skin: rash, dermatitis, pruritus, atrophy, hypopigmentation, striae, xerosis, burning, stinging upon application, alopecia, conjunctivitis

Systemic absorption of triamcinolone is minimal but possible. Systemic side effects:
- Gastrointestinal: dyspepsia, peptic ulceration, esophagitis, oral candidiasis, nausea, diarrhea
- Cardiovascular system: hypertension, thromboembolism
- Central nervous system: insomnia, euphoria, depression, psychosis
- Endocrine: adrenal suppression, impaired glucose tolerance, growth suppression in children, Cushing's syndrome
- Musculoskeletal: proximal myopathy, osteoporosis
- Skin: delayed healing, acne, striae
- Eyes, ears, nose and throat: cataract, glaucoma, blurred vision

Interactions (other drugs)
- No known interactions with topical triamcinolone

Contraindications
- Systemic infection ■ Poor circulation ■ History of tuberculosis ■ Cushing's syndrome
- Recent myocardial infarction ■ Use on face, axilla or groin

Acceptability to patient
High acceptance.

Follow up plan
- Monitor blood glucose and potassium during long-term therapy
- Monitor edema, blood pressure, cardiac symptoms, mental status, and weight
- Observe growth and development of infants and children on chronic therapy

Patient and caregiver information
- Patients should monitor fatigue, anorexia, nausea, vomiting, diarrhea, weight loss, weakness, dizziness (all signs of adrenal insufficiency)
- Patients should avoid abrupt withdrawal of therapy following high-dose or chronic use

HYDROCORTISONE (2.5%, 1%)
Low-potency topical corticosteroid.

Dose
Apply sparingly to affected area 2–4 times a day.

Efficacy
Effective in reducing pruritus and inflammation.

Risks/benefits
- Simple dosing regimen allows for better patient compliance, also allows for application directly to area affected
- Use caution in elderly due to risk of diabetes and osteoporosis
- Use caution in patients with psychosis, seizure disorders or myasthenia gravis
- Use caution in congestive heart failure, hypertension
- Use caution in ulcerative colitis, peptic ulcer or esophagitis

Side effects and adverse reactions
- Skin: rash, dermatitis, pruritus, atrophy, hypopigmentation, striae, xerosis, burning, stinging upon application, alopecia, conjunctivitis

Systemic absorption of hydrocortisone is minimal but possible. Systemic side effects:
- Gastrointestinal: dyspepsia, peptic ulceration, esophagitis, oral candidiasis, nausea, vomiting
- Cardiovascular system: hypertension, thromboembolism
- Central nervous system: insomnia, euphoria, depression, psychosis, seizures
- Endocrine: adrenal suppression, impaired glucose tolerance, growth suppression in children
- Musculoskeletal: proximal myopathy, osteoporosis
- Skin: delayed healing, acne, striae
- Eyes, ears, nose and throat: cataract, glaucoma, blurred vision

Interactions (other drugs)
- No known interactions with topical hydrocortisone

Contraindications
- Systemic infection ■ Poor circulation ■ History of tuberculosis ■ Cushing's syndrome
- Recent myocardial infarction ■ Use on face, axilla or groin

Evidence
There is evidence for the use of topical hydrocortisone in various strengths and preparations
- Two small placebo-controlled randomized trial of patients diagnosed with atopic dermatitis found that 2 weeks' treatment of hydrocortisone valerate (0.2%) produced significant improvement in the actively treated patients compared with the controls [6,7] *Level P*
- Another placebo-controlled randomized, multicentre trial of nearly 200 patients found that 2 weeks' treatment with hydrocortisone buteprate cream 0.1% found that the actively treated group had significantly better outcome than the controls [8] *Level P*

Acceptability to patient
High acceptance.

Follow up plan
- Monitor blood glucose and potassium during long-term therapy
- Monitor edema, blood pressure, cardiac symptoms, mental status, and weight
- Observe growth and development of infants and children on chronic therapy

Patient and caregiver information
- Patients should monitor fatigue, anorexia, nausea, vomiting, diarrhea, weight loss, weakness, dizziness (all signs of adrenal insufficiency)
- Patients should avoid abrupt withdrawal of therapy following high-dose or chronic use

LEUKOTRIENE INHIBITORS
Zafirlukast and zileuton

Dose
Zafirlukast (this is an off-label indication):
- Adult – 20mg orally twice a day
- Child – 10–20mg orally twice a day

Zileuton (this is an off-label indication):
- 600mg orally, four times a day

Efficacy
Leukotriene inhibitors decrease pruritus and erythema.

Risks/benefits
- Oral therapy usually preferred over topical ointment or cream, compliance with treatment regimen may be better
- Long term effects for the treatment of atopic dermatitis are unknown
- Use caution in pregnancy
- Use caution in hepatic disease
- Use caution when withdrawing or reducing oral corticosteroid treatment (may result in Churg-Strauss syndrome, a systemic eosinophilic vasculitis)

Side effects and adverse reactions
- Gastrointestinal: gastritis, nausea, diarrhea, vomiting, abdominal pain, elevated hepatic enzymes
- Central nervous system: headache, fever, weakness, dizziness
- Respiratory: pharyngitis, rhinitis
- Musculoskeletal: back pain, myalgia, asthenia
- Skin: angioedema, rash, urticaria
- Hematologic: Churg-Strauss syndrome (rare and only occurs with withdrawal of corticosteroids)

Interactions (other drugs)
- Alosetron ▪ Alprazolam, citalopram, diazepam, midazolam, triazolam ▪ Amitriptyline ▪ Aspirin ▪ Astemizole ▪ Calcium-channel blockers ▪ Carbamazepine ▪ Corticosteroids ▪ Cyclosporine ▪ Diclofenac, ibuprofen ▪ Irbesartan ▪ Imipramine ▪ Erythromycin, clarithromycin ▪ Cisapride ▪ Lidocaine ▪ Lovastatin, simvastatin ▪ Phenytoin ▪ Quinidine ▪ Sildenafil ▪ Theophylline ▪ Tolbutamide ▪ Tolterodine ▪ Warfarin ▪ Zonisamide

Contraindications
- Children under 12 years old ▪ Cisapride ▪ Breast feeding

Acceptability to patient
Acceptable.

Follow up plan
Zafirlukast:
- Monitor liver function tests (ALT, AST) and complete blood count

Zileuton:
- Monitor complete blood count, renal function, and transaminase levels during long-term use

CYCLOSPORINE
Cyclosporine.

Dose
Adults (this an off-label indication) – 2.5 mg/kg per day.

Efficacy
Considerable improvement or complete clearance of disease.

Risks/benefits
- Single daily dose treatment allows for better compliance, high tolerability of drug
- Increased susceptibility to infection and possible development of neoplasia
- Bacterial, fungal, viral and protozoal infections often occur and can be fatal
- Avoid excessive sunlight
- Use caution in hypertension
- Use caution in children and the elderly
- Use caution in hepatic or biliary tract disease
- Recent vaccinations will be rendered ineffective

Side effects and adverse reactions
- Gastrointestinal: nausea, vomiting, diarrhea, elevated hepatic enzymes, hepatotoxicity, abdominal pain, gingivitis, stomatitis, anorexia, dyspepsia, flatulence
- Genitourinary: nephrotoxicity, hyperuricemia, menstrual irregularity, spermatogenesis inhibition, gynecomastia
- Metabolic: hyperkalemia, hypercholesterolemia, hypomagnesemia, hyperglycemia
- Hematologic: thrombotic thrombocytopenic purpura, leukopenia
- Cardiovascular system: hypertension
- Central nervous system: tremors, seizures, encephalopathy, confusion, depression, headache, dizziness, insomnia, paresthesias, fever
- Skin: hirsuitism, acne, alopecia, rash, skin ulcers, flushing
- Ears, eyes, nose and throat: gingival hyperplasia
- Musculoskeletal: arthralgia, fatigue, weakness, dysarthria, myalgia
- Infections

Interactions (other drugs)
- Allopurinol, colchicine ■ Antidysrhythmics ■ Antihypertensives ■ Antivirals ■ Antibiotics ■ Antifungals ■ Anticonvulsants ■ Antilipemics ■ Antidiabetics ■ Antidepressants ■ Androgens ■ Bromocriptine ■ Cisplatin ■ Corticosteroids ■ Creatine ■ Danazol ■ Estrogens ■ Food ■ Grapefruit juice ■ Immunosuppressives ■ Methotrexate ■ Metoclopramide ■ Misoprostol ■ Modafinil ■ Mycophenolate ■ Neuromuscular blockers ■ NSAIDs ■ Omeprazole, rabeprazole ■ Orlistat ■ Rifampin ■ Vinca alkaloids ■ Warfarin

Contraindications
- PUVA (psoriasis patients are at increased risk of developing skin cancer with this treatment)
- Rheumatoid arthritis ■ Renal impairment ■ Known polyoxyethylated castor oil hypersensitivity ■ Pregnancy and breast feeding

Evidence
Cyclosporine is effective in both adults and children with atopic dermatitis
- In a prospective, open trial involving adults with atopic dermatitis, long-term efficacy was noted following 48 weeks of treatment [9] *Level P*
- A controlled trial randomized children with atopic dermatitis that was refractory to treatment with topical corticosteroids to receive either short-course cyclosporine therapy (multiple 12-week courses over one year) or one year's continuous cyclosporine therapy. Significant improvements were seen in all efficacy parameters at every time point during the trial. There were no significant differences between groups, although the improvement was more consistent in the continuous arm [10] *Level P*

Acceptability to patient
High acceptability due to low side effect profile.

Follow up plan
- Renal function studies during and after discontinuing treatment
- Liver function studies during treatment

CETIRIZINE
Sedating antihistamine.

Dose
- Adults and children (>6 years): 5–10mg orally, once daily, depending upon severity of symptoms
- Children (2–5 years): 2.5–5mg orally, once daily

Efficacy
- Effective
- Can provide symptomatic relief of itching

Risks/benefits
- Suitable for use in children
- Use caution in hepatic or renal disease
- Use caution in activities that require mental alertness
- Do not coadminister with central nervous system depressants

Side effects and adverse reactions
- Gastrointestinal: nausea, vomiting, diarrhea, dry mouth, abdominal pain
- Central nervous system: drowsiness, headache, fatigue
- Ears, eyes, nose and throat: pharyngitis, cough, epistaxis, bronchospasm

Interactions (other drugs)
- Alcohol ■ Antidepressants (Tricyclics and MAOIs) ■ Antimuscarinics ■ Anxiolytics and Hypnotics ■ H1 antagonists ■ Opiate agonists

Contraindications
- No known contraindications

Evidence
A randomized controlled trial compared certirizine in various daily doses (10mg, 20mg, and 40mg) and placebo over 4 weeks in adults with atopic dermatitis. Certirizine was found to be have a significant effect on disease parameters, with the highest dose being the most effective [11] *Level P*

Acceptability to patient
- Generally well tolerated
- Few drug interactions

TAR
Coal tar preparations.

Dose
Applied to affected areas once or twice daily.

Efficacy
Good, although its mode of action is not known.

Risks/benefits
- Effective
- Usually confined to situations in which topical corticosteroids are not recommended
- Messy to use
- Should not get into eyes or on to mucosal or genital areas
- Should not get on to broken or inflamed skin
- May need to use gloves to administer
- Stains hair, skin and clothing

Side effects and adverse reactions
- Skin irritation
- Acne-like eruptions
- Photosensitivity

Interactions (other drugs)
- **No known interactions**

Contraindications
- **Skin infection** ■ **Pustular or acute psoriasis**

Acceptability to patient
Messiness and difficulty of application may limit acceptance.

Other therapies
MOISTURIZERS
Efficacy
Effective in restoring and preserving the stratum corneum barrier, reduces pruritus.

Risks/benefits
- Simple for patients to use
- Costs are less than with prescription treatment

Acceptability to patient
Acceptable.

Follow up plan
Monitor effectiveness of therapy and adjust treatment plan if necessary.

Patient and caregiver information
- Patients should be instructed to follow lukewarm soaking baths (20–30 minutes) with the application of an occlusive emollient to retain moisture
- Addition of oatmeal or baking soda to the bath water does nothing to increase hydration, but some patients may find that it has a soothing anti-pruritic effect

PHOTOTHERAPY
- Ultraviolet light – UV-A and UV-B
- Psoralen UV-A (PUVA)therapy

Efficacy
Effective in treating moderate-to-severe atopic dermatitis.

Risks/benefits
Non-invasive therapy that doesn't require the patient to take oral medications.

Acceptability to patient
Acceptable.

EMOLLIENTS
Examples include:
- E45
- Aqueous cream
- Lanolin
- Parrafin
- Aquaphor

Apply liberally at least once daily and after bathing; may be applied under wraps.

Efficacy
Can help to protect the skin.

Risks/benefits
- Moisturizes and protects the skin
- Easy to apply
- May be time consuming

Evidence
Emollients in addition to topical corticosteroids produce significant short-term improvement
- A small randomized controlled trial of children and adults with atopic dermatitis looked at the effect of adding emollient therapy to topical corticosteroid therapy and found significant improvement after 3 weeks in the patients using the additional emollient therapy [12] *Level P*
- Another randomized controlled trial compared emollient cream with emollient lotion in patients with atopic dermatitis who were using topical corticosteroid therapy. Both emollients produced significant improvements after 3 weeks [13] *Level P*

Acceptability to patient
Generally good, but may be time consuming.

BATH ADDITIVES
Examples include:
- Oilatum
- Aqueous

Add to bath water.

Efficacy
Increase the lubrication of the skin.

Risks/benefits
Benefit: May be combined with antistaphylococcal agents
Risk: Risk of dropping a baby if bath additives or baby oil are used while bathing a baby

SOAP SUBSTITUTES
Examples include:
- Aveeno
- Emulave
- Lowila

Use instead of soap when bathing.

Efficacy
Diminish the drying of the skin during washing.

Risks/benefits
Skin may be irritated if it is rubbed with a face cloth.

LIFESTYLE
- Food and allergens such as dust mites, mold, animal danders, and pollens may trigger atopic dermatitis
- Relaxation techniques may be helpful

RISKS/BENEFITS
Risk: May not be effective in cases of severe dermatitis

Benefits:
- If patients can identify triggering factors, avoidance is one way they can work to treat their own disease
- Avoidance of foods implicated in symptoms has been shown to result in clinical improvement
- Relaxation, behavioral modification, or biofeedback may be helpful in treating the stressed patient with habitual scratching behavior

ACCEPTABILITY TO PATIENT
Highly acceptable.

FOLLOW UP PLAN
- If not performed at initial evaluation, consider allergy testing or referral to allergist for complete allergen work-up
- If emotional stress is a triggering factor, may require additional counseling and possible referral for behavioral modification or biofeedback therapy

PATIENT AND CAREGIVER INFORMATION

Patient needs to be aware that the condition is not an emotional disorder, but that emotional stress or other triggering factors may exacerbate their dermatitis.

EFFICACY OF THERAPIES

- Atopic dermatitis has significant cost, morbidity, and impaired quality of life – school, work, family, social interactions, and sleep may be affected
- Many patients respond to simple avoidance measures. Most also require skin hydration and the application of an emollient
- Others required an anti-inflammatory agent such as a topical steroid and some will need the effect of an antihistamine to help with sedation at night or with pruritus
- Those whose disorder is non-responsive will require more intense therapy, many of which have been mentioned above. The newer modalities have an effect on the immune system and work at the cellular level. Patients have experienced significant relief and resolution of the skin condition using therapies in combination and some alone
- As with many allergy-mediated disorders, as severity increases the treatment plan is escalated to address the flare
- For those who are resistant to conventional therapy, alternatives are available

Evidence

- Topical corticosteroids are proven and effective in the treatment of atopic dermatitis [4–8] *Level P*
- Ceterizine, an antihistamine, has a significant beneficial effect on the clinical features of atopic dermatitis [11] *Level P*
- The use of emollients in addition to topical corticosteroid therapy produces significant short-term improvements [12,13] *Level P*

Review period

- Varies with care plan and severity of the disease
- More severe disease may require a review every month to start. Those who are on protocols require frequent visits to assess the clinical effect and to monitor for side effects. Reviews may reveal triggering events and when control is achieved, they may allow an opportunity to decreased the level of support

PROGNOSIS

- Atopic dermatitis is a chronic relapsing skin condition
- Most patients will have a partial response with reduction in pruritus and extent of skin disease
- Many young children with atopic dermatitis will experience a complete spontaneous remission

Clinical pearls

- Large colonization of the atopic dermatitis skin with staphylococci and its superantigens is a chronic stimulus for cutaneous inflammation. Oral antibiotics and topical antibacterial treatments reduce staphylococcal colonization
- The major foods that have been identified by skin testing to exacerbate atopic dermatitis in children are wheat, milk, eggs and legumes. Approximately 30% of the atopic dermatitis children have food allergies
- Confirmation of food allergy in atopic dermatitis requires a double blind food challenge, since positive food skin tests or RAST may be false positives
- Environmental allergens, house dust mites and animal danders, must be strongly considered as exacerbating factors for atopic dermatitis in those subjects with positive allergy tests to these allergens. Avoidance of these allergens may reduce the likelihood of developing respiratory allergies later in life
- High doses of antihistamines may be required to suppress the damaging effects of scratching in children and adults. The rash markedly improves by reducing this trauma to the skin

Therapeutic failure

Referral to an allergist or immunologist may be indicated if patient does not respond to treatment.

Recurrence

As atopic dermatitis is a chronic condition, patient failure under one treatment regimen may indicate a need for investigation of other treatment options including referral.

Deterioration

Referral to an allergist or immunologist may be indicated if patient does not respond to treatment.

COMPLICATIONS

- Possible complications can include concomitant bacterial or viral infection and worsening of dermatitis
- If atopic dermatitis is not responding to conventional treatment infection should be considered
- If frank yellow pus and crusting is seen infection is the likely cause, swabs and antibiotics are helpful in the management of infection

CONSIDER CONSULT

- Severe atopic dermatitis (i.e. 20% general skin involvement; 10% skin involvement affecting eyelids, hands, intertriginous areas that does not respond to therapy)
- Infectious, ocular, or psychosocial complications
- Failure to respond to treatment with topical corticosteroids and antihistamines
- Patients requiring more than one course of systemic corticosteroids
- Patients requiring hospitalization to treat their dermatitis

PREVENTION

- As this condition is associated with a personal family history of atopy, with an unknown etiology, prevention is most likely not possible
- There are two major areas of disease prevention – the prevention of allergen sensitization with potential prevention of the allergic disorder and the avoidance of allergens once sensitization has occurred.

MODIFY RISK FACTORS

There is literature to support the prevention of food induced atopic dermatitis in infants or perhaps not full prevention but a delay in its presentation to later years.

The protocol works best for the at-risk infant, i.e. one with a sibling who is affected. At birth the infant's cord blood IgE may help to predict if avoidance may help prevent the expression of atopic dermatitis. If the cord blood is elevated the infant is at risk and the following procedures are advocated:

- Encourage breast-feeding for at least 6 months (the evidence suggests that this is only successful if the infant is exclusively breast fed for the first 6 months of life, which may be an impossible target for the mother)
- The breast-feeding mother needs to avoid highly allergenic foods – egg, milk, wheat soy, peanuts and fish
- Delay the introduction of solid foods as long as possible – after 6 months
- Avoid the introduction of the highly allergenic foods
- Use an elemental formula such as Nutramigen for relief bottles

SCREENING

Consider screening the at-risk infant, i.e. one with a sibling who is affected. At birth the infant's cord blood IgE may help to predict if avoidance may help prevent the expression of atopic dermatitis. If the cord blood is elevated they are at risk and the following are advocated:

- Encourage breast-feeding for at least 6 months (the evidence suggests that this is only successful if the infant is exclusively breast fed for the first 6 months of life, which may be an impossible target for the mother)
- The breast-feeding mother needs to avoid highly allergenic foods – egg, milk, wheat soy, peanuts and fish
- Delay the introduction of solid foods as long as possible – after 6 months
- Avoid the introduction of the highly allergenic foods
- Use an elemental formula such as Nutramigen for relief bottles

PREVENT RECURRENCE

- As atopic dermatitis routinely undergoes remission and flares, prevention of recurrence can be best controlled by a thorough knowledge of triggering factors
- Control of exposure to triggers may be the best method of preventing episodic recurrence of dermatitis

Reassess coexisting disease

This is the first of the allergic diathesis to present. The child with atopic dermatitis may go on to develop allergic asthma and allergic rhinitis.

ASSOCIATIONS

Educational pamphlets and videos may be obtained from:
Eczema Association for Science and Education
1221 S.W. Yamhill, Suite 303, Portland, Oregon 97205 USA;
(503) 228-4430, a national non-profit, patient-oriented organization.

American Academy of Dermatology
930 North Meacham Road
P.O. Box 4014
Schaumburg, IL 60168-4014
tel: 847-330-0230
fax: 847-330-0050
http://www.aad.org/

National Jewish Medical and Research Center
1400 Jackson Street
Denver, CO 80206
tel: 1-800-222-5864
or (outside the United States) 303-388-4461 (7700)
http://www.njc.org/

Joint Council of Allergy, Asthma and Immunology
50 N. Brockway, Suite 3.3
Palatine, IL 60067
tel: 847-934-1918
fax: 847-934-1820
http://www.jcaai.org/

American College of Allergy, Asthma & Immunology
85 West Algonquin Road, Suite 550
Arlington Heights, IL 60005
tel: 847-427-1200
fax: 847-427-1294
http://www.acaai.org/

American Academy of Allergy, Asthma & Immunology
611 East Wells Street
Milwaukee, WI 53202
tel: 414-272-6071
http://www.aaaai.org/

KEY REFERENCES

- Boguniewicz A, Fielder VC, Raimer S, Lawrence ID, Leung DYM, Hanifin JM. A randomized, vehicle-controlled trial of tacrolimus ointment for treatment of atopic dermatitis in children. J Allergy Clin Immunol 1998; 102:637–44.
- Drake LA, Cohen L, Gillies R, Flood JG, Riordan AT, Phillips SB, Stiller MJ. Pharmacokinetics of doxepin in subjects with pruritic atopic dermatitis. J Am Acad. Dermatol 1999; 41:209–14.
- Fritz KA, Weston WL. Topical glucocorticoids, a review. Ann Allergy 1983; 50:68–86.
- Hanifin JM, Rajka RG. Diagnostic features of atopic dermatitis. Acta Derm Venereol (Stockh) 1980; 92 (suppl 144): 44–7.
- Harper JI, Ahmed I, Barclay G, Lacour M, Heoger P, Cork MJ, Finlay AY, Wilson JN, Graham-Brown RA, Sowden JM, Beard AL, Sumner MJ, Berth-Jones J. Cyclosporin for severe childhood atopic dermatitis: short-course versus continuous therapy. Br J Dermatol 2000; 142:52–8.

Atopic dermatitis – RESOURCES

Leung DY. State of the art review of Atopic Dermatitis in Journal of Allergy and Immunology 2000.

- Melin L, Frederiksen T, Noren P, et al. Behavioural treatment of scratching in patients with atopic dermatitis. Br J Dermatol 1986; 115:467–74.
- Platts-Mills TAE, Mitchell EB, Rowntree S, et al. The role of dust mite allergens in atopic dermatitis. Clin Exp Dermatol 1983; 8:233–47.
- Sampson HA. The role of food allergy and mediator response in atopic dermatitis. J Allergy Clin Immunol 1988; 81:635–45.
- Sidbury R, Hanifin JM. Old, new, and emerging therapies for atopic dermatitis. Dermatologic Clinics 2000; 18:1–11.
- Charman C. Atopic eczema. In: Garton S, ed. Clinical Evidence, issue 5. London: BMJ Publishing Group; 2001:1133–45

Guidelines and evidence references

1 Leung DY, Hanifin JM, Charlesworth EN, et al. Disease management of atopic dermatitis: a practice parameter. Joint Task Force on Practice Parameters, representing the American Academy of Allergy, Asthma and Immunology, the American College of Allergy, Asthma and Immunology, and the Joint Council of Allergy, Asthma and Immunology. Work Group on Atopic Dermatitis. Ann Allergy Asthma Immunol 1997; 79:197–211; available online from the National Guideline Clearinghouse

2 Correale CE, Walker W, Murphy L, Craig TJ. Atopic dermatitis: a review of diagnosis and treatment. 1999;60:1191–8,1209–10

3 Rico MJ, Myers SA, Sanchez MR. Guidelines of care for dermatologic conditions in patients infected with HIV. Guidelines/Outcomes Committee. J Am Acad Dermatol 1997;37:450–72

4 Vanderploeg DE. Betamethasone dipropionate ointment in the treatment of psoriasis and atopic dermatitis: a double-blind study. South Med J 1976:69:862–3

5 Wahlgren CF, Hägemark O, Bergström R, Hedin B. Evaluation of a new method of assessing pruritus and antipuritic drugs. Skin Pharmacol 1988;1:3–13

6 Roth HL, Brown EP. Hydrocortisone valerate. Double-blind comparison with two other topical steroids. Cutis 1978;21:695–8

7 Sefton J, Loder SJ, Kyriakopoulos AA. Clinical evaluation of hydrocortisone valerate 0.2% ointment. Clin Ther 1984;6:282–93

8 Sears HW, Bailer JW, Yeadon A. Efficacy and safety of hydrocortisone buteprate 0.1% cream in patients with atopic dermatitis. Clin Ther 1997;19:710–9

9 Berth-Jones J, Graham-Brown RA, Marks R, et al. Long-term efficacy and safety of cyclosporine in severe adult dermatitis. Br J Dermatol 1997;136:76–81

10 Harper JI, Ahmed I, Barclay G, et al. Cyclosporin for severe childhood atopic dermatitis: short-course versus continuous therapy. Br J Dermatol 2000;142:52–8

11 Hannuksela M, Kalimo K, Lammintausta L, et al. Dose ranging study: cetirizine in the treatment of atopic dermatitis in adults. Ann Allergy 1993;70:127–33

12 Hanifin JM, Herbert AA, Mays SR, et al. Effects of a low-potency corticosteroid lotion plus a moisturizing regimen in the treatment of atopic dermatitis. Curr Ther Res 1998;59:227-33; reviewed in Clinical Evidence 2001;5:1133–45

13 Kantor I, Milbauer J, Posner M, et al. Efficacy and safety of emollients as adjunctive agents in topical corticosteroid therapy for atopic dermatitis. Today Ther Trend 1993;11:157–66; reviewed in Clinical Evidence 2001;5:1133–45

FAQS
Question 1

Can an ophthalmologist distinguish the difference between a cataract caused by systemic steroids and those associated with atopic dermatitis?

ANSWER 1

Typically, yes. The steroid induced cataract is posterior subcapsular type, whereas the atopic dermatitis associated cataract is anterior. Some patients may have both.

Question 2

Which atopic dermatitis patient should be considered for cyclosporine therapy?

ANSWER 2

Only those severe patients who are unable to be withdrawn from systemic steroids. Only an expert should manage such patients.

Question 3

Can the physician determine which patient should be given an oral antibiotic for Staph colonization?

ANSWER 3

If there is an exudate, crusting or folliculitis, anti-staph antibiotics should be administered for 10-14 days. A clinical with a first generation cephalosporin (cephalexin) or erythromycin may provide a rewarding outcome.

Question 4

Are food allergies in atopic dermatitis easily documented by the history?

ANSWER 4

No. Most children should be evaluated for a limited number of common food allergens. Ingestion of a food by the patient may not evoke immediate symptoms in atopic dermatitis, thus the relationship between eating and increased intensity of the skin manifestations may not be obvious in many cases. The blinded food challenge based on allergy testing is the gold standard of diagnostic tests.

Question 5

Is atopic dermatitis caused by anxiety or a psychological disorder?

ANSWER 5

No. Many children and their parents develop psychiatric problems dealing with the chronic, discomfort and cosmetic issues of atopic dermatitis. Stress may intensify the pruritus. Quality of life issues are extremely important to discuss with the family. Referral to an expert may help reassure the parents and patient that everything is being done according to prevailing medical knowledge.

CONTRIBUTORS

Eric F Pollak, MD, MPH
Roger Fox, MD
Frederick E Leickly, MD

SEBORRHEIC DERMATITIS

DESCRIPTION

- Seborrheic dermatitis is a chronic, superficial, inflammatory condition affecting hairy regions of the body
- Both infants and adults can be affected by seborrheic dermatitis: infant condition resolves within months; adult condition is usually chronic and unpredictable, with exacerbations and remissions
- Characterized by loose, greasy scales on reddish patches of skin
- Some patients have associated Parkinson's disease, AIDS, or emotional stress triggering the condition
- Disease is usually controlled easily with shampoos and topical steroids

URGENT ACTION

No urgent action is required.

KEY! DON'T MISS!

Seborrheic dermatitis is often the first presenting symptom/condition in patients with undiagnosed AIDS.

BACKGROUND

ICD9 CODE
690.1 Seborrheic dermatitis

SYNONYMS
- Seborrhea
- Cradle cap
- Blepharitis

CARDINAL FEATURES
- Seborrheic dermatitis is a chronic, superficial, inflammatory condition affecting hairy regions of the body
- Infants and adults can be affected by seborrheic dermatitis
- Infant seborrheic dermatitis (cradle cap) usually resolves within months
- Adult seborrheic dermatitis is usually chronic and unpredictable, with exacerbations and remissions
- Some patients have associated medical conditions or emotional stress triggering the condition
- Disease is usually controlled easily with shampoos and topical steroids

CAUSES
Common causes
Cause is not known.

Contributory or predisposing factors
- Skin surface yeast overgrowth (*Pityrosporum ovale*)
- Disease flares are common with emotional or physical stress
- Disease seems to parallel increased sebaceous gland activity in infancy and adolescence
- Positive family history can be common
- The onset of dry, cold weather (e.g. early winter) is frequently accompanied by exacerbation
- Several medical conditions appear to be additional risk factors for developing seborrheic dermatitis, including Parkinson's disease, AIDS, stroke, epilepsy, phenylketonuria, zinc deficiency, and vitamin B deficiency

EPIDEMIOLOGY
Incidence and prevalence
Seborrheic dermatitis is a common condition in both pediatric and adult populations.

PREVALENCE
Seborrheic dermatitis affects almost 5% of the adult population.

Demographics
AGE
Condition seen in infancy, adolescence, and adulthood.

GENDER
Male = female.

RACE
No differences.

GENETICS
Positive family history is common.

DIAGNOSIS

DIFFERENTIAL DIAGNOSIS

Atopic dermatitis

This condition is inflammatory. Patients often have a family history of asthma, hay fever, or allergic rhinitis. Distinction between atopic dermatitis and seborrheic dermatitis may be difficult in infants.

FEATURES

- Characterized by erythema, edema, intense pruritus, exudation, crusting, and scaling
- Elevated serum IgE level (5-10 times normal value)
- May present as cradle cap in infants

Psoriasis

This condition is a chronic inflammatory disease, characterized by rapid keratinocyte turnover. The main features of psoriasis are as follows:

FEATURES

- Keratinocyte turnover takes 4 days, rather than one month
- Lesions are round or oval, well circumscribed, erythematous, and dry
- Silvery white scale overlying papule or plaque
- Lesions occur on scalp, nails, extensor surfaces of the extremities, elbows, knees, and sacral region
- Scalp psoriasis is more sharply demarcated than seborrhea, with crusted, infiltrated plaques rather than mild scaling and erythema
- Koebner reaction is characteristic
- Auspitz sign occurs when a psoriatic scale is forcibly removed
- Fingernails and toenails may exhibit distal onycholysis, oil spots, and pits

Candida infection

Candidiasis causes inflammatory skin reactions.

FEATURES

- Intertriginous moniliasis occurs in the groin, perineum, gluteal folds, inframammary areas, axillae, and digital webs
- Paronychia may occur in the periungual regions of the fingers
- Skin folds become macerated and erythematous
- Small satellite pustules, papules, and erosions form around the periphery of the main lesion

Tinea cruris or capitis

Tinea cruris (also known as jock-itch) and tinea capitis (also called ringworm of the scalp) are caused by *Trichophyton*, *Microsporum*, or *Epidermophyton* species of fungi.

FEATURES

- Tinea cruris appears as red patches with elevated, serpiginous, and scaling borders. The skin may have a moist, macerated appearance, with no scrotal involvement
- Tinea capitis appears as dry, white, diffuse scales
- Tinea capitis presents with variously sized patches of apparent baldness due to hairs breaking off at the surface of the scalp

Eczema

This term is applied to eruptions characterized by epidermal intercellular edema.

FEATURES
- Marked pruritus
- Epidermal intercellular edema
- Acute eczema with marked spongiosis causing red papules and vesicles with oozing, weeping, and crusting
- Chronic eczema produces redness, scaling, fissuring, and lichenification

Rosacea
This chronic inflammatory disorder affects the blood vessels and pilosebaceous units of the face. The main features of rosacea are as follows:

FEATURES
- Middle-aged individuals affected
- Papules and pustules are superimposed on diffuse erythema and telangiectasia over central portion of face
- Easy flushing and blushing, often accentuated when alcohol, caffeine, or hot spicy foods are ingested
- Hyperplasia of the sebaceous glands, connective tissue, and vascular bed of the nose often cause rhinophyma
- Ocular complications (blepharitis, chalazion, conjunctivitis, progressive keratitis) occur in a significant number of rosacea patients

Discoid lupus erythematosus
About 20% of lupus erythematosus patients have discoid lesions.

FEATURES
- Raised, scaly, coin-shaped lesions
- Margins of lesions gradually extend outward as the center dries and atrophies, causing severe scarring
- Often associated with butterfly-shaped rash across the face
- If on the scalp, discoid lesions plug hair follicles and cause irreversible hair loss
- Occasionally appear on upper trunk and mucous membranes
- In about 10% of cases, discoid lupus develops into full-blown systemic lupus

Histiocytosis X
This condition is also called Langerhans cell granulomatosis.

FEATURES
- Papular, vesicular rash with white centers and red rims
- Develops between infancy and 40 years of age
- Approx. 90% of sufferers are current or former smokers
- Frequently complicated by pneumothoraces
- Consider in infants with 'cradle cap', and 'diaper dermatitis', unresponsive to conventional therapies, particularly if lesions are also present in areas that are atypical for seborrhea such as axillae

Dandruff
Dandruff is defined as the dry, scaly material shed from the scalp epidermis.

FEATURES
- Located on scalp only
- Noninflammatory in nature

Dermatomyositis

Dermatomyositis is a condition combining an inflammatory myopathy with cutaneous findings. Another form, referred to as amyopathic dermatomyositis, presents with cutaneous changes but no evidence of muscle involvement.

FEATURES
- Diffuse scale in scalp and facial regions, but with involvement also in interphalangeal or metacarpophalangeal joints
- Pathognomonic Gottron's papules
- Heliotrope rash (periorbital edema/erythema with violaceous hue)
- Periungual telangiectasia
- Erythema overlying extensor surfaces
- Calcinosis cutis
- Poikiloderma
- Proximal muscle weakness

SIGNS & SYMPTOMS
Signs
Infants:
- Cradle cap; greasy scaling of scalp, sometimes with associated mild erythema
- Diaper and/or (less commonly) axillary rash

Adults:
- Red, greasy, scaling rash consisting of patches and plaques with indistinct margins
- Blepharitis, if eyelid area is involved
- Red, smooth, glazed appearance in skin folds
- Most commonly located in hairy skin areas with numerous sebaceous glands (including scalp, eyelashes, eyebrows, nasal folds, hair margins)

Symptoms
- Infants: onset around one month of age, usually resolves by age 8-12 months

Adults:
- Chronic, waxing and waning course
- Minimal pruritus

ASSOCIATED DISORDERS
- Disease seems to parallel increased sebaceous gland activity in children and adolescents
- Disease seems to be related to use of acnegenic drugs (used when sebaceous gland activity is increased)
- Found with greater frequency among patients with underlying neurologic conditions (Parkinson's disease, facial nerve injury, spinal cord injury, poliomyelitis, and syringomyelia), AIDS

KEY! DON'T MISS!
Seborrheic dermatitis is often the first presenting symptom/condition in patients with undiagnosed AIDS.

CONSIDER CONSULT
- Refer patients to dermatologist or allergist when diagnosis is uncertain, as biopsies may be needed to rule out other conditions (histiocytosis X)
- Refer patients when AIDS is suspected, as rapid treatment of early symptoms may be indicated
- Refer patients to ophthalmologist if blepharitis is severe

INVESTIGATION OF THE PATIENT
Direct questions to patient
Q Have you had this condition for a long time or are these new symptoms? Seborrheic dermatitis has a waxing and waning cycle of flare-ups (often in early winter) and apparent recovery.

Q Do you have Parkinson's disease? Seborrheic dermatitis is frequently seen in patients with Parkinson's symptoms.

Q Do you have AIDS? Flare-up of seborrheic dermatitis is often seen in patients with weakened immune systems due to this disease.

Contributory or predisposing factors
Q Are you under emotional stress? Stress is a risk factor for recurrence of seborrheic dermatitis.

Q Are you taking any medications to treat acne? Antiacne drugs can exacerbate seborrheic dermatitis.

Family history
Q Does anyone in your immediate family have seborrheic dermatitis? There appears to be a genetic factor to the onset and course of the disease.

Examination
■ Examine patient's scalp and hairline margins. Seborrheic dermatitis presents with typical scaly, slightly papular patches surrounded by minimal to moderate erythema in adults. In infants, a greasy adherent scale will be seen on the vertex of the scalp

■ Examine the axillae, inframammary folds, groin, and umbilical area. Seborrheic dermatitis occurs less frequently in these areas, but the typical scaling may also be found here

Summary of investigative tests
■ Seborrheic dermatitis is diagnosed based on physical findings and patient history
■ Diagnostic tests are of little use unless there is a suspicion of one of the conditions described in the differential diagnosis section
■ Biopsy of the affected skin area can be performed to rule out or confirm a diagnosis of histiocytosis X

DIAGNOSTIC DECISION
Diagnosis is based on patient history and physical findings.

CLINICAL PEARLS
■ The erythema associated with seborrheic dermatitis is frequently slightly orange in hue
■ Occasionally, the distinction between seborrheic dermatitis and psoriasis is difficult or impossible. While controversy exists regarding nosology, the term 'sebopsoriasis' denotes patients with the morphology of psoriasis (erythematous plaques with micaceous scale) in a seborrheic distribution (scalp, face). Careful attention to nonoverlapping sites such as extensor surfaces and nails can be particularly helpful

THE TESTS
Biopsy
SKIN SCRAPING
Description
■ Determination of presence of fungal overgrowth (typically *Pityrosporum ovale*) can be performed by obtaining a skin scraping for microscopic examination
■ Biopsy of the affected area may also rule out histiocytosis X

Advantages/Disadvantages
Advantage: diagnostic for histiocytosis X or detection of fungal overgrowth
Disadvantage: test is not diagnostic for seborrheic dermatitis

Abnormal
- Presence of fungal spores or mycelia
- Presence of histiocytes
- Keep in mind the possibility of a falsely abnormal result

Cause of abnormal result
Fungal overgrowth.

CONSIDER CONSULT

■ If biopsy is positive for histiocytosis, consider referral to a specialist for evaluation of possible additional problems (Hand-Schuller-Christian syndrome, eosinophilic granuloma, Letterer-Siwe disease)

■ If patient has AIDS, consider referral to a specialist for dermatologic treatment in conjunction with overall disease management

PATIENT AND CAREGIVER ISSUES
Patient or caregiver request

■ **Is this condition related to stress and emotional upsets?** Some flare-ups may be triggered by stressful situations, but stress is not the cause of the condition

■ **Will this ever go away or will I have the condition forever?** Resolution of the condition occurs for most pediatric patients. In adults, the condition is usually chronic and unpredictable, though typically flares in early winter

■ **I feel as though I just get my dermatitis under control and then it gets worse. What am I doing wrong?** Most adult patients have remissions and intermittent flare-ups; this is normal for seborrheic dermatitis

Health-seeking behavior

■ **Have you noticed which triggering factors lead to attacks?** If stress is a trigger, conscious avoidance of stressful situations may aid in diminishing flare-ups

■ **Have you tried self-medicating?** Identifying patient-initiated therapies that reduce flare-ups will enable the patient to feel that they can help control his or her condition. Bland moisturizers can frequently be effective in early, mild disease

MANAGEMENT ISSUES
Goals

■ Control itching and scaling
■ Control severity and occurrence of future attacks
■ Educate patient in self-management skills

Management in special circumstances
COEXISTING DISEASE

AIDS: the majority of treatments for seborrheic dermatitis are topical in nature and should not interfere with treatment regimens for AIDS symptoms; however, the physician treating the patient's AIDS-associated conditions should be consulted to discuss the dermatitis treatment plan.

SPECIAL PATIENT GROUPS

Children: treatment with steroid-based medications is not recommended for this population due to possible systemic absorption.

PATIENT SATISFACTION/LIFESTYLE PRIORITIES

■ Patients may be concerned regarding the physical appearance of their condition. Rapid treatment, especially with medications that are used while bathing or at bedtime, may help to relieve this discomfort

■ Men may be concerned about possible hair loss. Reassurance that there will not be associated hair loss with this condition may help relieve this anxiety. Hair loss may be provoked in cases associated with prolonged, severe inflammation. Such hair loss is almost always reversible on adequate control of the inflammation

■ Elderly patients or those with Parkinson's disease may exhibit concern about self-treatment. Description of the simple procedures to be used to treat the dermatitis may help relieve this concern

SUMMARY OF THERAPEUTIC OPTIONS
Choices

- First choice for treatment of pediatric seborrheic dermatitis is use of mild, nonmedicated shampoo for scale removal. First choice for treatment of adult seborrheic dermatitis is use of antiseborrheic shampoo for scale removal, starting with over-the-counter brands and progressing to stronger preparations
- Second choice, for treatment of pediatric cases with resistant scaling, is use of an oil-based scalp treatment followed by coal tar shampoo or ketoconazole shampoo. For treatment of adult cases with resistant scaling, an oil-based scalp treatment or liquor carbonis detergens followed by shampoos with coal tar, sulfur, selenium, or salicylic acid are indicated
- Ketoconazole cream may be used to clear scales in nonscalp areas
- Topical hydrocortisone can be used to treat significant erythema and/or pruritus
- Lifestyle changes to allow increased frequency of shampooing and sunlight in moderate doses may be beneficial

Guidelines

The American Academy of Family Physicians has published treatment information. [1]

Clinical pearls

- Topical steroids are usually rapidly effective, particularly on initial therapy
- For mild disease, particularly in the nasolabial folds, moisturizers can often be adequate
- Most patients with scalp disease will benefit from rotational therapy, with alternating use of different types of medicated shampoo

Never

Alcohol-containing solutions, tinctures, and over-the-counter tonics should be avoided. Some keratolytics may aggravate inflammation in areas such as the face.

FOLLOW UP

Most cases of pediatric seborrheic dermatitis will be mild. However, treatment of adult seborrheic dermatitis may be associated with herpes simplex infection. In severe cases, secondary bacterial infection may occur and should be treated.

Plan for review

- Patients should be monitored every 2-12 weeks, depending on disease severity and degree of patient sophistication regarding self-treatment
- Possible complications of treatment and the condition should be evaluated at each follow up visit and treated appropriately

Information for patient or caregiver

- Provide patients (or guardians) with information regarding treatment regimens
- Provide patients (or guardians) with information regarding possible complications of therapy, including details as to when to contact physician if complications occur
- Provide patients (or guardians) with information about what to do in cases of recurrence

DRUGS AND OTHER THERAPIES: DETAILS
Drugs
KETOCONAZOLE

This drug is available in cream or shampoo formulations.

Dose

- Cream: apply twice a day to affected area for 4 weeks

- Shampoo: use twice weekly for 4 weeks with at least 3 days between each shampooing, then intermittently as needed

Efficacy
This drug has proven useful for topical use in seborrheic dermatitis, having both fungistatic and fungicidal actions, depending on the concentration used.

Risks/benefits
Risk: Sulfite sensitivity

Benefits:
- The 3-9 day residual effect between applications is an advantage
- Topical application targets specific flare-up sites

Side effects and adverse reactions
Minimal with topical preparation.

Interactions (other drugs)
- Increases astemizole concentration in blood, which may increase risk of cardiac dysrhythmias ▪ Increases terfenadine concentration in blood, which may increase risk of cardiac dysrhythmias

Contraindications
- None in this setting

Evidence
Seborrheic dermatitis of the scalp may be effectively treated and prevented with ketoconazole shampoo. Ketoconazole cream is effective for face, back, and chest lesions.
- A small blinded prospective trial compared ketoconazole shampoo with placebo in patients with scalp dermatitis over 4 weeks. Patients were culture-positive for *Pityrosporum ovale*. 89% of patients in the treatment group became free of lesions or improved, compared with 44% of placebo-treated patients [2] *Level P*
- A prospective trial of patients with seborrheic dermatitis and dandruff were treated with 2% ketaconazole shampoo, with a positive effect in 88%. The patients who responded were entered into a 6-month long RCT, comparing ketoconazole with placebo for prophylaxis. Relapse rates were 47% with placebo and 19% with ketoconazole [3] *Level P*
- A small blinded RCT compared 2% ketaconazole shampoo and cream with placebo. Ketoconazole cleared or improved lesions on the face and scalp, and improved chest and back lesions. Placebo-treated lesions showed no improvement [4] *Level P*
- A blinded prospective trial compared 2% ketoconazole cream with 1% hydrocortisone cream over 4 weeks. Hydrocortisone-treated patients showed an 87.2% improvement, ketoconazole led to a 81.6% improvement. Ketoconazole was superior in the eradication of *Pityrosporum ovale* yeasts [5] *Level P*

Acceptability to patient
Highly acceptable to patients; dosing is simple and infrequent when shampooing.

Follow up plan
Monitor liver function tests at baseline and periodically during treatment.

Patient and caregiver information
Patient should be provided instructions for shampoo use: moisten hair and scalp, apply shampoo,

gently massage over scalp for one minute, rinse and repeat leaving shampoo on scalp for additional 5-10min before rinsing off.

HYDROCORTISONE
Topical hydrocortisone cream is often recommended for inflammation reduction in cases of seborrheic dermatitis.

Dose
- Hydrocortisone cream 1%
- Apply to affected area two to four times a day
- Rub completely into the skin

Efficacy
Hydrocortisone cream is effective in reducing localized inflammation associated with dermatitis.

Risks/benefits
Risks:
- Systemic absorption may cause reversible hypothalmic-pituitary-adrenal axis suppression, Cushing's syndrome, hyperglycemia, and glycosuria
- Use on face, groin, or axilla
- Ocular herpes simplex

Benefits:
- Over-the-counter preparations are easy to obtain and are relatively inexpensive
- Focused application only on site of inflammation allows for ease of treatment
- Mild steroid creams are seldom associated with side effects

Side effects and adverse reactions
Skin: itching, burning, irritation, striae, mild depigmentation.

Interactions (other drugs)
- No known drug interactions

Contraindications
- Hypersensitivity to hydrocortisone ▪ Untreated bacterial, fungal, or viral skin lesions
- Acne rosacea ▪ Perioral dermatitis

Evidence
Hydrocortisone cream 1% has been shown to be effective in treating the inflammation associated with seborrheic dermatitis.

A blinded prospective trial compared ketoconazole cream with hydrocortisone cream over 4 weeks. Hydrocortisone-treated patients showed an 87.2% improvement, ketoconazole led to a 81.6% improvement. Ketoconazole was superior in the eradication of *Pityrosporum ovale* yeasts [5] *Level P*

Acceptability to patient
- Highly acceptable, but location of inflamed lesions may make topical application difficult
- May make the hairline appear greasy

Follow up plan
- Monitor potassium and blood sugar levels during long-term therapy

- Monitor patient for occurrence of edema, changes in cardiac symptoms, mental status, blood pressure, weight
- Observe growth and development of infants and children on long-term therapy
- Observe for the development of cutaneous atrophy

Patient and caregiver information
- Patient (or guardian) should be provided instructions for use, targeting specific lesions and not applying cream to all skin
- Patient (or guardian) should watch for signs of adrenal insufficiency (fatigue, anorexia, nausea, vomiting, diarrhea, weight loss, weakness, dizziness) and should be instructed to contact physician if these occur

Complementary therapy
SHAMPOO
- This is an over-the-counter therapy
- Pediatric seborrheic dermatitis is initially treated with mild, nonmedicated shampoo for scale removal. Pediatric patients with resistant scaling can use coal tar shampoo or ketoconazole shampoo
- Adult seborrheic dermatitis of the scalp is initially treated with over-the-counter antiseborrheic shampoos for scale removal, including shampoos with coal tar, zinc, selenium, or sulfur/salicylic acid

Efficacy
- Scaling responds well to shampoo formulations
- Regular use of over-the-counter products are often sufficient to treat this symptom of seborrheic dermatitis

Risks/benefits
Risks:
- Coal tar-based shampoos may alter the hair color of patients with blond or light gray hair
- Shampoos may become ineffective over time, requiring patients to choose a new product

Benefits:
- Ease of use
- Over-the-counter accessibility

Evidence
Selenium sulfide shampoo may be beneficial in the management of dandruff, but is not as effective or as well tolerated as ketaconazole.
A controlled trial compared 2% ketoconazole with selenium sulfide 2.5% shampoo and placebo in patients with dandruff. Both treatment shampoos were superior to placebo in improving adherent dandruff. Ketoconazole was significantly better than selenium sulfide by day 8 of treatment. Irritation and itching were reduced in the treatment groups compared with the placebo group. Selenium sulfide-treated patients experienced more adverse effects [6] *Level P*

Acceptability to patient
Patients may find this therapy acceptable due to the ease of use and accessibility of products. However, patients may be dissatisfied with shampoo odor and the products may become ineffective over time, requiring patients to use several different shampoos over the course of treatment. Many patients benefit from 'rotational therapy' in which they rotate shampoos from application to application or from week to week. A typical regime would be selenium sulfide one week, zinc the next, and so on.

Follow up plan
Patients should be monitored every 2-12 weeks, depending on disease severity and degree of patient sophistication regarding self-treatment.

Patient and caregiver information
- Provide patients (or guardians) with information regarding need to be compliant with shampooing regime, and possible need to change product brands due to ineffectiveness over time
- Provide patients (or guardians) with information about what to do in cases of recurrence

Other therapies
OIL-BASED SCALP TREATMENT
- Pediatric patients with thick scaling can be treated using applications of warm olive or mineral oil, washed off several hours later with detergent (such as dishwashing liquid) and a soft bristle toothbrush, followed by a bland emollient such as petrolatum
- Adult patients with thick scaling can be treated using application of 10% liquor carbonis detergens in a mild oil to the scalp at bedtime, covering the head with a shower cap, and then shampooing with detergent (such as dishwashing liquid) in the morning. This procedure should be performed nightly for 1-3 weeks
- Adult patients may also use fluocinolone applied over the entire dampened scalp and occluded with a shower cap. This treatment is repeated each night for 1-3 weeks until itching and erythema are controlled

Efficacy
Thick scales can be removed easily following oil application, especially when a brush or rough cloth is used to scrub the scalp.

Risks/benefits
Benefit: removes unsightly scaling from scalp, allowing for exposure of unaffected skin.

Acceptability to patient
Patients may find the process distasteful due to the overnight aspect of treatment and the need to shampoo with dishwashing liquid.

Follow up plan
Patients should be monitored every 2-12 weeks, depending on disease severity and degree of patient sophistication regarding self-treatment.

Patient and caregiver information
Provide patients (or guardians) with information regarding need to be compliant with treatment regime.

LIQUOR CARBONIS DETERGENS
Efficacy
Thick scales can be removed easily following oil application, especially when a brush or rough cloth is used to scrub the scalp.

Risks/benefits
Benefit: removes unsightly scaling from scalp, allowing for exposure of unaffected skin.

Acceptability to patient
Patients may find the process distasteful due to the overnight aspect of treatment and the need to shampoo with dishwashing liquid. Some also find the smell objectionable.

Follow up plan
Patients should be monitored every 2-12 weeks, depending on disease severity and degree of patient sophistication regarding self-treatment.

Patient and caregiver information
Provide patients (or guardians) with information regarding need to be compliant with treatment regime.

LIFESTYLE

■ Increased frequency of shampooing may be beneficial
■ Sunlight in moderate doses may also be helpful

RISKS/BENEFITS
Benefits:
■ Scalp cleanliness may reduce erythema and itching
■ Sunlight may aid in reducing skin discomfort

ACCEPTABILITY TO PATIENT
Highly acceptable, unless patient has mobility difficulty that would make frequent shampooing problematic.

PATIENT AND CAREGIVER INFORMATION
Caution patient regarding overexposure to sunlight without skin protection.

EFFICACY OF THERAPIES

- In infants, seborrheic dermatitis usually remits after 6-8 months; with treatment the patient should have resolution within days
- Even in adults undergoing treatment, seborrheic dermatitis is a chronic condition that has cycles of relapse and remission, lasting for months or years
- Judgments regarding efficacy should be made on a clinical basis. Most patients respond quickly to treatment; however, efficacy can be variable within patient populations

Evidence

- Seborrheic dermatitis of the scalp has been effectively treated and prevented with 2% ketoconazole shampoo [2,3] *Level P*
- Use of 2% ketoconazole cream has proven effective in treating seborrheic dermatitis of the face, scalp, and trunk [4] *Level P*
- Hydrocortisone and ketoconazole may effectively treat seborrheic dermatitis lesions. Ketoconazole is superior in the eradication of *Pityrosporum ovale* yeasts [5] *Level P*
- Selenium sulfide shampoo may be beneficial in the management of dandruff, but is not as effective or as well-tolerated as ketaconazole [6] *Level P*
- The therapies not supported by clinical trial data are recommended based on consensus of opinion of experts in the area

Review period

- Consider review of treatment strategies 3-4 weeks into the treatment regime
- There should be a gradual decline in symptoms, scale production, and erythema during this period

PROGNOSIS

- In infants, seborrheic dermatitis usually remits after 6-8 months
- Adult seborrheic dermatitis is a chronic condition, with exacerbations and remissions. Control of symptoms is usually easily performed using shampoos and topical steroids

Clinical pearls

- Seborrheic dermatitis is likely to remit in child patients and likely to be chronically relapsing in adults
- While seborrheic dermatitis can occasionally be severe and extensive, such cases are very rare
- Psychosocial functioning may be impaired to a greater extent than may be immediately apparent. Attention to this aspect of patient care should be paid

Therapeutic failure

- If atypical or resistant cases of scalp scaling occur, fungal cultures and potassium hydroxide examination are indicated to further define the condition
- Biopsy to exclude Langerhans cell histiocytosis should be considered in refractory cases

Recurrence

In adults, the chronic nature of seborrheic dermatitis indicates that exacerbations will occur, and should be treated with the drugs and over-the-counter preparations used at the original diagnosis.

Deterioration

- In cases of pediatric seborrheic dermatitis, if nonmedicated shampoo is ineffective, may use coal tar shampoo or ketoconazole shampoo
- In both pediatric and adult cases of seborrheic dermatitis, worsening of the condition while under treatment may indicate the need for referral to a dermatologist or rheumatologist for further investigation into the nature of the disease

COMPLICATIONS

- Secondary infections may occur with flare-ups; a short course of treatment with antibiotics may be needed
- Skin atrophy/striae or glaucoma are possible from long-term use of fluoroninated corticosteroids on the face or around the eyes
- Photosensitivity can occur when tar-based shampoos are used
- Herpes keratitis, a rare complication of herpes simplex, may occur if steroids are used around the eyes

CONSIDER CONSULT

- In both pediatric and adult cases of seborrheic dermatitis, worsening of the condition while under treatment may indicate the need for referral to a dermatologist for further investigation into the nature of the disease

PREVENTION

Techniques for prevention of seborrheic dermatitis are not currently known.

MODIFY RISK FACTORS
SCREENING

Screening for detection of seborrheic dermatitis is not indicated due to the common and chronic nature of this dermatologic condition.

PREVENT RECURRENCE

Methods for prevention of recurrence are not known, but modification of some correlated risk factors may reduce rate of recurrence.

Reassess coexisting disease

INTERACTION ALERT
- Disease flare-ups appear to parallel use of some acnegenic or antiacne drugs
- Changes in drug regimes may reduce potential for flares

PATIENT SATISFACTION/LIFESTYLE PRIORITIES
- Emotional stress appears to parallel disease flare-ups
- Attempts to reduce emotional stress may reduce frequency of recurrence

ASSOCIATIONS

American Skin Association
346 Park Avenue South, 4th Floor
New York, NY 10010
Tel: (212) 889-4858
Fax: (212) 889-4959
http://www.skinassn.org

American Academy of Dermatology
930 N Meacham Road
PO Box 4014
Schaumburg, IL 60168-4014
Tel: (847) 330-0230
Fax: (847) 330-0050
http://www.aad.org

KEY REFERENCES

- Robson KJ, Piette WW. Cutaneous manifestations of systemic diseases. Med Clin North Am 1998;82:1359-1379
- Friedman SJ, Shellow WVR. Management of seborrheic dermatitis. In: Goroll AH, May LA, Mulley AG Jr, eds. Primary care medicine, 3rd edn. Philadelphia: Lippincott, 1995, p909-910
- Habif TP. Clinical dermatology, 3rd edn. St. Louis, MO: Mosby, 1996, p214-218
- Berger R, Gilchrest BA. Skin disorders. In: Duthie EH Jr, Katz PR, eds. Practice of geriatrics, 3rd edn. Philadelphia: WB Saunders, 1998, chapter 43
- Rico MJ, Myers SA, Sanchez MR. The Guidelines/Outcomes Committee. Guidelines of care for dermatologic conditions in patients infected with HIV. J Am Acad Dermatol 1997;37:450-72
- Faergemann J. Treatment of seborrhoeic dermatitis of the scalp with ketoconazole shampoo. A double-blind study. Acta Derm Venereol 1990;70:171-172
- Peter RU, Richarz-Barthauer U. Successful treatment and prophylaxis of scalp seborrhoeic dermatitis and dandruff with 2% ketoconazole shampoo: results of a multicentre, double-blind, placebo-controlled trial. Br J Dermatol 1995;132:441-445
- Green CA, Farr PM, Shuster S. Treatment of seborrhoeic dermatitis with ketoconazole: II. Response of seborrhoeic dermatitis of the face, scalp and trunk to topical ketoconazole. Br J Dermatol 1987;116:217-221
- Katsambas A, Antoniou C, Frangoili E, et al. A double-blind trial of treatment of seborrheic dermatitis with 2% ketoconazole cream compared with 1% hydrocortisone cream. Br J Dermatol 1989;121:353-357
- Taieb A, Legrain V, Palmier C, et al. Topical ketoconazole for infantile seborrhoeic dermatitis. Dermatologica 1990;181:26-32
- Ferrera PC, Dupree ML, Verdile VP. Dermatologic problems encountered in the emergency department. Am J Emerg Med 1996;14:588-601

Evidence references and guidelines

1 The American Academy of Family Physicians has published treatment information. Johnson B, Nunley JR. Treatment of seborrheic dermatitis. American Family Physician, 2000.
2 Faergemann J. Treatment of seborrhoeic dermatitis of the scalp with ketoconazole shampoo. A double-blind study. Acta Derm Venereol 1990;70:171-172. Medline
3 Peter RU, Richarz-Barthauer U. Sucessful treatment and prophylaxis of scalp seborrhoeic dermatitis and dandruff with 2% ketoconazole shampoo: results of a multicentre, double-blind, placebo-controlled trial. Br J Dermatol 1995;132:441-445. Medline
4 Green CA, Farr PM, Shuster S. Treatment of seborrhoeic dermatitis with ketoconazole: II. Response of seborrhoeic dermatitis of the face, scalp and trunk to topical ketoconazole. Br J Dermatol 1987;116:217-21. Medline
5 Katsambas A, Antoniou C, Frangoili E, et al. A double-blind trial of treatment of seborrhoeic dermatitis with 2% ketoconazole cream compared with 1% hydrocortisone cream. Br J Dermatol 1989;121:353-357. Medline
6 Danby FW, Maddin WS, Margesson LJ, Rosenthal D. A randomized, double-blind, placebo-controlled trial of ketoconazole 2% shampoo versus selenium sulfide 2.5% shampoo in the treatment of moderate to severe dandruff. J Am Acad Dermatol 1993;29:1008-1012. Medline

FAQS

Question 1

Is it ever appropriate to use topical steroids when treating infants?

ANSWER 1

Yes; however, the threshold needs to be higher due to increased tendency to cutaneous atrophy, suppression of the hypothalamic-pituitary-adrenal axis (due to increased absorption and increased surface area to body volume). Attempts to minimize these risks through limiting the duration of use and the percent of the body treated are required.

Question 2

Is the scalp always involved?

ANSWER 2

While the scalp and face are most commonly affected, many adults may have chest involvement only.

Question 3

My patient's condition improved with an over-the-counter shampoo for a few months, then recurred and was unresponsive. What's the next step?

ANSWER 3

Try rotational shampoo therapy. Rotate between two or more types of shampoos (i.e. tar, selenium, zinc-based or ketoconazole shampoos) with each application or weekly.

Question 4

Given the role of *Pityrosporum ovale*, is this condition contagious?

ANSWER 4

The organism is ubiquitous. Attempts to quarantine or permanently eradicate the organism will not be productive.

Question 5

My patient with seborrheic dermatitis has developed nail deformities. Are they related?

ANSWER 5

Nail defects are not seen in seborrheic dermatitis. The possibility of coexistent disease or rethinking the diagnosis should be considered. Conditions that more typically can involve the scalp (with or without other sites of skin involvement) include dermatophyte infection, psoriasis, lichen planus with lichen planopilaris.

CONTRIBUTORS

Gordon H Baustian, MD
Seth R Stevens, MD
Richard Averitte, MD

ERYTHEMA MULTIFORME

DESCRIPTION

- Target lesions caused by the centrifugal spread of red maculopapules with a purpuric, vesicular, or papular center
- Target lesions are symmetric
- 1–3cm in diameter
- Present mainly on hands, feet, extensor surface of forearms and legs
- Urticarial papules, vesical, and bullae in severe disease

URGENT ACTION

Hospital admission in cases of Stevens-Johnson syndrome.

KEY! DON'T MISS!

The underlying cause, especially herpes simplex virus infection, should be determined because treatment is needed.

ICD9 CODE
695.1 Erythema multiforme

SYNONYMS
EM

CARDINAL FEATURES
- Target lesions caused by the centrifugal spread of red maculopapules with a purpuric, vesicular, or papular center
- Symmetric lesions
- 1–3cm in diameter
- Mainly on hands, feet, and extensor surface of forearms and legs
- In severe form, can be on the trunk and in the oral cavity
- Urticarial papules, vesical, and bullae in severe disease
- Individual lesions heal without scarring in 1–2 weeks
- Stevens-Johnson syndrome is a severe bullous form with fever, pneumonitis, renal failure, eye ulcers, and lesions occurring in the mouth and genital area

CAUSES
Common causes
- Immune complex formation and subsequent deposition in microvasculature may play a role in the pathogenesis of erythema multiforme
- The majority of cases follow outbreaks of herpes simplex virus infection
- Other causative agents include drugs (barbiturates, sulfonamides), infections (mycoplasma), and collagen diseases
- In >50% of patients, no specific cause is identified

Rare causes
Orf.

Serious causes
Causes of Stevens-Johnson syndrome include:
- Drugs (barbiturates, sulfonamides, penicillins, phenytoin)
- Infections (mycoplasma, herpes simplex)

Contributory or predisposing factors
Connective tissue diseases.

EPIDEMIOLOGY
Incidence and prevalence
Erythema multiforme is rare.

Demographics
AGE
Predominant age: 20–40 years.

GENDER
Males and females are equally affected.

DIAGNOSIS

DIFFERENTIAL DIAGNOSIS
Contact dermatitis
Contact dermatitis is an inflammation of the skin caused by irritant chemicals in the environment.

FEATURES
- Dry, erythematous, fissured skin
- Vesicles and blisters can be present in severe forms
- Asymmetric lesion pattern, depending on exposure site
- History of exposure to irritant chemical

Chronic urticaria
Urticaria is a pruritic rash involving the epidermis with hives that occur on contact with an allergen.

FEATURES
- Raised red and white plaques that change in size and shape with time
- Annular configuration with central pallor
- History of allergen exposure

Secondary syphilis
Distinguishing features of manifestations of secondary syphilis are as follows:

FEATURES
- Maculopapular lesions on palms and soles
- Mucocutaneous lesions on skin
- Generalized lymphadenopathy
- Mucous patch lesion on oral and genital mucosa

Pityriasis rosea
Pityriasis rosea is a common, self-limiting skin eruption of unknown origin.

FEATURES
- Initial lesion is the 'herald' patch
- 5mm pink oval lesions over trunk
- Symmetric distribution
- Most patients are asymptomatic

Pemphigus vulgaris
Pemphigus vulgaris is an intraepidermal, blistering skin disorder characterized by the formation of flaccid blisters.

FEATURES
- Oral mucosal lesions tend to form first
- Generalized bullous eruption within a few months
- Lesions are fragile and rupture easily, leaving denuded painful lesions
- Not pruritic

SIGNS & SYMPTOMS
Signs
- Target lesions caused by the centrifugal spread of red maculopapules with a purpuric, vesicular, or papular center

- Symmetric lesions
- 1–3cm in diameter
- Mainly on hands, feet, and extensor surface of forearms and legs
- In severe form, can be on the trunk and in the oral cavity
- Urticarial papules, vesical, and bullae in severe disease
- Individual lesions heal without scarring in 1–2 weeks
- A severe bullous form can occur (Stevens-Johnson syndrome) with fever, pneumonitis, renal failure, eye ulcers, and lesions occurring in the mouth and genital area
- There may be signs due to the underlying cause of erythema multiforme

Symptoms

- Lesions are generally symptom-free
- Stevens-Johnson syndrome can cause fever, and lesions in the mouth, genital area, and eye may be painful

KEY! DON'T MISS!

The underlying cause, especially herpes simplex virus infection, should be determined because treatment is needed.

INVESTIGATION OF THE PATIENT
Direct questions to patient

Q For how long have you had the lesions? Erythema multiforme is acute in onset.

Q Where are the lesions? Normally the lesions are present on the hands, feet, legs, and forearms.

Q Are the lesions irritative? Erythema multiforme is normally symptom-free.

Q Do you have any lesions in the mouth, genital areas, or eyes? Suggestive of Stevens-Johnson syndrome.

Contributory or predisposing factors

Q Have you recently had an infection? Erythema multiforme is associated with herpes simplex virus and mycoplasmal infections.

Q Are you taking any medication? Erythema multiforme is associated with barbiturates, penicillins, sulfonamides, and phenytoin.

Examination

- Check whether lesions are of the 'target' appearance. Erythema multiforme lesions are classic in appearance
- Check whether there are lesions on the hands, feet, legs, and forearms. These are the usual sites of lesions
- Check whether mucosal surfaces are involved. Stevens-Johnson syndrome involves two or more mucosal surfaces (including the oral cavity, the genital area, and the eyes)
- Check for systemic features. Stevens-Johnson syndrome includes clinical features of fever, renal failure, and pneumonitis

Summary of investigative tests

- White blood cell count to exclude infection
- Antinuclear antibodies to exclude connective tissue disease
- Viral culture for herpes simplex virus
- Chest X-ray for pneumonitis in Stevens-Johnson syndrome
- Skin biopsy when diagnosis is unclear

DIAGNOSTIC DECISION
Primarily, the diagnosis is based upon morphology of lesions (i.e. the 'target' appearance) coupled with history. Ultimately, the diagnosis is confirmed with characteristic histology observed with routine hematoxylin and eosin staining of a skin biopsy.

CLINICAL PEARLS
Severe itching suggests urticaria.

THE TESTS
Body fluids
WHITE BLOOD CELL COUNT
Description
Venous blood sample.

Advantages/Disadvantages
Advantages:
- Quick and reliable
- Readily available, inexpensive test

Disadvantage: Nonspecific

Normal
3200–9800 white blood cells/mm^3 (3.2–9.8x10^9/L).

Abnormal
>9800 white blood cells/mm^3 (>9.8x10^9/L).

Cause of abnormal result
Infection and inflammation.

Drugs, disorders and other factors that may alter results
- Corticosteroids
- Immunocompromise
- Disease states or drugs that alter systemic immunity may result in expression of an atypical inflammatory response or inability to mount a response. Hence alteration of test parameters may be encountered by many immune-altering causes. However, laboratory abnormalities are infrequently encountered in erythema multiforme

ANTINUCLEAR ANTIBODIES
Description
Venous blood sample.

Advantages/Disadvantages
Advantages:
- Quick and reliable
- Readily available, inexpensive test

Normal
<1:20 titer.

Abnormal
>1:20 titer.

Cause of abnormal result
- Connective tissue disease
- Tuberculosis
- Disease states or drugs that alter systemic immunity may result in expression of an atypical inflammatory response or inability to mount a response. Hence alteration of test parameters may be encountered by many immune-altering causes. However, laboratory abnormalities are infrequently encountered in erythema multiforme

Drugs, disorders and other factors that may alter results
Drugs such as phenytoin, methyldopa, penicillin, and thiazides.

VIRAL CULTURE
Description
Culture fluid from vesicle.

Advantages/Disadvantages
Advantage: gold standard
Disadvantage: takes up to 72h for positive result

Normal
Negative.

Abnormal
Positive culture.

Cause of abnormal result
Herpes simplex virus infection. Any cells infected with viral genome will demonstrate histology with viral changes.

Drugs, disorders and other factors that may alter results
The viral culture is more likely to be positive with more viral load (early vesicular lesions or first episode of herpes simplex).

Biopsy
SKIN BIOPSY
Description
- A biopsy of the skin lesion
- Reserved for situations in which the diagnosis is in doubt or the lesions are not classic in appearance

Advantages/Disadvantages
Disadvantage: can lead to scarring at site of biopsy.

Normal
Normal skin architecture.

Abnormal
Vasculitis, hemorrhage, and inflammation in the epidermis and dermis.

Cause of abnormal result
Erythema multiforme. In this case an 'abnormal result' is a positive finding, which assists in the diagnosis of erythema multiforme. The etiology of the abnormal histology is not clear; however, it is due to a cell-mediated immune reaction against keratinocytes.

Imaging
CHEST X-RAY
Advantages/Disadvantages
Advantage: quick, relatively inexpensive, and readily available
Disadvantage: equivalent to one year of background radiation

Normal
Clear lung fields.

Abnormal
Patchy changes in the lung fields.

Cause of abnormal result
Pneumonitis in Stevens-Johnson syndrome.

CONSIDER CONSULT

- Patients should be referred if the severe form of erythema multiforme – Stevens-Johnson syndrome – is diagnosed

PATIENT AND CAREGIVER ISSUES
Patient or caregiver request

- Patients may be worried about adverse effects of corticosteroids. Therefore if corticosteroids are to be used, the patient needs to be reassured that these drugs will be required for short-term treatment only
- Patients need to be reassured that lesions are not infective and will usually resolve spontaneously

Health-seeking behavior

Patients may need to be advised of medications that can cause erythema multiforme, including penicillins, phenytoin, barbiturates, and sulfonamides.

MANAGEMENT ISSUES
Goals

- Remove or treat causal agent
- Mild cases do not need treatment, just reassurance
- Careful skin nursing, especially in Stevens-Johnson syndrome

Management in special circumstances

Patients with Stevens-Johnson syndrome should be referred to hospital for specialist nursing.

SUMMARY OF THERAPEUTIC OPTIONS
Choices

Prednisolone can be used to treat patients with many target lesions. However, controversy exists about the decision to use corticosteroids in the treatment of erythema multiforme. Treatment decisions about erythema multiforme should be referred to a dermatologist.

Clinical pearls

Corticosteroids for erythema multiforme minor may be useful. Their use in Stevens-Johnson syndrome is controversial. Proponents tend to argue for their use only early in the course of the disease (first 24–48h) for a short course (a few days). Opponents of corticosteroid use present data showing increased risk of death from infectious complications.

FOLLOW UP
Plan for review

The patient should be reviewed weekly to check that lesions are resolving.

Information for patient or caregiver

The patient should be reassured that the lesions:
- Will resolve spontaneously
- Will not scar
- Are not infectious
- Are not malignant

DRUGS AND OTHER THERAPIES: DETAILS
Drugs
PREDNISOLONE

Corticosteroid. Controversy exists about the decision to use corticosteroids in the treatment of erythema multiforme. Treatment decisions about erythema multiforme should be referred to a dermatologist.

Dose
Adult oral dose: 40–80mg/day for up to 3 weeks.

Efficacy
The role of systemic corticosteroids is controversial for the use of Stevens-Johnson syndrome.

Risks/benefits
Risks:
- Overwhelming septicemia if patient has an infection
- Loss of control of blood glucose in those with diabetes
- Prolonged use causes adrenal suppression
- Use caution in elderly due to risk of diabetes and osteoporosis
- Use caution in patients with psychosis, seizure disorders, or myasthenia gravis
- Use caution in congestive heart failure, hypertension, ulcerative colitis, peptic ulcer, or esophagitis

Side effects and adverse reactions
- Side effects are minimized by short duration of therapy
- Cardiovascular system: hypertension, thromboembolism
- Central nervous system: insomnia, euphoria, depression, psychosis
- Endocrine: adrenal suppression, impaired glucose tolerance, growth suppression in children
- Eyes, ears, nose, and throat: cataract, glaucoma, blurred vision
- Gastrointestinal: dyspepsia, peptic ulceration, esophagitis, oral candidiasis
- Musculoskeletal: proximal myopathy, osteoporosis
- Skin: delayed healing, acne, striae

Interactions (other drugs)
- Aminoglutethimide ■ Barbiturates ■ Cholestyramine ■ Clarithromycin, erythromycin
- Colestipol ■ Isoniazid ■ Ketoconazole ■ Nonsteroidal anti-inflammatory drugs (NSAIDs)
- Oral contraceptives ■ Rifampin ■ Salicylates ■ Troleandomycin

Contraindications
- Systemic infection
- Avoid live virus vaccines in those receiving immunosuppressive doses

Acceptability to patient
Generally reasonable, although patients may worry about side effects.

Follow up plan
The patient should be reviewed at least weekly to check that lesions are resolving.

Patient and caregiver information
Short courses of corticosteroids are not associated with the adverse effects that are sometimes reported in the news media.

EFFICACY OF THERAPIES
Treatment efficacy is highly variable. Treating the underlying disorder or discontinuing triggering medications ensures the highest rate of success.

PROGNOSIS
- The rash of erythema multiforme evolves over a 2-week period
- The rash resolves within 3–4 weeks without scarring
- Stevens-Johnson syndrome has up to 10% mortality rate
- Scarring and corneal abnormalities occur in 20% of Stevens-Johnson cases

Clinical pearls
- Skin pain without obvious cause should raise suspicion of evolving severe elements of the spectrum: Stevens-Johnson syndrome or toxic epidermal necrolysis
- If urethral involvement is more than trivial in a male patient, placement of a Foley catheter should be considered to obviate urinary retention/bladder rupture
- Ophthalmology should be involved in eye care to reduce risk of corneal scarring in patients with ocular involvement

Therapeutic failure
Refer to a specialist if the lesions are not resolving or are not responding to prednisolone.

Recurrence
The risk of recurrence of erythema multiforme is high (>30%).

Deterioration
Refer for specialist treatment if the condition deteriorates.

COMPLICATIONS
- Stevens-Johnson syndrome has up to 10% mortality rate
- Scarring and corneal abnormalities occur in 20% of Stevens-Johnson cases

CONSIDER CONSULT
- Refer for specialist treatment if the condition deteriorates

PREVENTION

RISK FACTORS
- **Previous infections:** herpes simplex virus
- **Previous medication use:** barbiturates, phenytoin, penicillins, or sulfonamides
- Although these factors are causes, the probability that they will initiate erythema multiforme is low and difficult to predict

MODIFY RISK FACTORS
Lifestyle and wellness
SEXUAL BEHAVIOR
Use barrier contraception to avoid infection with herpes simplex virus.

DRUG HISTORY
Patients who have a history of erythema multiforme should avoid medications that cause the condition, including:
- Penicillins
- Phenytoin
- Barbiturates
- Sulfonamides

PREVENT RECURRENCE
The risk of recurrence of erythema multiforme exceeds 30%. Recurrence can be prevented by avoiding causal factors, including:
- Penicillins
- Phenytoin
- Barbiturates
- Sulfonamides
- Herpes simplex virus infection

Reassess coexisting disease
Connective tissue disorders need to be monitored because these can lead to recurrences of erythema multiforme.

PATIENT SATISFACTION/LIFESTYLE PRIORITIES
- Patient satisfaction in avoiding the causative agents will be enhanced if the recurrence of erythema multiforme is reduced to the minimum
- The recurrence of this disorder is high, exceeding 30%

KEY REFERENCES

- Revuz J. New advances in severe adverse drug reactions. Dermatol Clin 2001;19(4):697–709
- Eisen ER, Fish J, Shear NH. Management of drug-induced toxic epidermal necrolysis. J Cutan Med Surg 2000;4(2):96–102
- Leaute-Labreze C, Lamireau T, Chawki D, et al. Diagnosis, classification, and management of erythema multiforme and Stevens-Johnson syndrome. Arch Dis Child 2000;83(4):347–52
- Garcia-Doval I, LeCleach L, Bocquet H, et al. Toxic epidermal necrolysis and Stevens-Johnson syndrome: does early withdrawal of causative drugs decrease the risk of death? Arch Dermatol 2000;136(3):323–7
- Burton J. Essentials of dermatology, 3rd edn. New York: Churchill Livingstone, 1990
- Vickers C . Modern management of common skin diseases. New York: Churchill Livingstone, 1986

FAQS
Question 1
How much evaluation should be done for a patient who presents with erythema multiforme if a drug rash is not implicated?

ANSWER 1
Such patients should be evaluated for *Mycoplasma pneumoniae* or herpes simplex infection and treated as indicated. If the erythema multiforme is recurrent, herpes simplex prophylaxis should be considered since there may be subclinical infection that is driving the erythema multiforme.

Question 2
Why is the use of corticosteroids controversial in Stevens-Johnson syndrome?

ANSWER 2
There is little evidence that corticosteroids are beneficial in Stevens-Johnson syndrome, characterized by case series from allergy and pediatric centers, which, when scrutinized, showed that the severity of disease was extremely low (e.g. few patients had any blisters) and that the benefit from corticosteroids was of questionable value (e.g. a few less days of fever). On the other hand, there are several case series of more severely affected patients with significant blistering and erosion in which the rate of sepsis and resultant mortality rate was significantly elevated by concomitant corticosteroids. One should also recognize that a fairly common setting for Stevens-Johnson syndrome is the brain surgery patient who is simultaneously placed on systemic corticosteroids and Dilantin. In these settings, it has been shown that corticosteroids do not prevent (let alone treat) Stevens-Johnson syndrome.

CONTRIBUTORS
Dennis F Saver, MD
Seth R Stevens, MD
Richard Averitte, MD

ERYTHEMA NODOSUM

DESCRIPTION

- Acute onset of tender, red nodules
- Nodules are 1–4 inches (25.4–101.6mm) in diameter
- Nodules occur typically on shins, thighs, and forearms
- Fever, arthralgia, and malaise usually precede the tender nodules

URGENT ACTION

Erythema nodosum can be caused by bacterial infections, including meningococcal and streptococcal infections. These need urgent antibiotic treatment.

KEY! DON'T MISS!

The cause of erythema nodosum must be ascertained to determine if it is serious; causes include:

- Lymphoma
- Ankylosing spondylosis and reactive arthropathies
- Sarcoidosis
- Tuberculosis
- Streptococcal infection
- Meningococcal infection
- Hepatitis B virus
- Cytomegalovirus

BACKGROUND

ICD9 CODE
695.2 Erythema nodosum

CARDINAL FEATURES
- Acute tender, erythematous, nodular skin eruptions
- Fever, arthralgia, and malaise usually precede the tender nodules
- Nodules erupt without ulceration mainly on anterior aspects of legs
- Other sites include the backs of legs, thighs, neck, face, and forearms
- Usually between five and 10 nodules, each up to 4 inches (101.6mm) in diameter
- Nodules may become fluctuant, but they never suppurate
- Slow regression over several weeks to resemble contusions
- The nodules usually disappear within 6 weeks, but they may recur
- Signs of the underlying disease may be present

CAUSES
Common causes
The nodules result from an exaggerated reaction between an antigen and a cell-mediated immune mechanism leading to granuloma formation. Causative agents include:
- Sarcoidosis
- Pregnancy
- Lymphoma
- Ankylosing spondylosis and reactive arthropathies
- Tuberculosis
- Streptococcal infection
- Salmonella enteritis
- *Chlamydia* pneumonia
- *Mycoplasma* pneumonia
- Meningococcal infection
- Gonorrhea
- Syphilis
- Epstein-Barr virus
- Hepatitis B virus
- Cytomegalovirus
- Histoplasmosis
- Drugs (sulfonamides, penicillins, oral contraceptives, aspirin, prazosin)

Rare causes
- *Yersinia* enteritis bacterial infection
- Psittacosis
- Lymphogranuloma venereum
- Tularemia
- Cat-scratch fever
- Coccidioidomycosis
- Blastomycosis
- *Trichophyton verrucosum* infection
- Bromide
- Gold salts

Serious causes
- Lymphoma
- Ankylosing spondylosis and reactive arthropathies

- Tuberculosis
- Streptococcal infection
- Salmonella enteritis
- *Chlamydia* pneumonia
- *Mycoplasma* pneumonia
- Meningococcal infection
- Hepatitis B virus
- Cytomegalovirus

Contributory or predisposing factors

Patients with human leukocyte antigen (HLA) B8 are more likely to have cell-mediated hypersensitivity reactions.

EPIDEMIOLOGY
Incidence and prevalence

Erythema nodosum is a rare disorder.

INCIDENCE
0.02–0.03 cases/1000 patients/year.

Demographics
AGE
Peak age is 25–40 years.

GENDER
The ratio of cases in females to males is 4:1.

GENETICS
The presence of HLA B8 is associated with an increased risk of erythema nodosum.

DIFFERENTIAL DIAGNOSIS
Insect bites
Insect bites are common.

FEATURES
- Usually itchy, mild, and on exposed parts of the body
- Urticarial lesions with a central punctum
- Occur in groups
- Usually regress in 2–3 days

Post-traumatic ecchymosis
Ecchymoses are larger purpuric lesions >0.04 inch (>3mm), and are typical after trauma.

FEATURES
- History of trauma to site of lesion
- Usually resolve within 2 weeks
- Resemble late-stage erythema nodosum nodules
- Lesions can occur anywhere on the body

Erythema multiforme
Erythema multiforme causes 'target' lesions, usually on the limbs, in association with drugs, infections, and collagen disorders.

FEATURES
- Symmetrical target lesions with central blister
- Lesions occur on limbs, soles, and palms
- Stevens-Johnson syndrome may occur: mouth, genital, and eye ulcers with fever

SIGNS & SYMPTOMS
Signs
- Acute, tender, erythematous, nodular skin eruptions
- Fever, arthralgia, and malaise usually precede the tender nodules
- Lymphadenopathy
- Nodules erupt without ulceration, mainly on anterior aspects of legs
- Other sites include the backs of legs, thighs, neck, face, and forearms
- Usually between five and 10 nodules, each up to 4 inches (101.6mm) in diameter
- Nodules may become fluctuant, but they never suppurate
- Nodules slowly regress over several weeks to resemble contusions
- Nodules usually disappear within 6 weeks but may recur
- Signs of the underlying disease may be present

Symptoms
- Acute, tender, red nodules
- Fever, joint pains, and malaise usually precede the tender nodules
- Nodules most commonly occur on the shins
- Other sites include the backs of legs, thighs, neck, face, and forearms

KEY! DON'T MISS!
The cause of erythema nodosum must be ascertained to determine if it is serious; causes include:
- Lymphoma
- Ankylosing spondylosis and reactive arthropathies
- Sarcoidosis

- Tuberculosis
- Streptococcal infection
- Meningococcal infection
- Hepatitis B virus
- Cytomegalovirus

CONSIDER CONSULT

- If the diagnosis is in doubt
- If the underlying cause needs to be determined or evaluated

INVESTIGATION OF THE PATIENT
Direct questions to patient

Q **Are you pregnant?** Erythema nodosum can be associated with pregnancy.

Q **Are you taking medication?** Oral contraceptives, aspirin, prazosin, gold, sulfonamides, bromide, and penicillins can cause erythema nodosum.

Q **Have you any other illnesses?** Sarcoidosis, lymphoma, reactive arthropathies, and ankylosing spondylosis can cause erythema nodosum. Often, nondescript 'viral syndromes' precede erythema nodosum.

Q **Do you have (or have you recently had) an infection?** Certain infections are linked to erythema nodosum.

Q **How long have you had these nodules?** Usually the nodules last only up to 6 weeks.

Contributory or predisposing factors

Do you know whether you or your family carry the human leukocyte antigen (HLA) B8? This antigen is known to exhibit hypersensitive interaction between antigen and the cell-mediated immune mechanism leading to granuloma formation.

Examination

- **Are there tender, red nodules?** These are present in erythema nodosum
- **Are the nodules on the shins?** This is the most likely site
- **Are the nodules up to 4 inches (101.6mm) in diameter with no ulceration?** Indicative of erythema nodosum
- **Are there systemic features, including fever, lymphadenopathy, and arthralgia?** All can be present in erythema nodosum
- **Are there clinical features that are associated with the possible causes of erythema nodosum?** Infections and sarcoidosis can cause erythema nodosum

Summary of investigative tests

Most tests are directed toward finding the underlying cause:

- ESR is raised in infection
- White cell count is raised in infection
- Throat swab and antistreptolysin O titer indicate streptococcal infection
- Chest X-ray looks for sarcoidosis and tuberculosis
- Skin biopsy can provide a definitive diagnosis of the nodules

DIAGNOSTIC DECISION

Diagnosis is based on morphology and histopathology.

CLINICAL PEARLS

- If lesions are ulcerated, consider other diagnoses
- If a biopsy is obtained, a portion should be sent for fungal, bacterial, and mycobacterial culture

THE TESTS
Body fluids
ESR
Description
Venous blood sample.

Advantages/Disadvantages
Advantages:
- Easy, readily available test
- Quick and accurate
- Inexpensive

Disadvantage: Nonspecifically raised when there is inflammation or infection

Normal
- Male: 0–15mm/h
- Female: 0–20mm/h

Abnormal
- Male: >15mm/h
- Female: >20mm/h

Cause of abnormal result
- Infection
- Inflammation
- Erythema nodosum

Drugs, disorders and other factors that may alter results
- Corticosteroids
- Immunocompromise

WHITE CELL COUNT
Description
Venous blood sample.

Advantages/Disadvantages
Advantages:
- Inexpensive
- Quick and reliable

Normal
3200–9800 white cells/mm^3 (3.2–9.8x10^9/L).

Abnormal
>9800 white cells/mm^3 (>9.8x10^9/L).

Cause of abnormal result
Infection and inflammation.

Drugs, disorders and other factors that may alter results
- Corticosteroids
- Immunocompromise

ANTISTREPTOLYSIN O TITER
Description
Venous blood sample.

Advantages/Disadvantages
Advantages:
- Easy to perform
- Quick and accurate

Disadvantages:
- Two samples needed, one each in the acute and convalescent phases of disease
- Not specific for streptococcal infection

Normal
<1600 Todd units (adults).

Abnormal
- >1600 Todd units (adult)
- A 4-fold increase in titer between acute and convalescent specimens is diagnostic of streptococcal infection

Cause of abnormal result
- Streptococcal infection
- Acute rheumatic fever
- Acute glomerulonephritis
- Increased levels of beta-lipoproteins

THROAT SWAB
Description
Swab of the pharyngeal area.

Advantages/Disadvantages
Advantage: Easy to perform

Disadvantage:
- Unpleasant for patient
- Does not distinguish between carrier state and streptococcal infection

Normal
No heavy growth of streptococci.

Abnormal
Culture of streptococcus grown from swab.

Cause of abnormal result
- Streptococcal infection
- Carrier of streptococcal bacteria

Biopsy
SKIN BIOPSY
Description
Removal of a nodule for analysis.

Advantages/Disadvantages
Advantage: provides definitive diagnosis if the nodule is due to erythema nodosum and the sample is adequate (biopsy must include subcutaneous fat).

Abnormal
- Early lesion: inflammation and hemorrhage in subcutaneous tissue
- Late lesion: giant cells and granulomas

Cause of abnormal result
- Erythema nodosum
- Vasculitis due to other causes
- Granuloma diseases

Imaging
CHEST X-RAY
Advantages/Disadvantages
Disadvantage: equivalent to one year background radiation dose.

Abnormal
Shadowing in the lung tissue.

Cause of abnormal result
- Tuberculosis
- Sarcoidosis
- Pneumonia

TREATMENT

CONSIDER CONSULT
- If there are severe nodular lesions
- If the underlying cause requires specialist management

IMMEDIATE ACTION
Erythema nodosum can be caused by bacterial infections, including meningococcal and streptococcal infections. These need urgent antibiotic treatment.

PATIENT AND CAREGIVER ISSUES
Patient or caregiver request
- Patients may be concerned about the side effects of corticosteroids; these concerns will need to be addressed
- Patients may be concerned that the nodules will cause long-term scarring; reassure that the nodules will resolve without scarring
- Patients may want to know the cause of the lesions. Investigations to exclude serious causes may be needed
- Patients may believe the nodules are due to malignancy. These concerns should be addressed, but the patient should wait for diagnosis to be confirmed by skin biopsy. However, any suspicion of lymphoma should be investigated
- Patients should be told that erythema nodosum is a self-limiting disease, especially when a causative agent is diagnosed and treated

Health-seeking behavior
How long have you had the nodules? Patients may take time to present, as they may believe that the nodules are due to bruising from minor trauma.

MANAGEMENT ISSUES
Goals
- To reduce the pain and inflammation of the nodules
- To treat the underlying causative disease
- To prevent further nodules occurring

Management in special circumstances

COEXISTING MEDICATION
Medications that can cause erythema nodosum, and will need to be discontinued include:
- Oral contraceptives
- Aspirin
- Prazosin
- Penicillins
- Gold salts
- Bromide
- Sulfonamides

SPECIAL PATIENT GROUPS
Pregnancy limits the medication available to treat the lesions.

PATIENT SATISFACTION/LIFESTYLE PRIORITIES
Compliance with corticosteroids may be poor, owing to the perceived side effect profile, so careful explanation and monitoring will be needed.

SUMMARY OF THERAPEUTIC OPTIONS
Choices
- Nonsteroidal anti-inflammatory drugs (NSAIDs) for pain (e.g. ibuprofen, naproxen)
- Systemic steroids (e.g. prednisolone) for severe cases of erythema nodosum
- Intralesional triamcinolone may be used; this is a specialist therapy

Clinical pearls
- Because erythema nodosum is usually self-limited, therapy is directed at eliminating underlying cause (if possible) or at short-term amelioration of pain
- Reassurance is usually required, since lesions can be quite painful and dramatic in appearance

FOLLOW UP
Plan for review
- The patient needs to be followed up at weekly intervals if the erythema nodosum is severe and the patient has been put on corticosteroids
- Mild erythema nodosum should be followed up at 2-week intervals to check for resolution of the nodules

Information for patient or caregiver
- The disease is self-limiting and resolves within 8 weeks
- The causative agent may be identified by laboratory tests
- The nodules are not malignant or infectious
- Treatment is to remove the symptoms, except in severe erythema nodosum

DRUGS AND OTHER THERAPIES: DETAILS
Drugs
IBUPROFEN
NSAID with analgesic effect.
Dose
- Adult oral dose: 200–600mg four times daily
- Child oral dose: 20–40mg/kg daily divided in four doses

Efficacy
Highly variable.

Risks/benefits
Risks:
- Use caution in elderly
- Use caution in hepatic, renal, and cardiac failure
- Use caution in bleeding disorders
- May cause severe allergic reactions including hives, facial swelling, asthma, shock

Side effects and adverse reactions
- Cardiovascular system: hypertension, peripheral edema
- Central nervous system: headache, dizziness, tinnitus
- Gastrointestinal: anorexia, nausea, dyspepsia, peptic ulceration, bleeding
- Genitourinary: nephrotoxicity
- Hematologic: blood cell disorders
- Hypersensitivity: rashes, bronchospasm, angioedema

Interactions (other drugs)
- Aminoglycosides
- Anticoagulants
- Antihypertensives
- Baclofen
- Corticosteroids
- Cyclosporine, tacrolimus
- Digoxin
- Diuretics
- Lithium
- Methotrexate
- Phenylpropanolamine
- Warfarin

Contraindications
- Peptic ulceration
- Hypersensitivity to any pain reliever or antipyretic (including NSAIDs)
- Coagulation defects
- Severe renal or hepatic disease

Acceptability to patient
Usually very acceptable. Can cause gastrointestinal upset and peptic acid disease.

Follow up plan
Patient should be seen every few weeks to monitor treatment.

Patient and caregiver information
- Take medication with food
- If gastrointestinal symptoms occur, stop the medication immediately

NAPROXEN
NSAID with analgesic effect.

Dose
- Adult oral dose: 250–500mg twice daily
- Child oral dose: 10mg/kg daily divided into two doses

Efficacy
Highly variable.

Risks/benefits
Risks:
- Risk of gastrointestinal ulceration, bleeding, and perforation
- Use caution with renal impairment
- Use caution with hypertension or cardiac conditions aggravated by fluid retention and edema
- Use caution with history of liver dysfunction
- Use caution with history of coagulation

Side effects and adverse reactions
- Cardiovascular system: congestive heart failure, dysrhythmias, edema, palpitations, dyspnea
- Central nervous system: headache, dizziness, drowsiness, vertigo
- Gastrointestinal: constipation, heartburn, diarrhea, vomiting, nausea, dyspepsia, peptic ulceration, stomatitis
- Genitourinary: acute renal failure
- Hematologic: thrombocytopenia
- Hypersensitivity: rashes, bronchospasm, angioedema
- Skin: pruritus, ecchymoses, sweating, purpura

Interactions (other drugs)
- Aminoglycosides
- Anticoagulants
- Antihypertensives
- Corticosteroids
- Cyclosporine
- Digoxin
- Diuretics
- Lithium
- Methotrexate
- Phenylpropanolamine
- Probenecid
- Triamterene

Contraindications
- Peptic ulceration
- Coagulation defects
- Hypersensitivity to NSAIDs
- Do not use naproxen and naproxen sodium concomitantly

Acceptability to patient
Usually highly acceptable, though gastrointestinal upset can limit tolerability.

Follow up plan
Patient should be seen every few weeks to monitor treatment.

Patient and caregiver information
- Take medication with food
- If gastrointestinal symptoms occur, stop the medication immediately

PREDNISOLONE
- Corticosteroid
- Suppresses cell-mediated hypersensitivity reaction that is causing the nodule formation
- For use in severe erythema nodosum

Dose
- Adult oral dose: 5–60mg/day
- Child oral dose: 0.1–2mg/kg/day

Efficacy
Variable, yet generally good.

Risks/benefits
Risks:
- Overwhelming septicemia if patient has an infection
- Loss of control of blood glucose in those with diabetes
- Prolonged use causes adrenal suppression
- Use caution in elderly due to risk of diabetes and osteoporosis
- Use caution in patients with psychosis, seizure disorders, or myasthenia gravis
- Use caution in congestive heart failure, hypertension
- Use caution in ulcerative colitis, peptic ulcer, or esophagitis

Side effects and adverse reactions
- Side effects are minimized by short duration of therapy
- Cardiovascular system: hypertension, thromboembolism
- Central nervous system: insomnia, euphoria, depression, psychosis
- Endocrine: adrenal suppression, impaired glucose tolerance, growth suppression in children
- Eyes, ears, nose, and throat: cataract, glaucoma, blurred vision
- Gastrointestinal: dyspepsia, peptic ulceration, esophagitis, oral candidiasis
- Musculoskeletal: proximal myopathy, osteoporosis
- Skin: delayed healing, acne, striae

Interactions (other drugs)
- Aminoglutethimide
- Barbiturates
- Cholestyramine
- Clarithromycin, erythromycin
- Colestipol
- Isoniazid
- Ketoconazole
- NSAIDs
- Oral contraceptives
- Rifampin
- Salicylates
- Troleandomycin

Contraindications
- Systemic infection ■ Avoid live virus vaccines in those receiving immunosuppressive doses

Follow up plan
Weekly follow up initially while on this medication to check for compliance and side effects.

Patient and caregiver information
- Patient needs to know the side effect profile of prednisolone
- Seek medical advice if concomitant disease is contracted while on this medication
- Do not stop corticosteroids abruptly; seek medical supervision when reducing the dose

EFFICACY OF THERAPIES

- Erythema nodosum is a self-limiting disease when the underlying causative agent has been removed or treated
- The nodules usually resolve within 8 weeks

PROGNOSIS

- Self-limiting disease when the underlying causative agent has been removed or treated
- The nodules usually resolve within 8 weeks

Therapeutic failure

Referral will be required if the nodules have not resolved within 8 weeks.

Recurrence

Referral will be required if the nodules recur.

Deterioration

Referral will be required if there is deterioration of erythema nodosum.

CONSIDER CONSULT

- For recurrent lesions

PREVENTION

RISK FACTORS

Avoiding the causative agents will prevent erythema nodosum, especially as a recurrence. Such causative agents include:

- Tuberculosis
- Streptococcal infection
- *Salmonella* enteritis
- *Chlamydia* pneumonia
- *Mycoplasma* pneumonia
- Meningococcal infection
- Gonorrhea
- Syphilis
- Epstein-Barr virus
- Hepatitis B virus
- Cytomegalovirus
- Histoplasmosis fungus
- Causative drugs (sulfonamides, penicillins, oral contraceptives, aspirin, prazosin)

MODIFY RISK FACTORS
Lifestyle and wellness
SEXUAL BEHAVIOR

Certain sexually transmitted diseases can cause erythema nodosum, including syphilis and gonorrhea. Barrier contraception will prevent such infections being contracted.

FAMILY HISTORY

The human leukocyte antigen (HLA) B8 is linked to hypersensitivity of the cell-mediated immune system, which can lead to nodule formation in erythema nodosum.

DRUG HISTORY

The following medications can cause erythema nodosum:

- Sulfonamides
- Penicillins
- Oral contraceptives
- Aspirin
- Prazosin

SCREENING

Screening for erythema nodosum is not appropriate.

PREVENT RECURRENCE

Avoiding the causative agents will help to prevent recurrence of erythema nodosum, especially as a recurrence. Such causative agents include:

- Tuberculosis
- Streptococcal infection
- *Salmonella* enteritis
- *Chlamydia* pneumonia
- *Mycoplasma* pneumonia
- Meningococcal infection
- Gonorrhea
- Syphilis
- Epstein-Barr virus
- Hepatitis B virus

- Cytomegalovirus
- Histoplasmosis fungus
- Causative drugs (sulfonamides, penicillins, oral contraceptives, aspirin, prazosin)

RESOURCES

KEY REFERENCES

- Vickers F. Modern management of common skin diseases. New York: Churchill Livingstone, 1986, p126–7
- Fry J, et al. Dermatology. MTP Press, 1985, p173–4
- Burton J. Essentials of dermatology. 3rd edn. New York: Churchill Livingstone, 1990, p200
- Tierney L, et al. Current medical diagnosis and treatment. Appleton and Lange, 1993, p111–2

FAQS
Question 1
My patient with erythema nodosum has lesions that have ulcerated. What should I do?

ANSWER 1
Ulceration of erythema nodosum is rare. Consideration of other entities must be made, particularly infection.

CONTRIBUTORS
Fred F Ferri, MD, FACP
Seth R Stevens, MD
Richard Averitte, MD

FOLLICULITIS

DESCRIPTION

- Inflammation of a hair follicle
- Caused by bacterial and viral infections, chemical irritation, or physical injury
- The scalp, face, legs, and trunk are most often affected
- May be superficial or deep in the hair follicle
- Responds to antiseptic washes, warm compresses, and topical antibiotics. Moderate and severe cases may require systemic antibiotic treatment

URGENT ACTION

Appropriate antibiotic therapy is required for patients who are immunosuppressed or have severe involvement.

KEY! DON'T MISS!

Interfollicular pustules in a sick (particularly immunocompromised) patient may appear to be a folliculitis, but may be a sign of septicemia.

ICD9 code

704.8 Other specified diseases of hair and hair follicles.

SYNONYMS

- Sycosis
- Sycosis barbae for deep folliculitis in a bearded area
- Bockart's impetigo for superficial folliculitis

CARDINAL FEATURES

- Inflammation of a hair follicle caused by bacterial and viral infections, chemical irritation, or physical injury
- The most common form of infectious folliculitis is staphylococcal folliculitis, occurring most commonly in diabetics
- Lesions generally consist of painful pustules surrounded by erythema with a central hair present
- Usually there is no fever or other systemic symptoms
- The scalp, face, legs, and trunk are most often affected
- May be superficial or deep in the hair follicle
- Pseudofolliculitis barbae is a condition typically presenting in African-American men, and which is located in the bearded areas secondary to shaving, ingrown hairs, and subsequent inflammation
- Usually responds to antiseptic washes, warm compresses, and topical antibiotics
- Moderate to severe cases require systemic antibiotic treatment

Subtypes of folliculitis include:
- Staphylococcal folliculitis
- Pseudomonas folliculitis
- Herpetic folliculitis
- Irritant folliculitis
- Molluscum contagiosum folliculitis
- Dermatophytic folliculitis
- Syphilitic folliculitis

CAUSES

Common causes

- Physical injury to the skin, which can lead to the introduction of bacteria
- Systemic corticosteroid therapy causing a steroid folliculitis
- Staphylococcus infection (superficial folliculitis, sycosis barbae)
- Gram-negative folliculitis (organisms include *Enterobacter*, *Proteus*, and *Klebsiella*) is seen with antibiotic use for the treatment of acne
- *Pseudomonas aeruginosa* in 'hot tub' folliculitis
- Irritant folliculitis is caused by chemical agents, e.g. tar, oil, cutting oils
- Folliculitis can be caused by syphilis
- Herpes is a serious cause of folliculitis leading to vesicles and pustules
- Molluscum contaginosum can lead to a folliculitis
- Fungal infections can cause dermatophytic dermatitis

Rare causes

Eosinophilic folliculitis in HIV positive patients.

Serious causes
- Folliculitis can be caused by syphilis
- Herpes is a serious cause of folliculitis
- Staphylococcus infection (superficial folliculitis, sycosis barbae) can lead to an extensive folliculitis

Contributory or predisposing factors
- Poor hygiene, obesity, perspiration, friction, and occlusion are contributing factors to folliculitis
- Systemic steroids used for the treatment of acne can give rise to steroid folliculitis
- AIDS patients are susceptible to eosinophilic folliculitis, which is extremely pruritic and typically presents on the trunk
- Diabetes mellitus is a risk factor for folliculitis
- Accutane treatment for acne predisposes the patient to staphylococcal folliculitis

EPIDEMIOLOGY
Demographics
AGE
All ages can be affected although it is most common during the postpubertal years.

GEOGRAPHY
Hot, humid, climates predispose to folliculitis.

DIFFERENTIAL DIAGNOSIS
Miliaria rubra
FEATURES

- Associated with sweat retention
- Vesicles and papules appear, with pruritus or prickling
- Flexures and areas rubbed by clothing are most affected

Impetigo
The main features of impetigo are as follows.

FEATURES

- Contagious pyoderma due to *Staphylococcus aureus* or group A streptococcus
- Begins as a weepy, scaly red patch that eventuates into a honey-crusted plaque
- Children usually affected on the face

Acne vulgaris
The main features of acne vulgaris are as follows.

FEATURES

- Inflammation of pilosebaceous glands; cause unknown
- Comedones, papules, and cysts form and can result in scarring
- Face, back, and chest mostly affected

Furunculosis
FEATURES

- Painful subcutaneous nodules due to Staphylococcus infection of hair follicles that spreads into the surrounding dermis
- Commonly seen in diabetics

Cellulitis
The main features of cellulitis are as follows.

FEATURES

- Locally tender, warm, edematous inflammation of deep subcutaneous tissue, due to bacterial infection
- Regional lymphadenopathy may be present
- Cellulitis due to staphylococcal infection usually restricted to lower limbs

SIGNS & SYMPTOMS
Signs

- Erythematous papules and perifollicular pustules
- The scalp, face, legs, and trunk are most often affected
- HIV patients may be febrile

Symptoms

- Often asymptomatic
- Itching and burning can occur
- Pustules form in hair follicles and may be pruritic
- Lesions often grouped

ASSOCIATED DISORDERS
- Furunculosis
- Cellulitis

KEY! DON'T MISS!
Interfollicular pustules in a sick (particularly immunocompromised) patient may appear to be a folliculitis, but may be a sign of septicemia.

CONSIDER CONSULT
- Referral is rarely required for correctly diagnosed folliculitis. If the question arises of the relationship of a folliculitis to systemic infection, referral to dermatology and/or infectious disease may be appropriate
- Refer patients who present with nonresponsive disease or those with atypical presentations

INVESTIGATION OF THE PATIENT
Direct questions to patient
Q Are you using oral steroids? Oral steroids can lead to folliculitis.

Q Have you recently been in a hot tub or whirlpool? Bacterial infections can occur leading to pseudomonal folliculitis.

Q Are you using any new cosmetics or creams? Chemicals in cosmetics and creams can be the cause of irritant folliculitis.

Q Do you come in contact with any chemicals or irritants in the workplace? Occupational chemicals can be the cause of irritant folliculitis.

Q Does the affected area itch and cause you to scratch at night? Pruritus is a common symptom of folliculitis.

Q Is the razor that you use to shave new or borrowed? Poor razor hygiene is a cause of pseudofolliculitis barbae.

Q Is the condition confined to one area of the body, or evident elsewhere? Folliculitis normally occurs on hair-bearing skin especially on the face, scalp, legs, and trunk.

Q Have you ever had this condition before? If so, how was it treated? Recurrent folliculitis is common; it can be a chronic condition that waxes and wanes.

Q Have you suffered from herpes, fungal infections, syphilis, or molluscum contagiosum? All these diseases can cause folliculitis.

Q Are you taking any medications? Drug reactions can mimic folliculitis; these include follicular drug eruptions and acute generalized exanthematous pustulosis.

Contributory or predisposing factors
- **Diabetes mellitus** is a common predisposing factor for folliculitis
- **Oral steroids** for the treatment of acne can give rise to steroid folliculitis
- **AIDS patients** are susceptible to eosinophilic folliculitis
- **Poor hygiene, hyperhidrosis, obesity, and friction** are all risk factors for folliculitis
- **Chronic occupational exposure to a chemical agent** can lead to folliculitis

Family history
Q Does any member of the family suffer from folliculitis due to herpes?

Q Are any family members known staphylococcal carriers? Household contacts of a staphylococcal carrier are at increased risk of this type of folliculitis.

Examination
- **Identify the type of lesion** – folliculitis is characterized by papules and pustules affecting hair follicles
- **Observe the anatomical location and distribution over the body** – the scalp, face, legs, and trunk are most often affected in patients with folliculitis

Summary of investigative tests

Diagnosis is normally made by the patient's history and physical examination; investigative tests are generally unnecessary. However, in refractory cases the following investigative tests should be performed:

- Syphilis serologic testing – useful to diagnose syphilitic folliculitis
- Gram staining and culture – may be used to identify the organisms causing the infection and to arrive at appropriate antibiotic therapy
- Fungal culture – useful to diagnose dermatophytic folliculitis
- Punch biopsy of an active lesion
- Potassium hydroxide microscopy – useful to diagnose fungal infections
- Viral cultures – useful to diagnose herpes folliculitis

DIAGNOSTIC DECISION

- Folliculitis is a clinical diagnosis
- Culture may be used to determine the causative organism(s)

The American Academy of Family Physicians has published the following, with information on folliculitis: O'Dell M. Skin and wound infections: An overview. American Family Physician, 1998.

CLINICAL PEARLS

Carefully examine pustules to determine that they are truly follicular in nature; evenly distributed pustules may appear to involve follicles but in fact may be interfollicular.

THE TESTS
Body fluids
SYPHILIS SEROLOGIC TESTING
Description
Blood sample taken for laboratory analysis for venereal disease reaction level.

Advantages/Disadvantages
Advantages:
- Identifies specific causal agent (syphilis)
- Relatively inexpensive test
- Not performed routinely
- Useful for diagnosing refractory cases

Normal
Negative.

Abnormal
Positive.

Drugs, disorders and other factors that may alter results
- Systemic lupus erythematosus
- Infectious mononucleosis
- HIV
- Atypical pneumonia
- Malaria

GRAM STAINING AND CULTURE
Description
- Follicular pustules are cultured using a number 15 blade to scrape off the entire pustule
- The pustule should be placed on a cotton swab of a transport medium kit

- The pustule is cultured for bacterial growth
- If bacteria are grown these are Gram-stained for identification

Advantages/Disadvantages
Advantages:
- Identifies specific causal agent
- Relatively inexpensive test
- Should be performed at initial visit in moderate to severe cases
- Useful for diagnosing refractory cases

Normal
No bacterial growth.

Abnormal
Bacterial growth – Gram-positive organisms.

Cause of abnormal result
- Gram-positive *Staphyloccocal* and *Streptococcal* organisms
- Gram-negative *Enterobacter*, *Proteus*, and *Klebsiella* organisms

Drugs, disorders and other factors that may alter results
Antibiotics.

FUNGAL CULTURE
Description
- Follicular pustules are cultured using a number 15 blade to scrape off the entire pustule
- The pustule should be placed on a cotton swab of a transport medium kit
- The pustule is then cultured for fungal organisms

Advantages/Disadvantages
Advantages:
- Identifies specific causal agent
- Relatively inexpensive test
- Useful for diagnosing refractory cases

Normal
No fungal growth.

Abnormal
Fungal elements cultured.

Cause of abnormal result
Dermatophytic infections including trichophyton and malassezia.

Biopsy
PUNCH BIOPSY OF SKIN LESION
Description
- A 4mm punch biopsy is performed after injection with 2–3cm^3 lidocaine with epinephrine
- Specimen is sent for pathology, and wound is sutured with 4.0 prolene
- Procedure is generally performed by a dermatologist

Advantages/Disadvantages
Advantages:
- Identifies histologic architecture

- Relatively inexpensive test
- Not performed routinely
- Allows direct visualization of the organism when present, or has the ability to visualize with special stains, although speciation may be difficult and antibiotic sensitivities are not revealed
- Useful for diagnosing refractory cases

Normal
Normal skin architecture.

Abnormal
Neutrophilic perifollicular infiltrates.

Cause of abnormal result
Eosinophilic folliculitis of HIV patients.

Drugs, disorders and other factors that may alter results
Antibiotics.

POTASSIUM HYDROXIDE MICROSCOPY
Description
- Follicular pustules are sampled using a number 15 blade to scrape off the entire pustule
- A small fragment from the pustule is then placed on a microscopic slide using wet mount preparation and potassium hydroxide
- The pustule is then observed using direct microscopy

Advantages/Disadvantages
Advantages:
- Identifies specific causal agent (dermatophytes)
- Relatively inexpensive test
- Not performed routinely
- Useful for diagnosing refractory cases

Normal
No dermatophyte visualized.

Abnormal
- Dermatophytes appear as translucent branching filaments (hyphae)
- Lines of separation appear at irregular intervals

Cause of abnormal result
Dermatophytic infections including trichophyton and malassezia.

VIRAL CULTURE FOR HERPES SIMPLEX
Description
- The pustules should be sampled during the early ulcerative stage with a swab
- The swab is cultured for viral growth

Advantages/Disadvantages
Advantages:
- Most definitive method for identifying herpes agent
- Relatively inexpensive test
- Not performed routinely
- Takes 1–2 days
- Useful for diagnosing refractory cases

Normal
No growth.

Abnormal
Viral growth.

TREATMENT

CONSIDER CONSULT
- Refer cases refractory to topical and oral antibiotics.

IMMEDIATE ACTION
Immunocompromised patients with an infectious etiology of the folliculitis require immediate treatment.

PATIENT AND CAREGIVER ISSUES
Health-seeking behavior
Does the patient remove his or her bathing suit immediately after swimming? Patients should take off wet or moist bathing suits immediately after use, and keep affected areas clean, dry, and cool.

MANAGEMENT ISSUES
Goals
- Eliminate the presenting infection
- Provide good patient education to prevent recurrence
- Prevent chemical irritants causing skin folliculitis

Management in special circumstances
COEXISTING DISEASE
- Patients with diabetes are more susceptible to delayed healing and possibly worsening of folliculitis
- It is important that the person with diabetes is under good glycemic control to reduce the chance of the infection becoming systemic
- Patients with HIV and those who are immunocompromised are susceptible to eosinophilic folliculitis

COEXISTING MEDICATION
- Accutane predisposes to staphylococcal infection of the face
- Oral steroid therapy predisposes to pustules on the face and back

PATIENT SATISFACTION/LIFESTYLE PRIORITIES
- Skin infections, especially facial, can lead to embarrassment
- Patients need a rapid and permanent resolution
- Patients need to understand how to avoid future occurrences by improving personal hygiene
- Close contact with an infected person can result in transmission of disease

SUMMARY OF THERAPEUTIC OPTIONS
Choices
- The first treatment is to prevent recurrence by eliminating the chemical or mechanical skin irritant
- Topical application of 2% mupirocin ointment can be used
- Dicloxacillin can be used to treat moderate to severe cases of *Staphylococcus aureus* folliculitis along with topical mupirocin
- Ciprofloxacin can be used in severe cases of pseudomonas folliculitis
- Syphilic folliculitis should be treated with penicillin
- Herpetic folliculitis can be treated with acyclovir

The American Academy of Family Physicians has published the following, with information on folliculitis: O'Dell M. Skin and wound infections: An overview. American Family Physician, 1998.

Never
Never use steroids to treat folliculitis.

FOLLOW UP
The patient will require follow up as folliculitis can become chronic.

Plan for review
A 6-week follow up appointment should be scheduled.

Information for patient or caregiver
Patients should be educated to:
- Use good personal hygiene
- Avoid sharing razors, towels, and washcloths

DRUGS AND OTHER THERAPIES: DETAILS
Drugs
MUPIROCIN
- Used topically for folliculitis
- Can be used in conjunction with oral antibiotics for folliculitis

Dose
2% mupirocin ointment applied to affected areas twice daily.

Risks/benefits
Risks:
- Pregnancy category B – should be used during pregnancy only if clearly indicated
- Inactive against *Enterobacteriaceae*, *Pseudomonas aeruginosa*, and fungi

Benefits:
- Easy to use
- Efficacy in mild to moderate disease without adjunctive therapy
- Useful adjunct to oral antibiotics in moderate to severe cases of folliculitis

Side effects and adverse reactions
- Skin: local adverse reactions have been reported, including burning, stinging, pain, itching
- Rarely, rash, nausea, erythema, dry skin, tenderness, swelling, contact dermatitis, and increased exudate (<1%)

Contraindications
- History of sensitivity reactions to any of its components

Acceptability to patient
Usually well tolerated, although some patients will experience hypersensitivity reactions and others will experience GI upset due to alteration of intestinal flora.

Follow up plan
Patients not showing a clinical response in 3–5 weeks should be re-evaluated.

Patient and caregiver information
Medicine should be taken as prescribed. If any side effects occur, the medication should be discontinued and the primary care physician should be contacted.

DICLOXACILLIN
Used for moderate to severe folliculitis.

Dose
250mg four times daily for 10 days.

Risks/benefits
Risks:
- Use caution in patients with a history of gastrointestinal disease eczema or asthma
- Use caution in breast-feeding

Benefit: Can be used with a topical agent, e.g. mupirocin

Side effects and adverse reactions
- Central nervous system: seizures, anxiety, lethargy
- Gastrointestinal: nausea, vomiting, diarrhea, pseudomembraneous colitis, abdominal discomfort, gastrointestinal bleeding, elevated hepatic enzymes
- Hematologic: thrombocytopenia, leukopenia, neutropenia
- Skin: purpura, rashes, vasculitis, exfoliative dermatitis, maculopapular rash, Stevens-Johnson syndrome

Interactions (other drugs)
- Aminoglycosides
- Chloramphenicol
- Macrolide antibiotics
- Methotrexate
- Oral contraceptives
- Probenecid
- Tetracycline antibiotics
- Warfarin

Contraindications
- Hypersensitivity to cephalosporins

Follow up plan
Patients should be reviewed within 6 weeks.

Patient and caregiver information
Should be taken with water on an empty stomach – one hour before or 2h after meals.

CIPROFLOXACIN
Active against pseudomonal folliculitis.

Dose
500mg orally twice daily for 7–10 days.

Risks/benefits
Risks:
- Not suitable for children or growing adolescents
- Caution in adolescents, during pregnancy, epilepsy, G6PD deficiency
- Use with caution in renal disease

Benefits:
- Active against pseudomonal folliculitis
- The safety and effectiveness of ciprofloxacin in pediatric patients and adolescents, pregnant women, and lactating women has not been established

Side effects and adverse reactions
- Central nervous system: anxiety, depression, dizziness, headache, seizures
- Eyes, ears, nose, and throat: visual disturbances
- Gastrointestinal: abdominal pain, altered liver function, anorexia, diarrhea, heartburn, vomiting
- Skin: photosensitivity, pruritus, rash

Interactions (other drugs)
- Antacids ■ Beta-blockers ■ Cyclosporine ■ Caffeine ■ Didanosine ■ Diazepam
- Mineral supplements (zinc, magnesium, calcium, aluminium, iron) ■ NSAIDs ■ Opiates
- Oral anticoagulants ■ Phenytoin ■ Theophylline ■ Warfarin

Contraindications
- Use is not recommended in children because arthropathy has developed in weightbearing joints of young animals ■ Pregnancy category B: compatible with breastfeeding

Follow up plan
Patients not showing a clinical response within 7–10 days should be re-evaluated.

Patient and caregiver information
- Patients taking other medications that may interact with ciproploxacin should be made aware of possible reactions
- Medicine should be taken as prescribed. If any side effects occur, the medication should be discontinued and the primary care physician should be contacted

PENICILLIN
- Used for folliculitis caused by syphilis
- Three doses, one week apart, is required
- Given as an intramuscular injection

Dose
Adult: 2.4 millionU intramuscularly as one treatment weekly for three weeks.

Efficacy
Effective in the treatment of syphilis.

Risks/benefits
Risks:
- Use with caution in patients allergic to cephalosporins
- Use with caution in patients with severe renal failure

Benefit: Effective against primary, secondary, and latent syphilis

Side effects and adverse reactions
- Central nervous system : seizures, depression, anxiety, fever
- Gastrointestinal: diarrhea, nausea, vomiting, abdominal pain, antibiotic-associated colitis
- Hematologic: bone marrow suppression, coagulation disorders
- Renal: interstitial nephritis
- Respiratory: anaphylaxis
- Skin: eythema multiforme, rash, urticaria

Interactions (other drugs)
- Chloramphenicol ■ Macrolide antibiotics ■ Methotrexate ■ Oral contraceptives
- Phenindione ■ Probenecid ■ Tetracyclines

Contraindications
- Hypersensitivity to cephalosporins

Acceptability to patient
One dose regimen requiring minimal compliance.

ACYCLOVIR
Used for herpetic folliculitis.

Dose
Oral dose: 200mg five times daily for 5 days.

Efficacy
Useful in treating folliculitis where the identified causal agent is the herpes simplex virus.

Risks/benefits
Risks:
- Use with caution in patients with hepatic and renal disease, seizure disorders, or other neurologic disease
- Use with caution in patients with dehydration and electrolyte imbalance
- Use with caution in pregnant women and nursing mothers

Benefits:
- Effective against the herpes virus
- Useful when the causal agent has been identified as the herpes simplex virus

Side effects and adverse reactions
- Central nervous system: headache, coma, confusion, seizures, hallucinations, tremor, dizziness, encephalopathy
- Gastrointestinal: nausea, vomiting, diarrhea, abdominal pain, elevated liver enzymes, hepatitis, anorexia, jaundice
- Genitourinary: crystalluria, renal toxicity
- Hematologic: leukopenia, thrombocytopenia, hemolytic uremic syndrome
- Skin: injection site reaction, phlebitis, alopecia, erythema, rash, pruritus, toxic epidermal necrolysis, Stevens-Johnson syndrome, photosensitivity, urticaria

Interactions (other drugs)
- Mycophenolate ■ Phenytoin, fosphenytoin ■ Probenecid ■ Zidovudine

Contraindications
- Children under 2 years old ■ Hypersensitivity or intolerance to acyclovir

Patient and caregiver information
Carefully wash area to prevent secondary bacterial infection.

OUTCOMES

EFFICACY OF THERAPIES

Severe cases of folliculitis require both topical and systemic treatment.Oral antibiotics and topical bactoban can be used in these patients.

Evidence

PDxMD are unable to cite evidence that meets our criteria for evidence.

Review period

Review required after one month.

PROGNOSIS

- Prognosis is generally good but recurrences do occur
- Recurrence is possible in *Staphylococcus* carriers and it may be necessary to treat family members who are also carriers
- Repeated treatment failure may justify investigation for diabetes mellitus, HIV, or other immunosuppressive conditions

Clinical pearls

- Carefully determine the follicular nature of the patient's problem. Evenly distributed interfollicular papules or pustules may simulate folliculitis
- Pseudofolliculitis barbae, commonly in the beard area of men of African descent, should be considered and treated with alternatives to shaving with razor blades
- Recalcitrant folliculitis should be cultured in the absence of antibiotic therapy

Therapeutic failure

Referral to a dermatologist is indicated if therapy fails.

Recurrence

- Referral to a dermatologist is indicated
- Resistant cases require follow up every 4 weeks until the condition has cleared

COMPLICATIONS

- Furuncule or carbuncle formation
- Scarring of the skin

CONSIDER CONSULT

- Refer if treatment fails

RISK FACTORS
- Diabetes is a risk factor for folliculitis
- Poor personal hygiene
- Sharing shaving materials

MODIFY RISK FACTORS
Lifestyle and wellness
Diabetes control is important in preventing folliculitis in patients with diabetes.

PREVENT RECURRENCE
Patients should be instructed to practice good hygiene and avoid sharing razors, towels, and washcloths. In cases where there is an offending agent in the workplace, avoidance should be stressed.

ASSOCIATIONS
American Academy of Dermatology
930 N Meacham Road
PO Box 4014
Schaumburg, IL 60168-4014
Tel: (847) 330-0230; (888) 462-DERM
Fax: (847) 330-0050
http://www.aad.org

KEY REFERENCES
- National Skin Centre. Available online: www.nsc.gov.sg
- HIV dent. Available online: www.hivdent.org
- Columbia University Health Sciences. Available online: http://cpmcnet.columbia.edu
- Beers MH, Berkow R. The Merck Manual of Diagnosis and Therapy, 17th edn. New Jersey: Merck, 1999, p 620–1
- Habif TP. Clinical Dermatology, 3rd edn. Philadelphia: Mosby, 1996
- Fitzpatrick TB. Color Atlas and Synopsis of Clinical Dermatology. New York: McGraw-Hill, 1983
- Barker LR. Principles of Ambulatory Medicine, 2nd edn. Baltimore: Williams & Wilkins, 1986
- Bates B. A Guide to Physical Examination, 3rd edn. Philadelphia: Lippincott, 1983
- Krup MA. Current Medical Diagnosis and Treatment. Los Altos: Lange Medical Publications, 1986

FAQS
Question 1
What is the difference between folliculitis and acne?

ANSWER 1
Folliculitis is an inflammation of the hair follicle, usually due to infection, although it can also be caused by an irritant. Acne is fundamentally a problem with epithelial differentiation, in which a failure of appropriate differentiation of follicular and perifollicular epithelial differentiation leads to the formation of a comedo that obstructs the outflow of lipids (predominantly sebum). The metabolic breakdown of these lipids by commensal bacteria is irritating and leads to inflammation.

Question 2
A patient has evenly spaced pustules on the skin, but closer inspection reveals that they do not particularly involve follicles. What could this be?

ANSWER 2
Pustules can arise for a variety of reasons. In immunocompromised individuals, septic emboli – particularly with Candida species – should be considered. In patients taking medications, pustular drug eruptions may be causative. A specific pustular drug eruption that can be accompanied by fever, lymphadenopathy, and evidence of internal organ (particularly liver) involvement is termed AGEP (acute generalized exanthematous pustulosis). Other pustular eruptions should be considered. Examples include pustular psoriasis, neutrophilic dermatoses such as Sweets syndrome, which is often accompanied by fever and leukocytosis and may be seen in a patient with inflammatory bowel disease, myelogenous dysplasia, or leukemia.

CONTRIBUTORS
Fred F Ferri, MD, FACP
Seth R Stevens, MD
Laurie GS Jacobson, MD

HERPES SIMPLEX

DESCRIPTION

- Herpes simplex is a viral infection caused by the herpes simplex virus (HSV)
- Pain, burning sensation, or paresthesia at the site of inoculation precedes appearance of painful, uniform-sized vesicles on an erythematous base
- Oral and labial lesions most common with HSV-1 infection, genital lesions with HSV-2 infection
- After primary infection, the virus remains latent in dorsal root ganglia
- Recurrence may be precipitated by local trauma, sunburn, fatigue, or stress and is at the site of initial infection
- Lesions heal without scarring

URGENT ACTION

- If dehydration is present, rehydrate as a matter of urgency
- If secondary infection is present, institute antibiotic therapy immediately
- If there is any suggestion of ocular involvement, refer to ophthalmologist
- If suspicion of neonatal herpes simplex, refer to expert pediatrician for treatment
- If eczema herpeticum is suspected (a rapid onset of diffuse cutaneous herpes simplex, usually seen in patients with underlying atopic dermatitis), urgent treatment with acyclovir is indicated
- If patients are HIV-positive or immunocompromised, urgent treatment with antivirals is also recommended because these patients may experience greater morbidity with HSV infections
- If signs or symptoms of herpes encephalitis or pneumonitis are present, intravenous antibiotics and appropriate monitoring are required
- If genital herpes is diagnosed, testing for other sexually transmitted diseases should be performed
- Active genital disease at the time of delivery predisposes to neonatal herpes and is an indication for cesarean section

KEY! DON'T MISS!

Secondary infection of skin lesions.

ICD9 CODE

- 054.9 Herpes simplex, any site
- 054.9 Herpes labialis
- 054.0 Eczema herpeticum
- 771.2 Neonatal herpes simplex

SYNONYMS

- Herpes labialis (cold sores) for infections on the lips
- Eczema herpeticum for rapidly spreading cutaneous herpes simplex infection beginning in eczematous areas, usually within atopic dermatitis lesions
- Herpes gladiatorum for cutaneous herpes simplex infections contracted through contact sports, particularly wrestling. Hallmark is unusual location (e.g. shoulder)
- Herpes digitalis for herpetic whitlow
- Herpes progenitalis, genital herpes for genital infections

CARDINAL FEATURES

Primary infections:

- Many are asymptomatic
- Symptoms appear 3–6 days after contact with the virus
- Pain, burning, or paresthesia at site of inoculation prior to appearance of lesions
- Fever, headache, and malaise are the systemic symptoms associated with infection
- Local lymphadenopathy may occur
- Groups of painful, uniform-sized vesicles on erythematous base appear
- Oral and labial lesions are more common with HSV-1, and genital lesions (herpes progenitalis, genital herpes) are more common with HSV-2
- Lesions last 2–6 weeks and heal without scarring (unless bacterial superinfection occurs)
- Following infection, the virus travels up peripheral nerves supplying the area and remains in a latent state in the dorsal root ganglia

Recurrent infections:

- Often precipitated by local trauma, sun exposure, tiredness, or fever
- Recurs at site of initial infection as virus travels down nerves
- Prodromal symptoms occur 2–24h after reactivation
- Groups of painful vesicles with erythematous base appear within 12h of reactivation
- Vesicles rupture in 2–4 days, leaving ulcers in oral or vaginal mucosa or crusts in cutaneous areas
- Lesions heal in 8–10 days
- Systemic symptoms are rare
- Recurrence is most frequent with genital HSV-2 infection
- Recurrence is least frequent with oral/labial HSV-2 infection

CAUSES

Common causes

Infection with HSV. This is a DNA virus that has two types: HSV-1 and HSV-2.

Contributory or predisposing factors

- Impaired immunity, either chronic or acute (e.g. HIV infection/AIDS); transplantation; tiredness; malnutrition; and stress
- Prior infection
- Occupation as a dentist or doctor (a risk factor for herpetic whitlow)
- Minor trauma and sun exposure can precipitate recurrences

EPIDEMIOLOGY
Incidence and prevalence
INCIDENCE

There is increased incidence over the past decades, which is associated with increased awareness of subclinical and asymptomatic genital herpes infections.

PREVALENCE

- 1–20% of adults excreting virus at any time
- Antibodies present in 30% in high social classes, almost 100% in lower social classes
- A large majority of HSV-2 infections are not clinically apparent

Demographics
AGE

All ages.

GENDER

Both sexes equally affected.

SOCIOECONOMIC STATUS

Presence of antibodies more frequent in lower socioeconomic classes.

DIFFERENTIAL DIAGNOSIS
Impetigo
Impetigo is a bacterial skin infection.

FEATURES
- Spreading, usually circular, pale, straw-colored vesicles that form crusts
- Larger lesions than herpes simplex vesicles
- May be a secondary infection of primary cutaneous herpes simplex

Herpangina
Herpangina is an infection caused by coxsackievirus.

FEATURES
- Vesicles mainly in tonsillar areas, soft palate, and uvula
- Lips are not affected
- Usually due to group A coxsackievirus infection

Aphthous stomatitis
Aphthous stomatitis is inflammation of the oral mucosa.

FEATURES
- More shallow and grayer than herpes simplex ulcers
- Usually on the gums at the front of the mouth

Herpes zoster
Herpes zoster is an infection characterized by a painful rash.

FEATURES
- Eruption usually in area of single dermatome
- Vesicles of varying size

Behçet's syndrome
Behçet's syndrome is a chronic disease of unknown cause.

FEATURES
- Aphthous-type ulceration in oral and genital regions
- Usually accompanied by other features not seen in herpes simplex infections, such as iritis, phlebitis, and pustule formation
- There may also be arthritis and nervous system involvement

Varicella (chickenpox)
Varicella is a common infection caused by a herpesvirus.

FEATURES
- Spots appear in crops all over the body over a number of days
- May itch, but usually not painful

Primary syphilis
Syphilis is a sexually transmitted disease.

FEATURES
- Primary chancre in anogenitalia; can be oral
- Usually single and painless

SIGNS & SYMPTOMS
Signs
Primary infections:
- Vesicles in pharynx and mouth are seen in gingivostomatitis/pharyngitis. Vesicles may be on soft palate, floor of mouth, and tongue – sometimes on lips and cheeks. Fever, cervical lymphadenopathy, and dehydration may be present
- Keratoconjunctivitis, blepharitis with vesicles on edge of lids, keratitis with dendritic corneal ulcers or punctate lesions may occur
- Herpetic whitlow is characterized by vesicles around fingertip and side of nail
- In eczema herpeticum, vesicular eruptions are seen in areas of atopic dermatitis. Usually on upper body, head, and neck. Severe constitutional symptoms are present. Local swelling, lymphadenopathy, weeping, and crusting
- Neonatal herpes simplex is characterized by cutaneous lesions, eye disease, jaundice, hepatosplenomegaly, encephalitis seizures, conjunctivitis, chorioretinitis, and intravascular coagulation
- Signs of genital herpes include fever, malaise, painful ulcers in genital region, and inguinal lymphadenopathy. Urinary retention may occur

Recurrent infections:
- Herpes labialis. Ulcerated lesions with crusting, often at lip margin. May occur on nose or cheek. Lymphadenopathy and swelling are common
- Recurrent eye infections. Blepharitis, conjunctivitis, keratitis, and uveitis are all seen
- Painful ulcers in the genital region are seen in recurrent genital herpes

Symptoms
- May be asymptomatic
- Fever
- Headache
- Localized itching, paresthesia, and pain in the area of infection
- Malaise
- Myalgia

ASSOCIATED DISORDERS
Erythema multiforme – some cases of recurrent herpes simplex are followed by erythema multiforme, with erythematous papules evolving into target lesions, mucosal crusting, and ulceration.

KEY! DON'T MISS!
Secondary infection of skin lesions.

CONSIDER CONSULT
- Severe constitutional illness
- Pneumonitis
- Encephalitis
- During pregnancy, particularly at delivery if active lesions are present
- Any eye involvement: refer immediately to ophthalmologist
- Refer for hospitalization if widespread disease is present
- Eczema herpeticum

INVESTIGATION OF THE PATIENT
Direct questions to patient
Q Have you been exposed to anybody with active herpes simplex infection? Because many shedders of the virus are asymptomatic, the answer will usually be negative.

Q Have you had herpes infections before? Recurrent infection is common.

Q Have you had unprotected sexual intercourse? Even if a condom is worn, contact of genital areas can transmit infection.

Q Have you felt generally unwell recently?

Q Is there itching/burning in affected areas?

Contributory or predisposing factors
Q Is there a history of recent fever, illness, stress, or tiredness? These factors may lead to a brief immunocompromise and precipitate infection or recurrence.

Q Is there any suspicion of immune compromise? Particularly in severe or atypical infections, always consider HIV infection.

Q Are there other risk factors? Sexual promiscuity, occupational exposure (sex workers, dentists).

Examination
- Examine for vesicles/ulcerated lesions, the hallmarks of herpes simplex infections. Ensure that there is no secondary infection of vesicles/ulcers
- Perform a general examination. If the patient is generally unwell, this suggests primary infection
- Examine for tender regional lymphadenopathy. More common in primary infection
- Examine the eyes. If there is evidence of ocular involvement, refer to ophthalmologist
- Examine hydration status. Dehydration may be caused by inability to drink because of painful oral lesions or by fluid or blood loss in eczema herpeticum and erythema multiforme major
- Test for other sexually transmitted diseases in cases of genital herpes

Summary of investigative tests
- Investigations are not always necessary for the diagnosis of herpes simplex
- Serology is used to detect presence of IgM antibodies and rise in IgG titers
- Tzanck smear from lesions is rapid but insensitive and nonspecific
- Viral culture is the gold standard but often too slow to be helpful with an ill patient when the diagnosis is in doubt
- Biopsy of the lesion may be helpful in difficult cases
- Papanicolaou's smear of cervix can detect asymptomatic female carriers
- Direct fluorescent antibody testing is used to detect viral antigens in specimen. Can distinguish between HSV-1 and HSV-2

DIAGNOSTIC DECISION
- The diagnosis may not be difficult and is often made from the clinical history and physical examination
- The main features are painful vesicular or ulcerative lesions with fever and malaise in primary infections
- When necessary, laboratory tests can be used to confirm the diagnosis

CLINICAL PEARLS
- Diagnosis can frequently be made by history of recurring blisters in the same location with prodromal symptoms
- There is a moderate amount of subjectivity to the Tzanck smear that is dependent on the skill of the cytologist and sampling error. Thus clinical-pathologic correlation is always critical

- Direct fluorescent antibody testing is dependent on adequate sampling. In the instance of a negative test result, one should be notified of the adequacy of the sample. Adequacy is determined by the number of keratinocytes from the viable epidermis (not just stratum corneum squames) present
- Sampling for Tzanck smear or direct fluorescent antibody testing should be from intact vesicles if possible, whereas sampling from crusted lesions will reduce sensitivity significantly; it is not reduced to zero

THE TESTS
Body fluids
SEROLOGY
Description
Cuffed venous blood sample.

Advantages/Disadvantages
Advantages:
- Simple test
- Relatively inexpensive

Disadvantages:
- Requires a second sample after 2–3 weeks
- Does not discriminate well between HSV-1 and HSV-2 infections

Normal
Absence of antibodies or less than four-fold rise in second sample.

Abnormal
- Presence of IgM antibodies or greater than four-fold rise in IgG antibodies in second sample
- Keep in mind the possibility of a false-positive result

Cause of abnormal result
Reaction of immune system to infection with herpes simplex virus.

VIRAL CULTURE
Description
Fluid from vesicles.

Advantages/Disadvantages
Advantages:
- Easy to obtain
- Very specific
- The gold standard investigation

Disadvantage : The time taken for virus to grow in culture makes this test less useful in ill patients in whom the diagnosis is in doubt or for monitoring recurrent disease toward the end of pregnancy

Normal
- No growth of virus
- Be aware of false-negative results

Abnormal
Growth of virus.

Cause of abnormal result
- Presence of virus in vesicles
- Failure to use specialized growth conditions
- Keep in mind the possibility of false-positive results

Biopsy
BIOPSY
Description
Biopsy tissue sample of vesicles/ulcers and the surrounding tissue.

Advantages/Disadvantages
Disadvantages:
- May be painful
- May not distinguish between herpes simplex and herpes zoster infections

Abnormal
- Reveals characteristic picture of multinucleated giant cells with nuclear eosinophilic inclusion bodies
- Keep in mind the possibility of a false-positive result

Cause of abnormal result
Infection with HSV.

Drugs, disorders and other factors that may alter results
Prior treatment with corticosteroid creams may distort the pathology of the lesions.

Special tests
TZANCK SMEAR
Description
Smear from the base of the lesion.

Advantages/Disadvantages
Advantages:
- Simple
- Rapid

Disadvantages:
- Not very sensitive
- Does not distinguish between herpes simplex and herpes zoster infections

Normal
Depends on circumstances.

Abnormal
- Presence of multinucleated giant cells with intranuclear eosinophilic inclusions
- Keep in mind the possibility of a false-positive result

Cause of abnormal result
Reaction to herpesvirus.

DIRECT FLUORESCENT ANTIBODY TEST

Description
Smear from the base of the lesion is stained with fluorescein-conjugated anti-herpes antibodies and examined under fluorescence microscopy.

Advantages/Disadvantages
Advantages:
- Simple
- Rapid
- Very sensitive
- Can distinguish among HSV-1, HSV-2, and varicella-zoster virus

Disadvantage: Requires special equipment and laboratory skills

Normal
Negative.

Abnormal
Positive (fluorescence in a characteristic pattern).

Cause of abnormal result
Binding of reagent to herpesvirus within specimen.

PAPANICOLAOU'S CERVICAL SMEAR

Description
Smear taken from cervix.

Advantages/Disadvantages
Advantages:
- Simple test
- Detects asymptomatic carriers of HSV
- May reveal other abnormalities

Disadvantage: Patients often find this examination unpleasant or embarrassing

Normal
Normal cervical cells.

Abnormal
Characteristic appearance of herpes simplex affected cells.

Cause of abnormal result
Infection with HSV.

CONSIDER CONSULT
- If suspicion of neonatal herpes simplex, refer to expert pediatrician for probable treatment with intravenous acyclovir
- If differential diagnosis unresolved

IMMEDIATE ACTION
- Assess patient for dehydration. If present, rehydrate as a matter of urgency
- Assess patient for presence of secondary infection. If likely to be present, institute antibiotic therapy immediately
- If any ocular involvement, refer to ophthalmologist

PATIENT AND CAREGIVER ISSUES

Patient or caregiver request
- Will I have this problem again? Recurrent episodes are common with HSV
- Is the condition contagious? The condition is caused by a virus and can be spread by close contact with others

Health-seeking behavior
- Have you delayed visiting the doctor because of fear/stigma associated with herpes infections?
- Has the diagnosis been obscured by the use of antifungals or steroid creams?

MANAGEMENT ISSUES
Goals
- Make rapid assessment as to urgent treatment of dehydration or secondary infection
- Make rapid assessment as to whether referral is needed
- Treat pain and swelling. This can be severe enough to cause acute retention of urine in genital herpes simplex infections
- Begin treatment with antivirals locally or systemically if indicated
- Consider presence of HIV/AIDS or other sexually transmitted diseases in patients with genital infections

Management in special circumstances
COEXISTING DISEASE
- HIV/AIDS may underlie HSV infections. Other opportunistic infections may coexist
- There may be other sexually transmitted diseases present in patients with genital herpes
- Debility/malnutrition due to other diseases must be treated

COEXISTING MEDICATION
Patients on immunosuppressant medication may require more aggressive management.

SPECIAL PATIENT GROUPS
- Herpes simplex in pregnancy and in the newborn require specialized management
- If genital herpes vesicles are present at the time of delivery, a cesarean section is indicated
- Newborns may require intravenous acyclovir

PATIENT SATISFACTION/LIFESTYLE PRIORITIES
- Pain may be severe and may compromise ability to work
- Systemic antivirals may shorten period of disease
- Risk factors for future reinfection must be addressed

SUMMARY OF THERAPEUTIC OPTIONS
Choices

- Acyclovir locally or systemically is usually the drug of first choice
- Penciclovir cream can be useful in recurrent herpes labialis
- Valacyclovir is converted to acyclovir and may be used in genital infections
- Famciclovir is sometimes useful in genital herpes. It is converted to penciclovir
- Foscarnet is given for acyclovir-resistant infections in immunocompromised patients
- Lysine and zinc supplementation may be effective in reducing recurrences

Guidelines

The American Academy of Family Physicians has published information on HSV infection [1]

Clinical pearls

- Can be present at more than one site
- Can be confused with herpes zoster
- Existence of recurrent zoster is controversial. Viral typing by culture or DFA can distinguish

Never

- Never ignore central nervous system or pulmonary symptoms in herpes patients, particularly if widespread lesions are present
- Never forget to search for other sexually transmitted diseases in patients with genital herpes
- Never ignore public health implications. Have sexual partners of patients with genital herpes examined for infection and treated as indicated

FOLLOW UP
Plan for review

- See patient as necessary to ensure satisfactory progress
- May need follow up in 2–3 weeks for second blood sample for antibody titers
- Diagnose and monitor associated conditions

Information for patient or caregiver

- Educate regarding modes of transmission
- Avoid contact with patients who have acute infections
- Frequent hand washing
- Avoid sexual risk behaviors
- Encourage use of condoms
- Avoid contact sports in herpes gladiatorum

DRUGS AND OTHER THERAPIES: DETAILS
Drugs
ACYCLOVIR
Dose

- In primary herpes simplex stomatitis, primary genital herpes, recurrent herpes labialis, and recurrent genital herpes, the usual dose is 200mg five times a day for 10 days
- In herpes labialis, the 5% aqueous cream is applied four times a day

Efficacy
Steady improvement should be seen except when the virus is resistant to acyclovir.

Risks/benefits
Risks:
- Use caution with hepatic and renal disease, dehydration, electrolyte imbalance, and seizure disorders or other neurologic disease
- Use caution with pregnancy and nursing mothers

Benefits:
- Effective drug
- Low incidence of side effects

Side effects and adverse reactions
- Central nervous system: headache, coma, confusion, seizures, hallucinations, tremor, dizziness, encephalopathy
- Gastrointestinal: nausea, vomiting, diarrhea, abdominal pain, elevated liver enzymes, hepatitis, anorexia, jaundice
- Genitourinary: crystalluria, renal toxicity
- Hematologic: leukopenia, thrombocytopenia, hemolytic uremic syndrome
- Skin: injection site reaction, phlebitis, alopecia, erythema, rash, pruritus, toxic epidermal necrolysis, Stevens-Johnson syndrome, photosensitivity, urticaria

Interactions (other drugs)
- Mycophenolate ■ Phenytoin, fosphenytoin ■ Probenecid ■ Zidovudine

Contraindications
- Children under 2 years of age ■ Hypersensitivity or intolerance to acyclovir

Evidence
Oral acyclovir is effective in the treatment of first episode and recurrent herpes labialis.
- A randomized controlled trial (RCT) compared oral acyclovir with placebo in the management of recurrent herpes labialis in adults. Symptoms were found to resolve more quickly (12.5 to 8.1 days) when acyclovir was commenced at the beginning of the attack when tingling symptoms are present. Acyclovir commenced after the vesicular rash appeared did not lead to faster resolution [2] *Level P*
- Oral acyclovir was compared with placebo in another RCT. Acyclovir was found to significantly reduce healing time and duration of pain when commenced within 12h of symptom onset [3] *Level P*
- An RCT compared oral acyclovir with placebo in the management of a first attack of herpes labialis in children. Acyclovir was found to significantly reduce the duration of pain and excess salivation [4] *Level P*
- An RCT of children with gingivostomatitis found that acyclovir reduced the healing time of herpes simplex lesions when compared with placebo [5] *Level P*

Topical acyclovir when combined with a liposomal carrier accelerates the healing time of herpes labialis.
- A small RCT compared 5% acyclovir cream vs 5% acyclovir in a liposomal carrier vs the carrier alone in the treatment of recurrent herpes labialis. Lesion crusting was faster in patients treated with acyclovir plus carrier vs carrier alone. There was no significant difference between acyclovir cream alone and the drug-free liposomal carrier [6] *Level P*

There is limited evidence for the use of oral acyclovir in the prevention of herpes labialis.
- An RCT found that prophylactic acyclovir significantly reduced the number and duration of attacks in people with a history of recurrent herpes labialis induced by ultraviolet (UV) light (acyclovir commenced 7 days before exposure) [7] *Level P*

- Another RCT found no difference when acyclovir (commenced the day before UV exposure) was compared with placebo in the prevention of herpes labialis [8] *Level P*
- A small RCT found that acyclovir treatment for 4 months (400mg twice daily) reduced clinical recurrences and culture positive recurrences [9] *Level P*

Evidence for the treatment of genital herpes with acyclovir is available.

Acceptability to patient
High apart from frequency of tablets.

Follow up plan
Monitor clinically to ensure recovery as planned.

Patient and caregiver information
Patients should be taught to recognize symptoms and report early for treatment.

PENCICLOVIR
Dose
In recurrent herpes labialis, use cream every 2h during the day.

Efficacy
Lesions should steadily improve over some days.

Risks/benefits
Risk: use caution in immunocompromised patients
Benefit: low incidence of side effects

Side effects and adverse reactions
- Side effects are rare
- Skin: reaction at application site, pruritus, rash

Interactions (other drugs)
- None listed

Contraindications
- Hypersensitivity to penciclovir

Evidence
There is evidence for the use of penciclovir in the management of recurrent herpes labialis.
- An RCT compared penciclovir cream with placebo in the management of herpes labialis. Penciclovir reduced the duration of pain and healing time [10] *Level P*
- A significant reduction in healing time was noted in another RCT when penciclovir was compared with placebo [11] *Level P*

Acceptability to patient
High.

Follow up plan
Monitor clinically to ensure recovery as planned.

Patient and caregiver information
Complete the full course of treatment as prescribed.

VALACYCLOVIR
This antiviral medication is used for genital herpes.

Dose
Dosage depends on the indication:
- Initial episode – 1g twice daily for 10 days
- Recurrent episodes – 500mg twice daily for 5 days
- Prevention of recurrent episodes – 500–1000mg daily

Efficacy
- Useful for treating the initial episode or recurrent episodes of genital herpes in adults
- May be useful for the prevention of recurrence

Risks/benefits
Risks:
- Use caution in renal and hepatic disease
- Use caution in the elderly and children
- Use caution in pregnancy and breastfeeding
- More expensive than acyclovir

Benefit: May shorten the course of disease

Side effects and adverse reactions
- Central nervous system: asthenia, headache, dizziness
- Gastrointestinal: nausea, vomiting, diarrhea, constipation, abdominal cramps, anorexia
- Hematologic: anemia, thrombocytopenia

Interactions (other drugs)
- Cimetidine ■ Probenecid

Contraindications
- Immunocompromised patients

Evidence
Evidence is available for the treatment of genital herpes with valacyclovir.

Acceptability to patient
- Generally acceptable in the short term
- Side effects may make suppression therapy unacceptable

Follow up plan
Follow up to ensure resolution of lesions.

Patient and caregiver information
Continue the full course of medication as prescribed.

FAMCICLOVIR
Antiviral medication used to treat genital herpes.

Dose
- Genital herpes: 125mg twice daily for 5 days

- Suppression of genital herpes: 250mg twice daily; if creatinine clearance is 20–39mL/min, use 125mg twice daily; if creatinine clearance is <20mL/min, use 125mg once daily

Efficacy

- Useful for treating the initial episode or recurrent episodes of genital herpes in adults
- May be useful for the prevention of recurrence

Risks/benefits

Risks:

- Use caution in children
- Use caution in renal disease
- Use caution in pregnancy and breastfeeding

Benefit: Probably as effective as acyclovir and easier to use

Side effects and adverse reactions

- Central nervous system: headache, dizziness, insomnia, somnolence, paresthesia
- Gastrointestinal: nausea, vomiting, diarrhea, constipation, abdominal pain, anorexia
- Respiratory: pharyngitis, sinusitis
- Skin: rash, pruritus

Interactions (other drugs)

- **Cimetidine** ■ **Digoxin** ■ **Probenecid** ■ **Theophylline**

Contraindications

- **Hypersensitivity or intolerance to famciclovir** ■ **Impaired renal function** ■ **Pregnancy category B**

Evidence

- An RCT compared famciclovir (three different doses commenced 48h after exposure to UV light) with placebo for the prevention of sunlight-induced herpes labialis. The size and duration of lesions were reduced with an increasing dose of famciclovir. The mean healing time was significantly reduced with a 500mg dose of famciclovir compared with placebo [12] *Level P*
- Evidence is available for the treatment of genital herpes with famciclovir

Acceptability to patient

- Generally acceptable in the short term
- Side effects may make suppression therapy unacceptable

Follow up plan

Follow up to ensure that treatment was adequate.

Patient and caregiver information

Take the full course of medication prescribed.

FOSCARNET

Foscarnet may be of value in treating herpes simplex infections that are resistant to other antiviral medications such as acyclovir. However, its side effect profile (including gastrointestinal side effects and nephrotoxicity) limits its utility.

Dose

40mg/kg intravenously at 1mg/kg/min two to three times a day.

Efficacy
Moderately effective in treating acyclovir-resistant mucocutaneous infections in immunocompromised patients.

Risks/benefits
Risks:
- Use caution in renal impairment, electrolyte disturbances, neurologic abnormalities, cardiac abnormalities, seizure disorders, and severe anemia
- Use caution in children and the elderly
- Relatively toxic but can be useful

Side effects and adverse reactions
- Cardiovascular system: cardiac failure, cardiac arrest, bradycardia, cardiomyopathy, dysrhythmias, ECG abnormalities, hypertension, hypotension, palpitations, phlebitis
- Central nervous system: seizures, fever, headache
- Eyes, ears, nose, and throat: conjunctivitis, eye pain, vision abnormalities
- Gastrointestinal: nausea, pancreatitis, diarrhea, vomiting, abdominal pain, anorexia, constipation, dyspepsia, dry mouth, dysphagia, flatulence, melena, rectal hemorrhage, ulcerative stomatitis
- Genitourinary: abnormal renal function, albuminuria, dysuria, nocturia, polyuria, urethral disorder, urinary retention, urinary tract infection
- Hematologic: anemia, granulocytopenia, thrombocytopenia, leukopenia, lymphadenopathy, platelet abnormalities, thrombosis, white blood cell abnormalities
- Metabolism: mineral and electrolyte imbalance, including hypokalemia, hypocalcemia, hypomagnesemia, hypophosphatemia, hyperphosphatemia
- Respiratory: coughing, dyspnea
- Skin: erythematous rash, facial edema, maculopapular rash, pruritus, seborrhea, skin discoloration, skin ulceration, sweating

Interactions (other drugs)
- Quinolones (slightly increased risk of seizures)

Contraindications
- Hypersensitivity or intolerance to foscarnet ▪ Pre-existing renal impairment

Acceptability to patient
Gastrointestinal side effects may make it less acceptable.

Follow up plan
Monitor clinically to ensure recovery as planned.

Patient and caregiver information
Report any perioral tingling, or limb paresthesias, which could indicate an electrolyte imbalance.

Complementary therapy
ZINC
Efficacy
Zinc is useful in inhibiting herpes simplex virus in vitro, and by enhancing cell-mediated immunity in vivo when given orally. In addition, topical zinc sulfate 0.01–0.025% solution may be effective in lessening HSV symptoms and in preventing recurrences.

Risks/benefits
Risks:
- Occasional gastrointestinal irritation, nausea and vomiting occur when taken orally in high doses (greater than 8 times the RDA)
- Doses higher than 15mg/day should be avoided in pregnant women
- Doses higher than 19mg/day should be avoided in nursing mothers during first 6 months, and 16mg/day during second 6 months
- High doses of zinc supplementation can result in copper deficiency

Interactions:
- **Bisphosphates (may decrease the absorption of both)** ■ **Quinolones (may decrease the absorption of both)** ■ **Penicillamine (may suppress absorption of zinc)** ■ **Tetracyclines (may decrease the absorption of both)**

Acceptability to patient
Most patients tolerate zinc orally and topically without difficulty.

Follow up plan
Monitor patient for signs of viral resolution or for any complications of HSV.

Patient and caregiver information
Oral dose of zinc is 25mg/day; topical solution 0.025% zinc sulfate applied three times daily.

LYSINE
Efficacy
Lysine has been shown to have antiviral activity in vitro due to antagonism of arginine metabolism, which is required in HSV replication. Studies which use fairly high doses of lysine (1g three times daily) along with arginine restriction in the diet (nuts, chocolate, gelatin) have shown reduction in HSV recurrence.

Risks/benefits
Benefits:
- Lysine supplementation/arginine restriction is not curative, but is effective in reducing recurrences
- There appears to be negligible toxicity to this regimen

Evidence
A double-blind RCT found that L-lysine monohydrochlorine, given as an oral dose of 1248mg daily, may decrease the recurrence rate of herpes simplex infection in immunocompetent patients. A dose of 624mg daily was not effective, and neither dose reduced the duration of symptoms when compared with placebo [13] *Level P*

Acceptability to patient
Usually quite acceptable.

Follow up plan
Normal follow up as per usual care.

Patient and caregiver information
Dose of lysine is 1000mg three times daily and avoidance of dietary arginine (nuts, chocolate, gelatin) in order to prevent recurrences, not to treat acute outbreaks.

EFFICACY OF THERAPIES

- Most primary and recurrent attacks of herpes simplex respond well to treatment, and recovery can be expected within about 10 days
- In immunocompromised patients, particularly if the virus is resistant to acyclovir, treatment may be much less effective
- Recurrences are common, but their frequency can be significantly reduced with longer-term treatment with antivirals

Evidence

- There is limited evidence from RCTs that oral acyclovir may be effective as a preventive agent against recurrent herpes labialis [14] *Level P*
- Symptoms of first attack or recurrent herpes labialis may resolve more quickly when acyclovir is commenced at the beginning of an attack (as found in RCTs) [14] *Level P*
- There is limited evidence for the use of topical antiviral agents in the treatment of herpes labialis [14] *Level P*

Review period

Patients should be seen after the first course of therapy to assess recovery.

PROGNOSIS

- Prognosis is excellent in most cases of primary and recurrent HSV infections
- The prognosis is worse for immunocompromised patients and in neonatal herpes simplex, particularly in herpes simplex encephalitis

Clinical pearls

- Consider secondary bacterial infection if delayed wound healing is a problem
- Let patients know that scarring can be a problem if herpes lesions are overly excoriated or if they become secondarily infected by bacteria

Therapeutic failure

- Foscarnet is given for acyclovir-resistant infections in immunocompromised patients
- Cidofovir (HPMPC) may also be useful in acyclovir-resistant, thymidine-kinase deficient infections
- Ganciclovir may have activity against HSV, although it is mainly for cytomegalovirus infections
- Trifluorothymidine as a topical treatment may also be useful for acyclovir-resistant HSV

Recurrence

Recurrence is common and can be treated again with antiviral medication.

Deterioration

The development of diffuse infection, herpes meningitis, or herpes encephalitis requires hospital admission (usually seen in immunocompromised hosts).

COMPLICATIONS

- In immunocompromised patients, generalized viremia, herpes pneumonia, meningitis, and encephalitis may occur
- Secondary infection in skin lesions (particularly impetigo)

CONSIDER CONSULT

- If recovery is slower than expected
- If frequent recurrences are difficult to control
- When HIV/AIDS or other predisposing factors are suspected
- Extensive fluid loss from skin lesions
- Significant secondary infection
- Dehydration from fluid loss or inability to drink
- CNS involvement

PREVENTION

RISK FACTORS
- Stress and lethargy: reduce resistance to infections
- HIV/AIDS: predisposes to many opportunistic infections
- Sexual promiscuity without the use of condoms: increases risks of viral transmission
- Occupational exposure: e.g. sex workers, dentists, doctors

MODIFY RISK FACTORS
Lifestyle and wellness
ALCOHOL AND DRUGS
Malnutrition is a predisposing factor and may be related to alcohol abuse.

DIET
Ensure that diet is adequate and balanced.

SEXUAL BEHAVIOR
All people should be made aware of the following protective measures:
- Reduce number of contacts
- Always use condoms
- Avoid contact with people known to be infected

IMMUNIZATION
No vaccine currently available.

CHEMOPROPHYLAXIS
Long-term treatment with antivirals can markedly reduce the recurrence rate.

SCREENING
- General population screening for herpes simplex is not useful because subclinical infection is very common and most episodes are trivial
- Screening for genital infections in the asymptomatic general population and in asymptomatic pregnant women has been considered by the United States Preventive Services Task Force, which concluded that neither group should be routinely screened

Guidelines
Screening for genital herpes simplex. US Preventive Services Task Force. [15]

PREVENT RECURRENCE
Recurrences may be prevented by avoidance measures and by taking antiviral therapy.

RESOURCES

ASSOCIATIONS

American Social Health Association
PO Box 13827
Research Triangle Park, NC 27709
Tel: 919-361-8400
Fax: 919-361-8425
http://www.ashastd.org

National Herpes Hotline
Tel: 919-361-8488
9a.m.-7p.m. EST Monday to Friday

American Herpes Foundation
Tel: 201-342-4441
Fax: 201-342-7555
http://www.herpes-foundation.org

For support groups/links, The Herpes Network http://www.herpes.net

KEY REFERENCES

- Infectious diseases. In: Beers MH, Berkow R, eds. The Merck manual of diagnosis and therapy, 17th edn. New Jersey: Merck, 1999
- Warts, herpes simplex and other viral infections, chapter 12. In: Habif TP. Clinical dermatology, 3rd edn. Philadelphia: Mosby, 1996
- Report of the US Preventive Services Task Force. Guide to clinical preventive services, 2nd edn. Baltimore MD: Williams and Wilkins, 1996
- Drug references: Available online: www.aidsinfonyc.org

Evidence references and guidelines

1 The American Academy of Family Physicians has published information on herpes simplex infection: Emmert DH. Treatment of common cutaneous herpes simplex virus infections. American Family Physician 2000;61:1697–1706
2 Spruance SL, Hammil ML, Hoge WS, et al. ACV prevents reactivation of herpes labialis in skiers. JAMA 1988;260:1597–1599. Reviewed in: Clinical Evidence 2001;6:1303–1308
3 Kaminester LH, Pariser RJ, Pariser, et al. A double-blind, placebo-controlled study of topical tetracaine in the treatment of herpes labialis. J Am Acad Dermatol 1999;41:996–1001. Reviewed in: Clinical Evidence 2001;6:1303–1308
4 Ducoulombier H, Cousin J, DeWilde A. Herpetic stomatitis-gingivitis in children: controlled trial of acyclovir versus placebo (in French). Ann Pediatr (Paris) 1988;35:212–216. Reviewed in: Clinical Evidence 2001;6:1303–1308
5 Amir J, Harel L, Smetana Z, Varsano I. Treatment of herpes simplex gingivostomatitis with aciclovir in children: a randomised double blind placebo controlled trial. BMJ 1997;314:1800–1803. Reviewed in: Clinical Evidence 2001;6:1303–1308
6 Horwitz E, Pisanty S, Czerninski R, et al. A clinical evaluation of a novel liposomal carrier for acyclovir in the topical treatment of recurrent herpes labialis. Oral Surg Oral Med Oral Pathol 1999;87:700–705. Reviewed in: Clinical Evidence 2001;6:1303–1308
7 Raborn GW, Martel AY, Grace MG, McGaw WT. Oral acyclovir in prevention of herpes labialis: a randomized, double-blind, placebo controlled trial. Oral Surg Oral Med Oral Pathol Oral Radiol Endod 1998;85:55–59. Reviewed in: Clinical Evidence 2001;6:1303–1308
8 Spruance SL, Stewart JC, Rowe NH, et al. Treatment of recurrent herpes simplex labialis with oral acyclovir. J Infect Dis 1990;161:185–190. Reviewed in: Clinical Evidence 2001;6:1303–1308
9 Raborn WG, McGraw WT, Grace M, et al. Oral acyclovir and herpes labialis: a randomized, double-blind, placebo-controlled study. J Am Dental Assoc 1987;115:38–42. Reviewed in: Clinical Evidence 2001;6:1303–1308
10 Spruance SL, Rea TL, Thoming C, et al. Penciclovir cream for the treatment of herpes simplex labialis. JAMA

1997;277:1374–1379. Reviewed in: Clinical Evidence 2001;6:1303–1308

11 Boon R, Goodman JJ, Martinez J, et al. Penciclovir cream for the treatment of sunlight-induced herpes simplex labialis: a randomized, double-blind, placebo-controlled trial. Penciclovir Cream Herpes Labialis Study Group. Clin Ther 2000;22:76–90. Reviewed in: Clinical Evidence 2001;6:1303–1308

12 Spruance SL, Rowe NH, Raborn GW, et al. Peroral famciclovir in the treatment of experimental ultraviolet radiation-induced herpes simplex labialis: a double-blind, dose-ranging, placebo-controlled, multicenter trial. J Infect Dis 1999;179:303–310. Reviewed in Clinical Evidence 2001;6:1303–1308

13 McClune MA, Perry HO, Muller SA, O'Fallon WM. Treatment of recurrent herpes simplex infections with L-lysine monohydrochloride. Cutis 1984;34:366–73

14 Worrall G. Herpes labialis: skin disorders. In: Clinical Evidence 2001;6:1303–1308. London: BMJ Publishing Group

15 Screening for genital herpes simplex. US Preventive Services Task Force. Guide to clinical preventive services, 2nd ed. Baltimore MD: Williams and Wilkins, 1996: 335–346. Available online at the National Guideline Clearinghouse

FAQS
Question 1
If typical lesions occur more than once in a location, does that preclude the diagnosis of zoster and clinch the diagnosis of herpes?

ANSWER 1
There remains controversy whether recurrent zoster occurs. If so, it is quite rare.

Question 2
Is it true that herpes never leaves a scar?

ANSWER 2
Strictly speaking, yes. However, traumatization (such as by scratching) or secondary bacterial infection can lead to scarring in areas of herpes infection.

Question 3
Must patients with disseminated herpes be hospitalized?

ANSWER 3
This is the standard of care. However, in some circumstances it may be acceptable to treat such patients orally with careful monitoring and close follow up.

Question 4
Is anogenital herpes in an infant or child *prima facie* evidence of sexual abuse?

ANSWER 4
This unfortunate circumstance must be considered. Viral typing can help determine if the child's infection is with HSV-1 or HSV-2. If HSV-1 is detected, the likelihood of abuse is reduced.

CONTRIBUTORS
Randolph L Pearson, MD
Jane L Murray, MD
Seth R Stevens, MD
Elma D Baron, MD

HERPES ZOSTER

DESCRIPTION

■ A painful, unilateral, dermatomal eruption, most commonly in the thoracic region
■ Occurs as a result of reactivation of the varicella zoster (chickenpox) virus, which is caused by suppression of the immune system (e.g. by immunosuppressive drugs, disease, or increasing age)
■ Can give rise to postherpetic neuralgia, especially in elderly patients

URGENT ACTION

■ Involvement of the nasociliary branch of the ophthalmic division of the trigeminal nerve (manifested by vesicles on the tip and side of the nose, swelling of the eyelid, or conjunctivitis) should prompt urgent referral to a specialist dermatologist or ophthalmologist
■ Disseminated zoster requires prompt evaluation, likely hospitalization for intravenous antiviral therapy, and monitoring. Evaluation for immunocompromise should be performed
■ Patients are contagious – contact with pregnant women who have not had chickenpox needs to be prevented

KEY! DON'T MISS!

■ Check for involvement of the nasociliary branch of the ophthalmic division of the trigeminal verve, manifested by vesicles on the tip and side of the nose, swelling of the eyelid, or conjunctivitis. If the patient is affected, refer to a specialist dermatologist or ophthalmologist
■ Ramsay Hunt syndrome, which leads to facial palsy. Vesicles on the pinna and external auditory canal are seen

ICD9 CODE
053.9 Herpes zoster, NOS

SYNONYMS
- Shingles
- Zoster

CARDINAL FEATURES
- Rash in dermatomal distribution, which is painful
- Pain, tingling, or itching sensation in the affected dermatome often precedes the rash
- Most commonly seen on the thorax
- May occur in the trigeminal region, the lumbar region, or on the limbs
- Rash is almost always unilateral and does not cross the midline
- Rash consists of irregularly sized vesicles on an erythematous base
- Patient is often generally unwell (e.g. malaise and fever)

CAUSES
Common causes
- Shingles is caused by reactivation of varicella zoster virus that has been dormant in the dorsal root ganglia following chickenpox
- The virus is reactivated when cell-mediated immunity is suppressed
- Common causes for reactivation include advancing age, pre-existing disease, and immunosuppressant drugs

Contributory or predisposing factors
- Previous chickenpox, caused by infection with the varicella virus, is always present
- Increasing age (>50 years)
- Immunocompromise (e.g. due to AIDS or immunosuppressant therapy)
- A history of chickenpox before 2 months of age
- Chemotherapy or radiotherapy
- Stress, such as other illness, trauma, or bereavement
- Spinal surgery
- Spinal cord radiation

EPIDEMIOLOGY
Incidence and prevalence
INCIDENCE
- 2 per 1000 of the general population per year
- 0.5–1.6 per 1000 of the population per year in those aged <20 years
- 11 per 1000 of the population per year in those aged >80 years

PREVALENCE
- 0.024 cases per 1000
- 0.086 cases of postherpetic neuralgia per 1000

FREQUENCY
- Shingles affects 10–20% of people at some stage during their life
- More common in immunocompromised patients (e.g. 50% of people with active Hodgkin's disease develop shingles)

Demographics

AGE
Incidence increases with age.

GENDER
Shingles is equally common in men and women.

RACE
No clinically significant difference between races.

SOCIOECONOMIC STATUS
More common in the undernourished.

DIFFERENTIAL DIAGNOSIS

- Differential diagnoses of the rash include herpes simplex virus infection, disseminated coxsackievirus infection, contact dermatitis, autoimmune bullous skin diseases, blistering bacterial infection
- Differential diagnoses of the pain include cholecystitis, pleuritic chest pain, myocardial infarction, pericarditis, renal colic, prolapsed disc

Herpes simplex virus infection
Herpes simplex is a viral disease. Recurrence is common.

FEATURES

- Less extensive rash than herpes zoster and nondermatomal in distribution
- Individual lesions of herpes simplex virus are all of the same size and tend to be smaller than those of herpes zoster
- Tend to be recurrent, unlike zoster

Disseminated coxsackievirus infections
Infection with coxsackievirus can lead to a rash.

FEATURES

- Maculopapular rash in nondermatomal distribution, often beginning on the face and body and later spreading to the limbs, especially the extensor surfaces
- Posterior cervical and occipital lymphadenopathy is common
- More likely to be confused with the rash of measles or rubella than with herpes zoster

Contact dermatitis
Contact dermatitis is related to contact with an antigenic or irritant substance or material. Patch testing may be needed to identify the precise antigen or irritant.

FEATURES
Nondermatomal rash, often in an unusual distribution with a clear-cut border.

Autoimmune bullous skin diseases

- Autoantibodies against epidermal or basement membrane zone proteins are responsible for blister formation
- Chronic, progressive disease course
- Immunohistology may be needed to establish correct diagnosis
- Examples include pemphigus vulgaris, pemphigoid group, and dermatitis herpetiformis

FEATURES

- Nondermatomal, often symmetrically distributed vesicles or bullae with clear content
- Involvement of mucous membranes is common
- Usually no prodromal symptoms
- Usually pain-free

Blistering bacterial skin infection (impetigo)
Caused by *Staphylococcus aureus* or *Streptococcus* strains. Mostly affects children; recent upper respiratory infection and fever in history. There is a risk of developing poststreptococcal glomerulonephritis after resolution of skin symptoms. The main features of impetigo are as follows.

FEATURES

Large vesicles with cloudy content on erythematous base.

Cholecystitis

In cholecystitis, the patient's history may reveal that eating a large or fatty meal precedes the onset of pain.

FEATURES

- Pain in the right upper quadrant of the abdomen
- Tenderness to palpation
- Guarding may be present
- Palpation may cause patient to stop breathing in suddenly (Murphy's sign)

Pleuritic chest pain

Inflammation of the pleura and lungs secondary to infection or pulmonary infarction are the usual causes.

FEATURES

Sharp, localized chest pain exacerbated or produced by deep inspiration and coughing.

Myocardial infarction

Diagnosis of myocardial infarction is based on history, muscle enzymes, and ECG findings.

FEATURES

- Pain is typically retrosternal and is often described as crushing
- Pain may radiate to the arms (most commonly the left arm) or to the jaw, neck, or shoulders
- Physical examination may reveal signs associated with cardiac disease

Pericarditis

Pericarditis is an inflammation of the pericardium, often related to viral infection.

FEATURES

- Pain in the chest that may radiate to the arms or back
- Pain is sharp and is often relieved with breathing in and by leaning forward
- Pericardial friction rub may be heard on auscultation

Renal colic

Often related to kidney stones.

FEATURES

- Pain in the abdomen or side, often of sudden onset
- Patient moves or writhes constantly in an attempt to relieve the pain
- Pain may radiate to the testes in men or the labium in women
- Urine may be bloodstained

Prolapsed disc

Pain in the back due to a prolapsed disc may be preceded by injury or trauma, which is often apparently minor.

FEATURES

- Back pain
- Pain often relieved by lying on the back with the hips flexed
- Neurologic signs may be present (e.g. weakness or change in sensation in the lower limbs, bowel or bladder dysfunction)

SIGNS & SYMPTOMS
Signs
- Closely grouped red papules, which rapidly become vesicular, appear in a continuous, uninterrupted band, generally in a single dermatome
- A few patients have some vesicles outside the affected dermatome
- Rash is almost always unilateral
- Appearance of the rash may be the first sign in children
- Lymph nodes draining the affected area may be enlarged and tender
- Vesicles become papular and/or hemorrhagic in 1–4 days
- Vesicles have a red base and are cloudy in appearance
- Vesicles are of different sizes
- Vesicles become umbilicated and then form crusts that fall off in about 3 weeks, generally leaving some scarring
- Unilateral facial nerve palsy in herpes zoster of the facial nerve (Ramsay Hunt syndrome)

Symptoms
- Malaise
- Headache
- Acute, knife-like pain (with tingling and itching) that occurs 3–5 days before the rash in the dermatome where the rash will appear
- Weakness
- Fever
- Acute loss of hearing, vertigo, and paralysis of the affected side of the face may occur in herpes zoster of the facial nerve (Ramsay Hunt syndrome)

ASSOCIATED DISORDERS
Chickenpox: patients with herpes zoster always have a history of previous chickenpox.

KEY! DON'T MISS!
- Check for involvement of the nasociliary branch of the ophthalmic division of the trigeminal nerve, manifested by vesicles on the tip and side of the nose, swelling of the eyelid, or conjunctivitis. If the patient is affected, refer to a specialist dermatologist or ophthalmologist
- Ramsay Hunt syndrome, which leads to facial palsy. Vesicles on the pinna and external auditory canal are seen

CONSIDER CONSULT
- Involvement of the nasociliary branch of the ophthalmic division of the trigeminal nerve (manifested by vesicles on the tip and side of the nose, swelling of the eyelid, or conjunctivitis) should prompt urgent referral to a specialist dermatologist or ophthalmologist
- Disseminated zoster requires prompt evaluation, likely hospitalization for intravenous antiviral therapy, and monitoring. Evaluation for immunocompromise should be performed
- Refer if herpes zoster is a complication of a pre-existing disorder that needs specialist assessment or management
- Refer if herpes zoster is in the distribution of the ophthalmic division of the trigeminal nerve and the eye is involved or threatened
- Refer if uncontrollable postherpetic neuralgia or other neurologic complications (e.g. palsy)

INVESTIGATION OF THE PATIENT
Direct questions to patient
Q Have you had chickenpox (varicella zoster infection)? Herpes zoster occurs only after a previous occurrence of varicella zoster infection (but patients may not always remember if they have had chickenpox).

Q Is the rash painful? Herpes zoster is usually extremely painful.

Q Was the rash preceded by acute, severe pain in the area in which it has subsequently appeared? Was there any itching or tingling? All these symptoms are common features of herpes zoster.

Q Have you felt tired, felt unwell, or had a headache? These are common nonspecific symptoms of herpes zoster.

Contributory or predisposing factors

Q Are you taking any immunosuppressive medication? Is there any reason to suspect immunocompromise or immunosuppression? Any condition that causes a decrease in cell-mediated immunity predisposes to herpes zoster.

Q Are you HIV-positive? HIV infection is a common predisposing factor for herpes zoster, especially when herpes zoster occurs in a younger person.

Q Do you have leukemia or lymphoma? These conditions predispose to herpes zoster.

Examination

Examine the:

- Skin of the affected area for a vesicular rash in dermatomal distribution, usually at the site of preceding pain
- Face for involvement of the nasociliary branch of the ophthalmic division of the trigeminal nerve (manifested by vesicles on the tip and side of the nose, swelling of the eyelid, or conjunctivitis)
- Mucous membranes in affected region for presence of blisters or erosions
- Regional lymph nodes for lymphadenopathy
- Entire cutaneous surface for evidence of disseminated disease

Summary of investigative tests

Usually, no laboratory tests are required. However, in cases of genuine diagnostic doubt, diagnostic testing may be useful, including the following:

- Direct antigen staining (monoclonal antibody testing)
- Tzanck test
- Serologic methods – varicella zoster (chickenpox) virus IgG antibody titer determination; titers rise in the course of the disease
- Viral culture from swab of lesion
- Viral DNA detection by polymerase chain reaction

DIAGNOSTIC DECISION

Diagnosis is almost always clinical, based on the history and the dermatomal distribution of the rash.

CLINICAL PEARLS

- Pain of zoster prior to onset of the rash may be confused with surgical abdomen, myocardial infarction, or renal or biliary disease. Appropriate consideration of the differential diagnosis is required
- Classically, zoster is considered dermatomal; however, spread to one or two adjacent ipsilateral dermatomes is not unusual and therefore do not exclude the diagnosis. Similarly, there may be modest crossing of the midline in zoster

THE TESTS
Body fluids
SEROLOGIC METHODS
Description

- Serologic blood test
- Testing for antibodies against varicella zoster virus present in blood sample
- Used mainly for establishing prior varicella zoster virus infection or for diagnosing primary varicella infections

Advantages/Disadvantages
Advantages:
- Easily accessible diagnostic sample
- High sensitivity, moderate specificity

Disadvantages:
- Only becomes positive after 3–7 days
- Not useful in determining recurrent varicella zoster virus infection (zoster)

Normal
No change or less than four times increase in antivaricella zoster virus titer.

Abnormal
Four times or greater increase in IgG antibody titer to varicella zoster virus.

Cause of abnormal result
Development of antivaricella zoster virus antibodies after infection.

Biopsy
TZANCK TEST
Description
- Scraping from the floor of a herpes zoster vesicle
- The scraping is put on a glass slide and stained with Wright's or Giemsa stain

Advantages/Disadvantages
Advantage: reliably identifies Tzanck cells (multinucleated giant cells), which are characteristic of herpes virus infections, although this reliability is dependent on the skill of the cytologist
Disadvantage: does not differentiate from other herpes virus infections

Abnormal
- The presence of any Tzanck cells (multinucleated giant cells) in the preparation
- Keep in mind the possibility of a false-positive result

Special tests
DIRECT ANTIGEN STAINING
Description
Cellular scrapings from the base of fresh lesions are submitted on slides to a laboratory specialized in antigen staining (instead of carrying out the staining procedure in the office).

Advantages/Disadvantages
Advantages:
- Confirms the presence of varicella zoster virus antigens and thus rules out other infective etiology
- Rapid test and result (within one day)
- Relatively inexpensive
- Highly sensitive and specific

Abnormal
- The presence of varicella zoster virus antigens, which stain positive with specific fluorescein-conjugated monoclonal antibodies
- Keep in mind the possibility of a false-positive result

Cause of abnormal result
Varicella zoster virus antigens.

Other tests
VIRAL CULTURE
Description
Culture of varicella zoster virus in laboratory from swab of vesicle, tissue, or body fluids.

Advantages/Disadvantages
Advantage: almost 100% specificity

Disadvantages:
- Less sensitive than other tests
- May require long time (up to 3 weeks) to obtain results

Normal
Varicella zoster virus cannot be cultured from sample.

Abnormal
Varicella zoster virus cultured from sample.

Cause of abnormal result
Presence of varicella zoster virus in sample.

Drugs, disorders and other factors that may alter results
Inadequate sampling can lead to a false-negative result.

VARICELLA ZOSTER VIRUS DNA POLYMERASE CHAIN REACTION
Description
Amplification and detection of a specific segment of varicella zoster virus DNA by polymerase chain reaction method from tissues or cerebrospinal and other body fluids.

Advantages/Disadvantages
Advantage: most sensitive, very specific method

Disadvantages:
- Very expensive, not widely available
- Used only in cases when other methods failed to provide valuable information

Abnormal
The specific DNA region can be amplified and detected from the sample.

Cause of abnormal result
Presence of varicella zoster virus DNA in sample.

CONSIDER CONSULT

- Patients with severe postherpetic neuralgic pain that does not respond to usual treatment may benefit from referral with a view to rhizotomy or sympathetic nerve block

IMMEDIATE ACTION

It is important, whenever possible, to begin antiretroviral treatment within 72h of the onset of rash because this speeds resolution of the rash and may reduce the likelihood of postherpetic neuralgia.

PATIENT AND CAREGIVER ISSUES
Patient or caregiver request

- **Will I have recurrent bouts of shingles?** Most people have herpes zoster only once
- **Is the condition contagious?** The virus that causes zoster can only be passed on to others who have not had chickenpox; they will then develop chickenpox, not zoster. This point is important particularly for pregnant women who have not been previously exposed (i.e. no history of having had chickenpox). It is much less contagious than chickenpox
- **Will I develop scars?** Infected blisters are more likely to cause scars

Health-seeking behavior

- **Have you waited too long before seeking treatment?** Since the initial symptoms of herpes zoster are often vague, delay in seeking treatment is likely. Such delay may limit the effectiveness of antiviral medication, which should ideally be given in the first 72h of an episode of herpes zoster
- **Have you used over-the-counter (OTC) analgesia?** Since the pain precedes the rash and the cause of the pain is often not recognized by the patient, the patient is likely to have used OTC analgesics
- **Have you used OTC treatments for the rash?** The patient may have used OTC creams or lotions for the rash in the hope that this will cure it

MANAGEMENT ISSUES
Goals

- Relieve pain
- Eradicate the rash and speed up recovery
- Prevent secondary bacterial infection
- Prevent or minimize postherpetic neuralgia

Management in special circumstances
COEXISTING DISEASE

Patients who are immunocompromised or immunosuppressed, including patients with HIV infection, are more likely to have severe disease and to develop postherpetic neuralgia. Such patients should therefore receive antiviral therapy and may require referral for intravenous antiviral therapy.

Causes of immunosuppression:

- HIV infection
- Organ transplantation
- Chemotherapy
- Lymphoid malignancy

COEXISTING MEDICATION

Patients who are taking immunosuppressant medication should receive antiviral therapy because they are more likely to have severe disease and develop postherpetic neuralgia.

SPECIAL PATIENT GROUPS

- Caution is needed in prescribing antiviral agents to pregnant patients
- Patients who are elderly (aged >60 years) are at greater risk of developing postherpetic neuralgia. Such patients should therefore receive antiviral therapy and possibly corticosteroids
- All three of the antivirals are excreted into breast milk, and their effect on infants is unknown. Although the risk appears to be very small, the risks and benefits of use in pregnant or breastfeeding women should be carefully considered

PATIENT SATISFACTION/LIFESTYLE PRIORITIES

- Most patients are likely to regard relief of pain as their main priority of treatment
- Advice on obtaining adequate rest may be difficult to heed for some patients

SUMMARY OF THERAPEUTIC OPTIONS
Choices

- First-choice drug in most patients is one of the oral antiviral agents that are effective against the herpes viruses (acyclovir, famciclovir, or valacyclovir). Early use (within 72h of onset of first symptoms) speeds up the process of reducing acute pain, rash, and inflammation. May also reduce the risk of postherpetic neuralgia or shorten its duration
- Prednisone for 2 weeks with reducing dose over a third week may be useful provided that there are no contraindications. It is especially useful in patients aged >50 years and is the treatment of choice in Ramsay Hunt syndrome (herpes zoster of the facial nerve)
- Analgesics (e.g. NSAIDs or codeine) should be used as indicated
- Wet compress with cold tap water to break vesicles
- Patients who develop disseminated zoster may need referral to a specialist for intravenous antiviral therapy. Consider referral for intravenous antiviral therapy in immunocompromised patients and immunosuppressed patients
- Some patients (especially transplant recipients and those with HIV infection) may develop acyclovir-resistant zoster. Such patients need referral to a specialist for intravenous foscarnet therapy
- Vidarabine is a topical antiviral agent used in the treatment of keratoconjunctivitis caused by herpes zoster
- Tricyclic antidepressants, particularly amitriptyline, are useful in the treatment of postherpetic neuralgia. This is an off-label indication
- Anticonvulsant medications (e.g. carbamazepine, clonazepam, phenytoin, topiramate) may also be tried in the case of postherpetic neuralgia not relieved by simple measures. This is an off-label indication and would usually be prescribed by a specialist once other medication has failed
- Patients who have severe pain that does not respond to usual treatment may benefit from referral to a specialist with a view to rhizotomy or sympathetic nerve block
- No real lifestyle restrictions are needed, but patients should avoid contact with children, pregnant women, and immunocompromised people

Guidelines

The American Academy of Family Physicians has published the following: Stankus SJ, Dlugopolski M, Packer D. Management of herpes zoster (shingles) and postherpetic neuralgia. Am Fam Physician 2000;61:2437–44 2447–8 [1]

Clinical pearls

- Oral therapy is adequate for most patients
- Care must be taken to provide intravenous therapy for those with disseminated zoster or who are at increased risk for such complication (i.e. immunocompromised for any reason)

Never

Never manage a patient who has involvement of the nasociliary branch of the ophthalmic division of the trigeminal nerve (manifested by vesicles on the tip and side of the nose, swelling of the eyelid, or conjunctivitis) without referring to a specialist dermatologist or ophthalmologist.

FOLLOW UP
Plan for review

- Patient monitoring is dependent on severity of symptoms and presence of coexisting disease
- Normally suggest return if rash has not subsided within 2–3 weeks or if pain relief is not adequate
- Re-evaluate if signs of CNS or pulmonary symptoms develop

Information for patient or caregiver

- Rash should subside within 2–3 weeks
- If other disorder arises, rash grows, or other unusual signs or symptoms (e.g. CNS, pulmonary) appear, the patient should come back to physician for review
- Warn the patient that pain during the rash and after it has subsided may be significant and should prompt return to physician for review
- Warn of potential for postherpetic neuralgia (suspect if pain persists for at least 4 weeks after the rash has disappeared)

DRUGS AND OTHER THERAPIES: DETAILS
Drugs
ACYCLOVIR
Antiviral treatment.

Dose

- 800mg five times daily for 7–10 days or until all external lesions are crusted
- Treatment should be started as early in the course of disease as possible, and preferably within 72h of the onset of symptoms

Efficacy

Effectively speeds up healing of the skin and prevents virus dissemination.

Risks/benefits

Risks:

- Use caution with hepatic and renal disease, dehydration, and electrolyte imbalance
- Use caution with pregnancy and nursing mothers
- Use caution in seizure disorders or other neurologic disease

Benefit: May reduce the risk of postherpetic neuralgia

Side effects and adverse reactions

- Central nervous system: headache, coma, confusion, seizures, hallucinations, tremor, dizziness, encephalopathy
- Gastrointestinal: nausea, vomiting, diarrhea, abdominal pain, elevated liver enzymes, hepatitis, anorexia, jaundice
- Genitourinary: crystalluria, renal toxicity
- Hematologic: leukopenia, thrombocytopenia, hemolytic uremic syndrome
- Skin: injection site reaction, phlebitis, alopecia, erythema, rash, pruritus, toxic epidermal necrolysis, Stevens–Johnson syndrome, photosensitivity, urticaria

Interactions (other drugs)
- Mycophenolate ■ Phenytoin, fosphenytoin ■ Probenecid ■ Zidovudine

Contraindications
- Children <2 years of age ■ Hypersensitivity or intolerance to acyclovir

Evidence
There is evidence that acyclovir is effective in the management of herpes zoster and the prevention of postherpetic neuralgia.
- In a double-blind, prospective trial, acyclovir was compared with placebo in the management of localized herpes zoster in immunocompetent patients. Acyclovir significantly shortened the time to full lesion crusting. No difference was noted between the groups for postherpetic neuralgia [2] *Level P*
- A systematic review found that postherpetic neuralgia prevalence at 6 months was significantly reduced when acyclovir treatment was given for at least 7 days during an acute attack of herpes zoster [3] *Level M*
- Another systematic review found that acyclovir treatment in general practice and inpatient settings did not significantly reduce pain secondary to postherpetic neuralgia at 6 months when compared with placebo [4] *Level M*

Acceptability to patient
- Generally well tolerated, although effect may not be as quick as patients would like or expect
- Dosing five times daily is difficult for some patients

Follow up plan
See patient again in 2–3 weeks or at end of treatment course.

Patient and caregiver information
Patient must be made aware of the importance of continuing the course for the full treatment period and of complying with the five times daily dosage regimen for the full benefit of the drug to be realized.

FAMCICLOVIR
Antiviral medication.
Dose
- 500mg three times daily for 7 days, started as early in the course of the disease as possible
- Reduce dose in renal impairment (if creatinine clearance is 40–59mL/min, give 500mg twice daily for 7 days; if creatinine clearance is 20–39mL/min, give 500mg once daily for 7 days)

Efficacy
- Effectively speeds up healing of the skin, prevents virus dissemination, and reduces acute pain
- Reduces the duration of postherpetic neuralgia

Risks/benefits
Risks:
- Use caution in children
- Use caution in renal disease
- Use caution in pregnancy and breastfeeding

Benefit: May reduce the duration of the disease and prevent complications

Side effects and adverse reactions
- Central nervous system: headache, dizziness, insomnia, somnolence, paresthesia
- Gastrointestinal: nausea, vomiting, diarrhea, constipation, abdominal pain, anorexia
- Respiratory: pharyngitis, sinusitis
- Skin: rash, pruritus

Interactions (other drugs)
- Cimetidine ▪ Digoxin ▪ Probenecid ▪ Theophylline

Contraindications
- Hypersensitivity or intolerance to famciclovir ▪ Impaired renal function
- Pregnancy category B

Evidence
Famciclovir may be effective in the treatment of herpes zoster and the reduction of pain duration.
A double-blind, randomized controlled trial (RCT) compared famciclovir (500mg and 750mg) with placebo in immunocompetent adults with herpes zoster. Famciclovir accelerated lesion healing and reduced the duration of viral shedding. Famciclovir recipients (both doses) had a significantly faster resolution of postherpetic neuralgia pain than placebo recipients [5] *Level P*

Acceptability to patient
- Generally well tolerated, although effect may not be as quick as patients would like or expect
- Dosage regimen (only once or three times daily) is an advantage over acyclovir

Follow up plan
See patient again in 2–3 weeks or at end of treatment course.

Patient and caregiver information
Patient must be made aware of the importance of continuing the course for the full treatment period and of complying with the dosage regimen for the full benefit of the drug to be realized.

VALACYCLOVIR
Antiviral medication.

Dose
- 1g three times daily for 7 days, started as early in the course of the disease as possible
- Reduce dose in renal impairment (if creatinine clearance is 30–49mL/min, give 1g twice daily for 7 days; if creatinine clearance is 10–29mL/min, give 1g once daily for 7 days)

Efficacy
- More effective than acyclovir for fast pain resolution and reducing the risk of postherpetic neuralgia
- Emerging in favor of acyclovir for its effectiveness against occurrence of postherpetic neuralgia

Risks/benefits
Risks:
- Use caution in renal and hepatic disease
- Use caution in the elderly and children
- Use caution in pregnancy and breastfeeding

Benefits:
- Pain control is achieved quickly
- Complications may be prevented

Side effects and adverse reactions
- Central nervous system: asthenia, headache, dizziness
- Gastrointestinal: nausea, vomiting, diarrhea, constipation, abdominal cramps, anorexia
- Hematologic: anemia, thrombocytopenia

Interactions (other drugs)
- **Cimetidine** ▪ **Probenecid**

Contraindications
- **Immunocompromised patients**

Evidence
There is evidence supporting valacyclovir use in the treatment of herpes zoster and postherpetic neuralgia.
- A double-blind RCT compared valacyclovir with famciclovir, commenced within 72 hours of rash appearance. Valacyclovir treatment was found to be comparable with famciclovir in accelerating the resolution of zoster-associated pain, rash healing, and postherpetic neuralgia [6] *Level P*
- An RCT compared valacyclovir (7– or 14-day treatment) with acyclovir (for 7 days) in the management of immunocompetent herpes zoster patients. Pain was reduced significantly faster in the valacyclovir-treated patients. Prevalence of pain secondary to postherpetic neuralgia was also reduced at 6 months in the valacyclovir group [7] *Level P*

Acceptability to patient
Generally well tolerated.

Follow up plan
See patient again in 2–3 weeks or at end of treatment course.

Patient and caregiver information
Patient must be made aware of the importance of continuing the course for the full treatment period and of complying with the dosage regimen for the full benefit of the drug to be realized.

PREDNISONE
Dose
60mg daily for 2 weeks followed by a reducing dose.

Efficacy
- Corticosteroids in combination with an antiviral agent probably reduce acute pain and improve quality of life in patients aged 50 years or older
- Its effect on postherpetic neuralgia is controversial
- Corticosteroids are considered especially useful in Ramsay Hunt syndrome (herpes zoster of the facial nerve)
- Corticosteroids in combination with an antiviral agent are also used for severe herpes zoster and when the eyes are affected or threatened

Risks/benefits
Risks:
- Use caution in congestive heart failure, diabetes mellitus

- Use caution in elderly
- Use caution in glaucoma, osteoporosis, hypertension (ophthalmic)
- Use caution in ulcerative colitis, renal disease, peptic ulcer

Benefit: Useful for patients with involvement of the trigeminal nerve

Side effects and adverse reactions
- Side effects are minimized by short duration of therapy
- Cardiovascular system: hypertension, thromboembolism
- Central nervous system: insomnia, euphoria, depression, psychosis, seizures
- Endocrine: adrenal suppression, impaired glucose tolerance, growth suppression in children
- Eyes, ears, nose, and throat: cataract, glaucoma, blurred vision
- Gastrointestinal: dyspepsia, peptic ulceration, esophagitis, oral candidiasis
- Musculoskeletal: proximal myopathy, osteoporosis
- Skin: delayed healing, acne, striae, fragile skin

Interactions (other drugs)
- Aminoglutethimide (increased clearance of prednisone) ■ Antidiabetics (hypoglycemic effect inhibited) ■ Antihypertensives (effects inhibited) ■ Barbiturates (increased clearance of prednisone) ■ Cardiac glycosides (toxicity increased) ■ Cholestyramine, colestipol (may reduce absorption of corticosteroids) ■ Clarithromycin, erythromycin, troleandomycin (may enhance steroid effect) ■ Cyclosporine (may increase levels of both drugs; may cause seizures) ■ Diuretics (effects inhibited) ■ Isoniazid (reduced plasma levels of isoniazid) ■ Ketoconazole ■ NSAIDs (increased risk of bleeding) ■ Oral contraceptives (enhanced effects of corticosteroids) ■ Rifampin (may inhibit hepatic clearance of prednisone) ■ Salicylates (increased clearance of salicylates) ■ Warfarin (alters clotting time)

Contraindications
- Systemic infection ■ Avoid live virus vaccines in those receiving immunosuppressive doses ■ History of tuberculosis ■ Cushing's syndrome ■ Recent myocardial infarction

Evidence
Prednisone may be effective in the management of acute herpes zoster when used in combination with antiviral medication.
- A double-blind RCT compared prednisone, acyclovir, and placebo in the management of localized herpes zoster in immunocompetent patients. Acyclovir plus prednisone was superior to placebo for speed of lesion healing, resolution of acute neuritis, and cessation of analgesic use. Acyclovir plus prednisone was not superior to either therapy alone or to placebo in the treatment of pain during the 6 months after disease onset [8] *Level P*
- An RCT compared acyclovir alone and in combination with prednisolone in the treatment of postherpetic neuralgia. No significant difference in the relief of symptoms was noted between the treatment groups [9] *Level P*

Acceptability to patient
- Short courses of prednisone are generally well tolerated
- Patients may be concerned because of popular conceptions of steroids as misused by athletes and because of possible side effects of long-term use of corticosteroids. Reassurance may be required
- Some patients may find the reducing dose confusing

Follow up plan
See patient again in 2–3 weeks or at end of course of treatment.

Patient and caregiver information
- Patient must be made aware of the importance of taking the full course of any prescribed antiviral medication as well as the prednisone
- Reasons for the reducing dose at the end of the treatment course should be explained
- The medication should not be stopped abruptly

NSAIDS
- Simple analgesics
- Many preparations available
- Available as OTC medication

Dose
Dose depends on specific drug.

Efficacy
Usually provides at least partial pain relief in herpes zoster.

Risks/benefits
Risks:
- Use caution in elderly
- Use caution in hepatic, renal, and cardiac failure
- Use caution in bleeding disorders
- There is no evidence that final outcome changed by NSAIDs

Benefits:
- Inexpensive
- Effective for mild to moderate pain

Side effects and adverse reactions
- Cardiovascular system: hypertension, peripheral edema, congestive heart failure
- Central nervous system: headache, dizziness, tinnitus, fever
- Gastrointestinal: anorexia, nausea, dyspepsia, peptic ulceration, bleeding
- Genitourinary: nephrotoxicity
- Hematologic: blood cell disorders
- Hypersensitivity: rashes, bronchospasm, angioedema
- Skin: pruritus, rash

Interactions (other drugs)
- Aminoglycosides ▪ Anticoagulants ▪ Antihypertensives ▪ Baclofen ▪ Corticosteroids
- Cyclosporine, tacrolimus ▪ Digoxin ▪ Diuretics ▪ Lithium ▪ Methotrexate
- Phenylpropanolamine ▪ Warfarin

Contraindications
- Peptic ulceration ▪ Hypersensitivity to NSAIDs ▪ Coagulation defects
- Severe renal or hepatic disease

Acceptability to patient
- Generally well tolerated
- Gastrointestinal side effects may be minimized by taking the drugs with milk or food

Follow up plan
Follow up to ensure pain relief is adequate.

Patient and caregiver information
Take with food or a glass of water.

CODEINE
- Many OTC preparations
- Often in combination with other analgesics

Dose
Adult: 15–60mg every 4h, as necessary.

Efficacy
Provides at least partial pain relief in most cases of herpes zoster.

Risks/benefits
Risks:
- Use caution in the elderly, pregnancy, and breastfeeding
- Use caution in renal and hepatic disease, Addison's disease, hypothyroidism, and gastrointestinal disease
- Use caution in recent head injury, in patients with a history of drug abuse, and in cardiac disease
- Small risk of dependency

Benefit: Provides adequate analgesia in the short-term

Side effects and adverse reactions
- Cardiovascular system: bradycardia, tachycardia, palpitations, hypotension
- Central nervous system: headache, drowsiness, dizziness, dysphoria, addiction
- Gastrointestinal: nausea and vomiting, constipation, diarrhea, paralytic ileus, abdominal cramps
- Respiratory: respiratory depression
- Skin: rashes, urticaria

Interactions (other drugs)
- Alcohol ■ Antidepressants (tricyclics and monamine oxidase inhibitors) ■ Antipsychotics ■ Anxiolytics and hypnotics ■ Cimetidine ■ Ciprofloxacin ■ Domperidone ■ Metoclopramide ■ Moclobemide ■ Ritonavir

Contraindications
- Colitis ■ Liver failure ■ Diarrhea secondary to poisoning or infectious diarrhea ■ Severe pulmonary disease or respiratory failure ■ Children

Evidence
There is conflicting evidence regarding the efficacy of codeine and related analgesics in postherpetic neuralgia.
- A double-blind RCT compared oxycodone with placebo in patients with postherpetic neuralgia. 67% of patients had a masked preference for oxycodone vs 11% for placebo [10] *Level P*
- A small double-blind RCT compared dextromethorphan (a codeine analog) with placebo for pain management in patients with postherpetic neuralgia. No significant benefit was found for the treatment group after 6 weeks of treatment [11] *Level P*

Acceptability to patient
- Usually tolerated
- Constipation and nausea are likely to be the most troublesome side effects for most patients

Follow up plan
Follow up to ensure pain relief is adequate.

Patient and caregiver information
- Codeine should only be used as an analgesic for a short period
- Nausea may be reduced by taking codeine with food

VIDARABINE
- Topical antiviral medication
- Usually prescribed by an ophthalmologist after specialist referral

Dose
- Initially, 0.5 inch of ointment to lower eyelid every 3h up to five times daily
- Once re-epithelialization has occurred, continue treatment twice daily for 7 days

Efficacy
Effective at promoting re-epithelialization in keratoconjunctivitis caused by herpes zoster.

Risks/benefits
Risks:
- Associated with negative adverse effects with long-term use, including liver problems and hypertension
- Use caution with impaired liver function

Benefit: The period of infection and the risk of complications are reduced

Side effects and adverse reactions
- Central nervous system: headache, insomnia
- Eyes, ears, nose, and throat: burning, photophobia, pain, stinging, temporary visual haze
- Gastrointestinal: nausea, vomiting, carbohydrate intolerance

Interactions (other drugs)
- There are no known interactions with topical application

Contraindications
- Systemic fungal infections ■ Known hypersensitivity to the drug

Acceptability to patient
Generally acceptable.

Follow up plan
Follow up by ophthalmologist is required.

Patient and caregiver information
Continue entire course of medication as prescribed.

AMITRIPTYLINE
- Tricyclic antidepressant
- This is an off-label indication

Dose
- 50–100mg before bed; dose can be increased gradually up to 200–300mg until side effects become intolerable
- Treatment should be continued for 3 months after pain of postherpetic neuralgia has ceased

Efficacy
- Can be effective at relieving the constant pain of postherpetic neuralgia
- The pain relief is independent of any effect on mood

Risks/benefits
Risks:
- May have withdrawal symptoms if stopped abruptly
- Should be discontinued several days before surgery
- May cause significant drowsiness that the patient must adapt to regarding dosing schedule and daytime 'hangover' drowsiness
- Patients often gain significant weight, even on low doses
- Can achieve symptom relief in lower doses than when used to treat depression; this can help reduce side effects and enhance compliance
- Use caution in narrow-angle glaucoma, hepatic and renal disease, Parkinson's disease, pre-existing seizure disorders, cardiac disease
- Use caution in carbamazepine hypersensitivity, respiratory depression, asthma, hypo – or hyperthyroidism, and diabetes mellitus
- Use caution in the elderly

Benefit: May relieve chronic pain when other medications are ineffective

Side effects and adverse reactions
- Cardiovascular system: ventricular tachycardia, orthostatic hypotension, palpitations, hypertension, myocardial infarction, stroke, congestive heart failure, PR and/or QT prolongation
- Central nervous system: drowsiness, sedation, dizziness, anxiety, confusion, tremor, pseudoparkinsonism, seizures, EEG changes, neuroleptic malignant syndrome
- Eyes, ears, nose, and throat: visual disturbances, mydriasis, dry mouth
- Gastrointestinal: nausea, vomiting, diarrhea, constipation, abdominal pain, dry mouth, jaundice, anorexia
- Genitourinary: sexual dysfunction, breast enlargement, galactorrhea, gynecomastia

Interactions (other drugs)
- Anticonvulsants (barbiturates, carbamazepine) ■ Antimuscarinics (atropine, phenothiazines, H$_1$ antagonists, other tricyclic antidepressants, clozapine, cyclobenzaprine disopyramide) ■ Cimetidine ■ Cisapride ■ Clonidine ■ Cocaine ■ Central nervous system depressants (e.g. entacapone, hypnotics, anxiolytics, ethanol, sedatives) ■ Disulfiram ■ Dofetilide ■ Guanabenz, guanfacine ■ Levodopa ■ Opiate agonists ■ Monoamine oxidase inhibitors ■ Selective serotonin reuptake inhibitors ■ St. John's Wort, Valerian ■ Sympathomimetics ■ Thyroid hormone ■ Tramadol

Contraindications
- Weigh risk and benefits of use in pregnant women or in women wishing to become pregnant ■ Acute recovery phase of myocardial infarction ■ Avoid using together with monoamine oxidase inhibitors ■ Dofetilide ■ Cisapride ■ Intravenous administration ■ Decreased gastrointestinal motility

Evidence
Amitriptyline may be effective for the management of postherpetic neuralgia pain.

- A double-blind RCT compared amitriptyline with placebo in the management of patients over 60 years of age with herpes zoster. Treatment with amitriptyline (commenced within 48h of rash appearance and continued for 90 days) was associated with an insignificant reduction in the prevalence of postherpetic neuralgia at 6 months [12] *Level P*
- A systematic review found that tricyclic antidepressants given for 3–6 weeks to patients with postherpetic neuralgia significantly reduced pain [13] *Level M*
- A small randomized, double-blind, crossover trial compared amitriptyline with nortriptyline in patients with postherpetic neuralgia. 67.7% of patients had at least a good response to amitriptyline or nortriptyline. There was no significant difference noted in efficacy between the two drugs. Adverse effects were more common with amitriptyline [14] *Level P*

Acceptability to patient
- Dry mouth and drowsiness are particularly likely to be problematic for patients
- The long time required for any treatment benefits may also limit compliance
- Must explain that the treatment is not for depression in this case

Follow up plan
Follow up to ensure adequate analgesia is achieved and side effects are being tolerated.

Patient and caregiver information
- Therapeutic effects may take a few weeks
- Driving may need to be avoided
- Avoid alcohol

Other therapies
WET COMPRESS
A wet compress with cold tap water applied for 20–40 min four to eight times daily.

Efficacy
Helps break vesicles.

Risks/benefits
Benefit: may provide some relief and speed resolution of the rash.

Acceptability to patient
Generally well accepted.

Follow up plan
Review patient in 2–3 weeks.

LIFESTYLE
- No real restrictions are needed, but patients should avoid contact with children, pregnant women, and immunocompromised people
- No special diet is required except in cases of malnourishment

ACCEPTABILITY TO PATIENT
Dietary modification may be difficult for some patients. Assistance may be required.

PATIENT AND CAREGIVER INFORMATION
Information on healthy eating or meal delivery services may be necessary for some patients (e.g. elderly patients who are undernourished).

EFFICACY OF THERAPIES

- Antiviral therapies may be useful in allowing faster rash healing and pain control if instituted within 48–72h of the onset of signs and symptoms. They also reduce the risk of developing postherpetic neuralgia
- Immunocompromised patients may not be treated as effectively with oral antiviral therapies and may require intravenous medication
- Corticosteroids and amitriptyline may be useful in pain relief and may improve quality of life
- In elderly patients and patients with eye involvement, very early treatment has been shown to be especially effective in reducing the occurrence and/or severity of postherpetic neuralgia

Evidence

- Acyclovir significantly reduces the time to full lesion crusting in herpes zoster infection [2] *Level P*
- Postherpetic neuralgia prevalence at 6 months may be significantly reduced when acyclovir treatment is given for at least 7 days during an acute attack of herpes zoster [3] *Level M*
- Famciclovir has been shown to accelerate lesion healing and reduce the duration of viral shedding. Famciclovir may significantly accelerate the resolution of postherpetic neuralgia pain when compared with placebo [5] *Level P*
- Valacyclovir treatment (commenced within 72h of rash appearance) has been found to be comparable with famciclovir in accelerating the resolution of zoster-associated pain, rash healing, and postherpetic neuralgia [6] *Level P*
- Valacyclovir has been shown to be superior to acyclovir for the speed of pain reduction. Prevalence of pain secondary to postherpetic neuralgia was also reduced at 6 months with valacyclovir [7] *Level P*
- Acyclovir plus prednisone may be superior to placebo for speed of lesion healing, resolution of acute neuritis, and cessation of analgesic use [8] *Level P*
- Early treatment of herpes zoster in elderly patients with amitriptyline (commenced within 48h of rash appearance and continued for 90 days) has been associated with an insignificant reduction in the prevalence of postherpetic neuralgia at 6 months [12] *Level P*
- A systematic review found that tricyclic antidepressants given for 3–6 weeks to patients with postherpetic neuralgia significantly reduced pain [13] *Level M*

Review period
Three weeks.

PROGNOSIS

- More than 70% of patients show full recovery
- Recovery can take 2–3 weeks in children and younger patients, and sometimes as much as 3–4 weeks in older (aged >50 years) patients

Clinical pearls

- Herpes zoster is contagious. Prevention of exposure of pregnant women without prior chickenpox should occur
- Modest extension across the midline or into adjacent ipsilateral dermatomes is common and does not rule out the diagnosis
- More extensive blistering suggests alternative diagnosis, although disseminated zoster needs to considered
- Prevention of secondary bacterial infection is important and will reduce risk of scarring

Therapeutic failure

- Failure of antiviral therapy is rare
- Therapy may not prevent postherpetic neuralgia
- Herpes zoster that fails to respond to antiviral treatment or that does not resolve spontaneously should prompt referral to a dermatologist or other appropriate specialist for further assessment and treatment
- Some patients (especially HIV-infected patients and transplant recipients) may develop acyclovir-resistant herpes zoster. Such patients should be referred; foscarnet is likely to be effective

Recurrence

- Most people have herpes zoster only once
- If recurrence occurs, it is most likely to be in the form of postherpetic neuralgia

Deterioration

- Deterioration should prompt a search for a predisposing factor such as immunocompromise
- Common causes of immunosuppression include HIV infection, lymphoid malignancy, and immunosuppressive treatment

COMPLICATIONS

- Postherpetic neuralgia occurs in 50% of those aged >60 years with herpes zoster; it rarely occurs in children or younger adults. It is said to occur when the pain of herpes zoster persists for >30 days
- Ocular involvement with facial herpes zoster
- Meningoencephalitis in elderly
- Secondary infection of the vesicles with *Staphylococcus aureus* or *Streptococcus pyogenes*
- Ramsay Hunt syndrome

PREVENTION

The elderly, children, pregnant women, and immunocompromised people should avoid contact with a person who has shingles.

MODIFY RISK FACTORS
Lifestyle and wellness
DIET
Dietary advice may be useful in poorly nourished patients.

PREVENT RECURRENCE
Consider symptomatic ganglionic block to avoid postherpetic neuralgia.

ASSOCIATIONS

American Academy of Dermatology
930 N. Meacham Road
PO Box 4014
Schaumburg, IL 60168-4014
Tel: 847-330-0230 or 888-462-DERM (3376)
Fax: 847-330-0050
http://www.aad.org

National Center for Infectious Diseases (NCID)
Centers for Disease Control and Prevention
1600 Clifton Road
Atlanta, GA 30333
Tel: 404-639-3311
Fax: 404-639 3120
http://www.cdc.gov

KEY REFERENCES

- Armstrong D, Cohen J. Infectious disease. Philadelphia: Mosby, 1999
- Furuta Y, Ohtani F, Zkwabata H, et al. High prevalence of varciella-zoster virus reactivation in herpes simplex virus seronegative patients with acute peripheral facial palsy. Clin Infect Dis 2000;30:529–33
- Galil K, Choo PW, Donahue JG, Platt R. The sequelae of herpes zoster. Arch Intern Med 1997;157:1209–13
- Gilden DH. Herpes zoster with postherpetic neuralgia: persisting pain and frustration. N Engl J Med 1994;330:932–4
- Gilden DH, Kleinschmidt-De Masters BK, LaGuardia JL, et al. Neurologic complications of the reactivation of varicella-zoster virus. N Engl J Med 2000;342:636–45
- Whitley RJ. Varicella-zoster virus. In: Mandell, Douglas, Bennet, eds. Principles and practice of infectious diseases, 5th edn. Philadelphia: Churchill Livingstone, 2000, p1580–5
- Wood MJ, Johnson RW, McKendrick MW, et al. A randomized trial of acyclovir for 7 or 21 days with or without prednisolone for the treatment of acute herpes zoster. N Engl J Med 1994;330:898–900

Evidence references

1 Stankus SJ, Dlugopolski M, Packer D. Management of herpes zoster (shingles) and postherpetic neuralgia. Am Fam Physician 2000;61:2437–44, 2447–8
2 Wassilew SW, Reimlinger S, Nasemann T, Jones D. Oral acyclovir for herpes zoster: a double-blind controlled trial in normal subjects. Br J Dermatol 1987 Oct;117(4):495–501. Medline
3 Jackson JL, Gibbons R, Meyer G, et al. The effect of treating herpes zoster with oral acyclovir in preventing postherpetic neuralgia: a meta-analysis. Arch Intern Med 1997;157:909–912. Reviewed in: Clinical Evidence 2001;5:554–562
4 Lancaster T, Silagi C, Gray S. Primary care management of acute herpes zoster: systematic review of evidence from randomized controlled trials. Br J Gen Pract 1995;45:39–45. Reviewed in: Clinical Evidence 2001;5:554–562
5 Tyring S, Barbarash RA, Nahlik JE, et al. Famciclovir for the treatment of acute herpes zoster: effects on acute disease and postherpetic neuralgia. A randomized, double-blind, placebo-controlled trial. Collaborative Famciclovir Herpes Zoster Study Group. Ann Intern Med 1995;123(2):89–96. Medline
6 Tyring SK, Beutner KR, Tucker BA, et al. Antiviral therapy for herpes zoster: randomized, controlled clinical trial of valaciclovir and famciclovir therapy in immunocompetent patients 50 years and older. Arch Fam Med 2000;9:863–9. Reviewed in: Clinical Evidence 2001;5:554–562
7 Beutner KR, Friedman DJ, Forszpaniak C, et al. Valaciclovir compared with acyclovir for improved therapy for herpes zoster in immunocompetent adults. Antimicrob Agents Chemother 1995;39:1546–53. Reviewed in: Clinical Evidence 2001;5:554–562
8 Whitley RJ, Weiss H, Gnann JW Jr, et al. Acyclovir with and without prednisone for the treatment of herpes zoster: a randomized, placebo-controlled trial. The National Institute of Allergy and Infectious Diseases Collaborative Antiviral Study Group. Ann Intern Med 1996;125:376–383 Reviewed in Clinical Evidence 2001;5:554–562

9   Wood MJ, Johnson RW, McKendrick MW, et al. A randomized trial of acyclovir for 7 days or 21 days with and
    without prednisolone for treatment of acute herpes zoster. N Engl J Med 1994;330:896–900. Reviewed in Clinical
    Evidence 2001;5:554–562
10 Watson CP, Vernich L, Chipman M, Reed K. Nortriptyline versus amitriptyline in postherpetic neuralgia: a
    randomized trial. Neurology 1998;51(4):1166–71. Medline
11 Nelson KA, Park KM, Robinovitz E, et al. High-dose oral dextromethorphan versus placebo in painful diabetic
    neuropathy and postherpetic neuralgia. Neurology 1997;48:1212–1218. Reviewed in: Clinical Evidence
    2001;5:554–562
12 Bowsher D. The effects of pre-emptive treatment of postherpetic neuralgia with amitriptyline: a randomized,
    double-blind, placebo-controlled trial. J Pain Symptom Manage 1997;13:327–31. Reviewed in Clinical Evidence
    2001;5:554–562
13 Volmink J, Lancaster T, Gray S, et al. Treatments for postherpetic neuralgia: a systematic review of randomized
    controlled trials. Fam Pract 1996;13:84–91. Reviewed in Clinical Evidence 2001;5:554–562
14 Watson CP, Babul N. Efficacy of oxycodone in neuropathic pain: a randomized trial in postherpetic neuralgia.
    Neurology 1998;50:1837–1841. Reviewed in: Clinical Evidence 2001;5:554–562

FAQS
Question 1
Is herpes zoster contagious?

ANSWER 1
Yes. Particular care must be taken to prevent infection in pregnant women.

Question 2
Does recurrence clinch the diagnosis of herpes simplex?

ANSWER 2
Rarely, herpes zoster can recur, although generally herpes simplex virus is much more likely. A direct fluorescent antibody testing culture can distinguish between the two.

Question 3
Will the lesions scar?

ANSWER 3
In most cases, without secondary bacterial infection, no. However, the likelihood increases with, for example, secondary infection and vigorous scratching.

Question 4
How severe can the pain of zoster be?

ANSWER 4
The pain can be quite severe, both acutely and chronically as postherpetic neuralgia. Acutely, this pain can mimic a surgical abdomen, renal colic, or myocardial infarction. Chronically, surgical transection of affected nerves may be required.

CONTRIBUTORS
Randolph L Pearson, MD
Seth R Stevens, MD
Rolland P Gyulai, MD, PhD

HIDRADENITIS SUPPURATIVA

DESCRIPTION

- Chronic suppurative disease of the apocrine glands
- The disease is caused by a defect in the terminal follicular epithelium
- Affects axillary, anogenital, breast, and scalp areas
- Disabling disease manifested by abscesses, fistulas, and scarring
- Unknown etiology
- Spontaneous resolution is rare
- Medical treatment is not definitive
- Wide local excision of the diseased skin is the treatment of choice

URGENT ACTION

Overwhelming sepsis in immunocompromised patients will require urgent intravenous antibiotics.

KEY! DON'T MISS!

Nonmelanoma skin cancers (particularly squamous cell carcinomas) can arise from hidradrenitis suppurativa-affected skin, so close follow up is required for all patients.

BACKGROUND

ICD9 CODE
705.83 Hidradenitis suppurativa

SYNONYMS
- Apocrine acne
- Acne inversa
- Verneuil's disease
- Pyodermia fistulans sinifica

CARDINAL FEATURES
- Suppurative disease of apocrine glands with inflammation of the terminal hair follicles of the intertriginal areas
- Affects axillary, anogenital, breast, and scalp areas
- Disabling disease manifested by abscesses, fistulas and scarring
- Disease is common but often the right diagnosis is missed
- Unknown etiology
- Spontaneous resolution is rare
- Medical treatment is not definitive
- Radical surgical wide excision is the treatment of choice

CAUSES
Common causes
- Etiology is not fully understood
- Excessive perspiration occurs in the obese and with athletes, which may lead to the apocrine glands becoming blocked (apocrine follicular occlusion)
- Secretions trapped in the glands force perspiration into the surrounding tissue
- This leads to inflammation and infection (infundibulofolliculitis)
- The primary event may, however, be infundibulofolliculitis with secondary involvement of the apocrine and eccrine sweat glands
- Over one-third of patients have a positive family history
- The clinical genetics of hidradenitis suppurativa are complex
- Genetic factors associated with HLA-A, HLA-B, or HLA-DRB1 alleles do not contribute significantly to hidradenitis suppurativa
- A familial form of hidradenitis suppurativa with autosomal inheritance has been reported
- It is likely to be a polygenic disease

Contributory or predisposing factors
- Use of chemical irritants, including deodorants and antiperspirants, seems to be a potential causal factor
- The disease is more common in women, and the use of the oral contraceptive pill and menstruation seem to be associated with both disease onset and recurrence. This suggests that hormonal factors may play a role
- The condition has a tendency to subside after menopause
- Disease activity may be related to stress
- Cigarette smoking has been implicated as a major triggering factor for hidradenitis suppurativa

EPIDEMIOLOGY
Incidence and prevalence
Relatively common skin disease but its diagnosis is often missed.

PREVALENCE

Actual prevalence not fully known because of missed diagnoses. Studies estimate the prevalence to be 10–40 per 1000 in industrialized countries.

Demographics

AGE

Average age of onset is in the second to third decade.

GENDER

Females are more commonly affected than males.

GENETICS

- Over one-third of patients have a positive family history
- The clinical genetics of hidradenitis suppurativa are complex
- Genetic factors associated with HLA-A, HLA-B or HLA-DRB1 alleles do not contribute significantly to hidradenitis suppurativa
- A familial form of hidradenitis suppurativa with autosomal inheritance has been reported
- It is likely to be a polygenic disease

DIFFERENTIAL DIAGNOSIS
Candidiasis
Candidiasis is a common skin infection due to candidial fungal species.

FEATURES
- Affects skin and oral mucosa
- Skin candidiasis affects warm moist areas (e.g. axilla and perineum)
- The rash consists of well-demarcated brick-red areas with peripheral scaling and satellite lesions
- Oral candidiasis produces white patches on the buccal mucosa
- Antifungal topical agents are effective, including nystatin

Cellulitis
Cellulitis is an acute infection of the skin usually caused by bacterial agents.

FEATURES
- Skin infection leading to erythema, warming, and tenderness of affected area
- Systemic features include fever, malaise, and circulatory shock
- Cellulitis can spread rapidly
- Cellulitis can be indolent in venous insufficiency
- Precipitating factors include immunosuppression, poor hygiene, recent surgery, and diabetes mellitus
- Oral antibiotics are indicated

Folliculitis
Folliculitis is an inflammation of the hair follicle as a result of infection, chemical irritants, or physical injury.

FEATURES
- Painful yellow pustules with a central hair
- Surrounding erythema
- Occurs on the face due to physical trauma of shaving (sycosis barbae)
- *Staphylococcus, Klebsiella, Proteus*, and *Candida* species are common causal agents
- Correct treatment depends on the causal agent, and involves topical and oral antibacterial and antifungal agents
- Sycosis barbae can be difficult to cure, and requires prolonged treatment and shaving with a clean razor

Carbuncle
Two or more confluent furuncles (boils) which are circumscribed perifollicular staphylococcal abscesses.

FEATURES
- Process begins in hair follicles
- Lesions undergo central necrosis and often rupture
- Drainage is purulent
- Predisposing factors include alcoholism, malnutrition, blood dyscrasias, disorders of neutrophil function, immunosuppression, AIDS, and diabetes

Tuberculosis

Infection of the skin caused by *Mycobacterium tuberculosis* or *M. bovis*. The main features of tuberculosis are as follows.

FEATURES

- Can be from an exogenous or endogenous source (pulmonary tuberculosis)
- Has a variety of clinical presentations from ulceration to nodules
- Associated or exacerbated by decreased immunity
- Requires intensive treatment with a multidrug regimen

Actinomycosis

A chronic, suppurative, granulomatous and fibrosing infection caused primarily by the bacterium *Actinomyces israelii*.

FEATURES

- Infection often spreads to adjacent tissues, forming cutaneous sinus tracts
- Associated with low-grade fever and mildly elevated white blood cell count
- Often presents in the cervicofacial region, called 'lumpy jaw'
- Treated with long-term high-dose penicillin and surgical debridement

Tularemia

Tularemia is an uncommon zoonotic infection caused by *Francisella tularensis*.

FEATURES

- Often affects the skin, in an ulcerative form
- Ulcers may be solitary or multiple
- Wild rabbits are the major source of infection from animals
- Biting ticks are the chief vectors, responsible for 90% of human infections in North America
- Often associated with local lymphadenopathy
- Streptomycin remains the treatment of choice

Cat scratch disease

Cat scratch disease is a cutaneous infection caused by *Bartonella henselae*.

FEATURES

- A benign and self-limited disease, lasting 6–12 weeks
- Presents with regional lymphadenopathy
- Skin lesions occur 3–10 days after primary cutaneous inoculation
- Commonly occurs following scratch from a kitten
- Usually no antimicrobial therapy is required

Lymphogranuloma venereum

Lymphogranuloma venereum is a systemic disease caused by the sexual transmission of specific serotypes of *Chlamydia trachomatis*.

FEATURES

- Presents as a small painless genital lesion after incubation period of 3–30 days
- Progresses into the inguinal syndrome consisting of painful inguinal lymphadenopathy
- Complications include fistula formation, fibrosis, lymphedema, and resultant elephantiasis
- Caused by serotypes L1, L2, L3 of *C. trachomatis*
- Treatment of choice is oral doxycycline

Granuloma inguinale

Anogenital and inguinal ulcerogranulomatous lesions caused by sexual transmission of *Calymmatobacterium granulomatis*. The main features of granuloma inguinale are as follows.

FEATURES
- Occurs primarily in tropical and subtropical regions of the world
- Genital nodules often erode to form painless ulcerations with a beefy red base
- Ulcerations spread by direct extension, giving the appearance of 'kissing lesions'
- Scarring and fibrosis may be prominent
- Treatment of choice is oral tetracycline

SIGNS & SYMPTOMS
Signs
- Multiple papules and pustules leading to recurrent boils
- Occurs in skin containing sweat glands, including the axillae, groin, perineum, breasts, and scalp
- The lesions are tender and can lead to restricted movement of the affected area
- Complications are common, including abscesses, fistulas, and scarring
- The disease has a significant clinical and social impact on the patient's life

Symptoms
- Patients may be embarrassed to present for medical advice due to the nature and site of the lesions, often in the groin and axillae
- Painful lesions, boils, and pustules in sweat gland areas, especially the axillae, groin, and perineum
- The lesions are recurrent and multiple, leading to chronicity
- The boils are painful and can lead to restriction of movement
- Boils can develop monthly but some patients can have long remissions
- Patients complain of the cosmetic impact of the disease and its complications, including abscesses, fistula formation, and scarring
- Extensive disease can prevent the patients from leading their normal working and social lives

ASSOCIATED DISORDERS
- Crohn's disease, an inflammatory bowel disease
- Spondyloarthropathy; case reports link this disease with hidradenitis suppurativa
- Dowling-Degos disease; the follicular occlusion of this disease may predipose to hidradenitis suppurativa
- Acne conglobata and dissecting cellulitis of the scalp, both of which are also caused by abnormal follicular occlusion

KEY! DON'T MISS!
Nonmelanoma skin cancers (particularly squamous cell carcinomas) can arise from hidradenitis suppurativa-affected skin, so close follow up is required for all patients.

INVESTIGATION OF THE PATIENT
Direct questions to patient
Q **How long have you noticed these lesions?** The patients may be embarrassed to present for medical advice due to the nature and site of the lesions, often in the genitalia and axillae.
Q **What areas of your body are affected?** The disease is classically in the axillae, groin, perineum, breasts, and scalp.
Q **How many recurrences of these boils have you had?** The disease is chronic, leading to multiple recurrences.

Q How has your life been affected? The disease can prevent the patients from leading their normal working and social lives.

Contributory or predisposing factors

Q Do you use deodorants and antiperspirants? Cosmetic and hygiene products are associated with the disease.

Q Do you find recurrences are linked with your monthly cycle? Menstruation is linked with recurrences of the disease.

Q Are you on any medication? The oral contraceptive pill is linked with the disease.

Q Are you athletic or do you sweat profusely? Excess perspiration is a potential causal agent of the infundofolliculitis.

Q Do you smoke? Smoking may be associated with exacerbations.

Family history

Q Do any of your family members suffer from this disease? Over one-third of patients have a positive family history.

Examination

- What are the nature of the lesions? The lesions include pustules and boils
- Are the lesions tender? The lesions are very tender, causing the patient much distress and restriction of movement
- Is there evidence of chronicity? Old scarring is characteristic of this disease
- What areas of the body are affected? The disease only affects apocrine glands, so it is evident in the axillae, groin, perineum, breasts, and scalp
- Are complications of the disease present? Abscesses, fistula, and scarring
- Are there any sinister lesions in the affected skin? Nonmelanoma skin carcinomas are associated with hidradenitis suppurativa

Summary of investigative tests

- Culture of exudate from boils or abscesses to determine the infective agent (if present) and its antibiotic sensitivity
- Skin biopsy of the affected area is mandatory for diagnosis
- Histology will be diagnostic of hidradenitis suppurativa
- Histology of the skin disease reveals the following: poral occlusion, epithelial cysts, apocrinitis, and epidermis-lined sinuses surrounded by dense plasma cell infiltration
- Complications, including abscesses, diffuse dermal inflammation, and pyogenic granuloma, will be confirmed

DIAGNOSTIC DECISION

These patients usually have severe disease and are fairly easily recognizable. Those with limited disease pose diagnostic dilemmas. The main decision point is distinguishing from recurrent, widespread carbuncles/ furuncles.

CLINICAL PEARLS

Patients are frequently embarrassed by hidradenitis suppurativa; thus the physician must be assertive to examine all pertinent areas to determine extent and nature of the disease.

THE TESTS
Body fluids
CULTURE OF EXUDATE
Description
- Culture of any exudate collected from the boils or abscesses
- The pus has to be collected and sent to a laboratory
- The laboratory will determine if an infective agent is present and its antibiotic sensitivity

Advantages/Disadvantages
Advantages:
- Easy to obtain the exudate
- Useful in determining the correct antibiotic treatment

Disadvantages:
- Culture growth and sensitivity testing takes >48h
- Not diagnostic of hidradenitis suppurativa

Abnormal
- Pathogenic and saphrophytic bacterial growth
- Often multiple pathogens present, especially staphyloccocal and streptococcal bacteria

Cause of abnormal result
Infected skin lesion characteristic of hidradenitis suppurativa.

Biopsy

SKIN BIOPSY
Description
- Skin biopsy of the lesion is essential
- Dermatology referral may be required to perform the procedure
- A cylindrical punch biopsy removes a fusiform excision of skin spanning the border between the clinically normal and abnormal areas
- The punch biopsy tool is pushed into the skin with a twisting action to cut a small core of skin and underlying fat
- The biopsy is then sent for histologic analysis using microscopy

Advantages/Disadvantages
Advantages:
- Easy to obtain and quick to perform
- Diagnostic of hidradenitis suppurativa

Disadvantages:
- Biopsy procedure is blind and may damage underlying structures such as blood vessels
- Can be painful and cause scarring so the patient must give full consent

Abnormal
- Histology of the skin disease reveals the following: poral occlusion, epithelial cysts, apocrinitis and epidermis-lined sinuses surrounded by dense plasma cell infiltration
- Complications, including abscesses, diffuse dermal inflammation, and pyogenic granuloma, will be confirmed

Cause of abnormal result
Hidradenitis suppurativa.

TREATMENT

CONSIDER CONSULT
- All cases of hidradenitis suppurativa should be referred to a dermatologist, as the disease is chronic and difficult to treat
- Surgical treatment is indicated in this disease because wide local excision is the treatment of choice

IMMEDIATE ACTION
- Overwhelming sepsis in an immunocompromised patient can be fatal
- Immediate intravenous antibiotics and systemic fluids are required

PATIENT AND CAREGIVER ISSUES
Patient or caregiver request
- **Is the treatment curative?** Medical treatment will not cure hidradenitis suppurativa, but surgical excision of the diseased skin or apocrine glands affords good cure rates
- **Do I need to take antibiotics?** Patients must be informed that repeated courses of antibiotics are necessary, especially in cases of severe disease with constant successions of new lesions
- **Will repeated courses of antibiotics affect my health?** Antibiotic compliance is important to treat the recurrent boils and should not adversely affect the patient's health
- **Does the steroid cream cause side effects?** Thinning of the skin and hypersensitivity are the main side effects. Since the steroid is used topically, it is unlikely to cause any systemic side effects

Health-seeking behavior
- The patient may have tried creams prior to seeking medical help, especially as the lesions are in potentially embarrassing areas of the body
- The lesions may be advanced at presentation due to the delay in seeking medical advice
- This can lead to fibrosis and severe scarring of the affected skin

MANAGEMENT ISSUES
Goals
- To treat the disease and reduce its impact on the patient's life
- Medical treatment has limited therapeutic effect
- Wide local excision is indicated for recurrent disease
- Treatment is needed to prevent complications

Management in special circumstances

COEXISTING DISEASE
- Diabetes may cause complications of hidradenitis suppurativa
- Isotretinoin causes glucose levels to fluctuate

SPECIAL PATIENT GROUPS
Pregnancy will contraindicate certain medications, including isotretinoin.

SUMMARY OF THERAPEUTIC OPTIONS
Choices
- Medical and surgical treatment are indicated for hidradenitis suppurativa
- Medical treatment can reduce recurrence and complications but is not curative
- Medical treatment can control the disease allowing for surgery
- Isotretinoin decreases sebaceous gland size and sebum production

- Topical and intralesional steroids (triamcinolone) treat inflammation by suppressing the migration of polymorphic leukocytes
- Antibiotics (tetracycline, minocycline) will treat boils and abscesses
- Surgery is usually indicated because spontaneous cure of the disease is rare. Wide local excision with split-thickness grafts can remove the diseased skin; alternatively, apocrine glands can be removed with fat, leaving dermis and epidermis relatively intact
- Radiotherapy has been used to good effect in hidradenitis suppurativa
- Laser therapy can be used to treat lesions of hidradenitis suppurativa

Clinical pearls
Early referral for surgical treatment should be made for any patient with disease that does not respond readily to oral agents.

FOLLOW UP
- Spontaneous resolution is rare
- Progressive disability due to recurrent succession of boils and complications
- Therefore, careful follow up is imperative, especially if the clinical and social impact of the disease is to be minimized

Plan for review
- Medical and surgical treatment requires close follow up
- Patient review enables the disease to be monitored for remission or relapse
- Complications are frequent and patients should be examined for abscesses, fistulas, new skin lesions, and the effects of scarring

Information for patient or caregiver
- Hidradenitis suppurativa is a chronic disease which needs careful follow up
- Treatment compliance is important to prevent relapses and complications
- Surgery will probably be required to prevent repeated relapses and complications

DRUGS AND OTHER THERAPIES: DETAILS
Drugs
ISOTRETINOIN
- Reduces the number of relapses
- Exact mechanism not known
- Decreases sebaceous gland size and inhibits gland activity, which reduces sebum production
- Side effects require dermatologist referral and follow up
- Expensive medication
- Full patient consent must be obtained prior to commencement of treatment

Dose
0.5–2mg/kg given in two divided doses daily for 15–20 weeks.

Efficacy
- More effective for mild disease than severe disease
- Clearance rates are less than 25%
- Isotretinoin can be used to reduce skin lesions prior to surgery

Risks/benefits
Risks:
- Can aggravate any ocular involvement
- Mucocutaneous irritation
- Pseudotumor cerebri

- Diminished night vision
- Musculoskeletal symptoms
- Hyperlipidemia

Benefits:
- Useful in severe cases and when standard antibiotic treatments are not effective
- Improvement in acne

Side effects and adverse reactions
- Eyes, ears, nose, and throat: conjunctivitis
- Gastrointestinal: abdominal pain
- Hematologic: hematuria, increase in serum lipids
- Musculoskeletal: arthralgias/myalgias
- Skin: dryness of skin, epidermal fragility, may exacerbate ocular involvement at higher doses, cheilitis/drying of mucosal membranes

Interactions (other drugs)
- **Vitamin A (enhances toxic effects)** ■ **Tetracycline, minocycline (associated with pseudotumor cerebri or papilledema)**

Contraindications
- **Pregnancy and breast-feeding** ■ **Renal or hepatic impairment** ■ **Hypervitaminosis A** ■ **Hyperlipidemia**

Acceptability to patient
- Effective treatment for hidradenitis suppurativa
- Isotretinoin causes severe dryness of the mucous membranes and conjunctiva

Follow up plan
- Blood tests are required while the patient is on isotretinoin: CBC with differential, platelet count, serum triglycerides (baseline and biweekly for 4 weeks), and liver enzymes
- The patient must be warned not to become pregnant while taking the medication. This is of paramount importance since isotretinoin is severely teratogenic, pregnancy category X

Patient and caregiver information
- Full patient consent must be obtained prior to commencement of treatment
- The patient must undergo careful follow up with blood monitoring
- The patient should practice two methods of birth control prior to, while on, and for one month after taking isotretinoin
- Pregnancy testing should be done 2 weeks before starting the treatment and isotretinoin should be started on day 2–3 of the next menstrual period
- The patient must stop the medication immediately if pregnancy is suspected
- Prolonged exposure to the sun should be avoided
- The medication should be taken with food
- The patient should avoid alcohol and vitamin A while taking isotretinoin
- Use caution when driving at night
- If visual difficulties occur, discontinue the drug and have an ophthalmologic examination

TRIAMCINOLONE
- Corticosteroid
- Can be administered topically, or injected intralesionally (10mg/mL)
- Intralesional treatments are more effective due to more efficient delivery of the corticosteroid
- Treats hidradenitis suppurativa effectively when used as an adjunctive treatment
- Decreases inflammation by suppressing the migration of polymorphonuclear leukocytes

Dose
- Adult topical dose: apply topically two or three times daily to the affected skin
- Adult intralesional dose: 10mg/mL strength

Efficacy
Useful to reduce inflammatory exacerbation.

Risks/benefits
Risks:
- Does not provide quick response; may take several hours for relief
- Risk of infection with intralesional injection
- Use caution in glomerulonephritis, ulcerative colitis, renal disease, AIDS, tuberculosis, ocular herpes simplex, live vaccines, viral and bacterial infections, diabetes mellitus, glaucoma, osteoporosis, hypertension, recent myocardial infarction
- Use caution in children and the elderly
- Use caution in psychosis
- Do not withdraw abruptly

Side effects and adverse reactions
- Side effects are minimized by short duration of therapy
- Cardiovascular system: hypertension, thromboembolism
- Central nervous system: insomnia, euphoria, depression, psychosis, seizures
- Endocrine: adrenal suppression, impaired glucose tolerance, growth suppression in children
- Eyes, ears, nose and throat: cataract, glaucoma, blurred vision
- Gastrointestinal: dyspepsia, peptic ulceration, esophagitis, oral candidiasis, nausea, vomiting
- Musculoskeletal: proximal myopathy, osteoporosis
- Skin: delayed healing, acne, striae

Interactions (other drugs)
- **Aminoglutethimide** ■ **Antidiabetics** ■ **Barbiturates** ■ **Carbamazepine** ■ **Cholestyramine** ■ **Cholinesterase inhibitors** ■ **Cyclosporine** ■ **Diuretics** ■ **Estrogens** ■ **Isoniazid** ■ **Isoproterenol** ■ **Nonsteroidal anti-inflammatory drugs** ■ **Phenytoin** ■ **Rifampin** ■ **Salicylates**

Contraindications
- **Local or systemic infection** ■ **Peptic ulcer** ■ **Pregnancy and breast-feeding**

Acceptability to patient
Topical treatment limits the side effects of steroids.

Patient and caregiver information
- The patient must be told that topical steroids have limited side effects
- Hypersensitivity may occur
- Prolonged use should be avoided to prevent skin thinning and systemic absorption

TETRACYCLINE
- Antibiotic used for infective exacerbations
- Treats susceptible bacterial infections of both Gram-positive and Gram-negative organisms and atypical organisms
- Therapy needs to be administered for at least 2 months

Dose
Adult oral dose: 250mg, four times daily, or 500mg, twice daily.

Efficacy
Useful for infective exacerbations, with activity against a wide spectrum of organisms.

Risks/benefits
Risks:
- Compliance can be a problem
- Use caution in patients with hepatic impairment
- Use caution with repeated or prolonged doses

Side effects and adverse reactions
- Cardiovascular system: pericarditis
- Central nervous system: headache, paresthesia, fever
- Gastrointestinal: abdominal pain, diarrhea, heartburn, hepatotoxicity, vomiting, nausea, dental staining, anorexia
- Genitourinary: polyuria, polydipsia, azotemia
- Hematologic: blood cell dyscrasias
- Skin: pruritus, rash, photosensitivity, changes in pigmentation, angioedema, stinging

Interactions (other drugs)
- Antacids ▪ Atovaquone ▪ Barbiturates ▪ Bismuth subsalicyclate ▪ Calcium, iron, magnesium, zinc ▪ Cephalosporins ▪ Cholesytramine, colestipol ▪ Carbamazepine ▪ Digoxin ▪ Ethanol ▪ Methoxyflurane ▪ Oral contraceptives ▪ Penicillins ▪ Phenytoin ▪ Quinapril ▪ Sodium bicarbonate ▪ Vitamin A ▪ Warfarin

Contraindications
- Pregnancy ▪ Nursing mothers ▪ Children less than 8 years ▪ Severe renal disease

Patient and caregiver information
- Photosensitivity may occur with prolonged exposure to sunlight
- Patients should not become pregnant while taking this medication

MINOCYCLINE
- Antibiotic
- Useful as an oral treatment for hidradenitis suppurativa
- Treats Gram-negative and Gram-positive organisms; treats infections caused by *Rickettsia*, *Chlamydia*, and mycoplasmas
- Treatment needs to be administered for at least 2 months
- Expensive medication

Dose
Adult oral dose: 100mg, twice daily, or 50mg, four times daily, for at least 2 months.

Efficacy
Useful to treat infective exacerbation.

Risks/benefits
Risks:
- Use of this drug may result in overgrowth of nonsusceptible organisms, including fungi. If superinfection occurs, the antibiotic should be discontinued
- Risk of pseudotumor cerebri (benign intracranial hypertension) in adults
- Risk of bulging fontanelles in infants
- Photosensitivity manifested by an exaggerated sunburn reaction has been observed

Side effects and adverse reactions
- Cardiovascular system: pericarditis
- Central nervous system: bulging fontanelles in infants and benign intracranial hypertension (pseudotumor cerebri) in adults, headache, anaphylaxis
- Gastrointestinal: anorexia, nausea, vomiting, diarrhea, glossitis, dysphagia, enterocolitis, esophagitis, and esophageal ulcerations
- Metabolic: pancreatitis, inflammatory lesions (with candidal overgrowth) in the anogenital region, increases in liver enzymes, hepatitis and liver failure
- Musculoskeletal: polyarthralgia
- Skin: maculopapular erythematous rashes, exfoliative dermatitis, erythema multiforme, Stevens-Johnson syndrome, photosensitivity, pigmentation of the skin and mucous membranes, urticaria, angioneurotic edema, anaphylactoid purpura, exacerbation of systemic lupus erythematosus, pulmonary infiltrates with eosinophilia. Transient lupus-like syndrome has also been reported with the capsules
- Hematologic: hemolytic anemia, thrombocytopenia, neutropenia and eosinophilia have been reported.
- Other: with prolonged treatment, brown-black microscopic discoloration of the thyroid glands

Interactions (other drugs)
- Methoxyflurane (has been reported to result in fatal renal toxicity) ■ Anticoagulants (may depress plasma prothrombin activity) ■ Penicillin (bactericidal action may be reduced) ■ Oral contraceptives (may reduce effectiveness of contraceptives) ■ Antacids containing aluminum, calcium, or magnesium, and iron-containing preparations (may impair absorption of minocycline)

Contraindications
- Children under 8 years of age ■ Pregnancy and lactation ■ Hypersensitivity to any of the tetracyclines

Patient and caregiver information
- Photosensitivity may occur with prolonged exposure to sunlight
- Treatment must stop if the patient becomes pregnant

Surgical therapy
- Surgery is regarded as the definitive treatment for hidradenitis suppurativa
- Isotretinoin can reduce the disease activity to allow for surgical treatment
- Spontaneous resolution is rare and progressive disability is the rule with hidradenitis suppurativa
- Excision of the diseased tissue with split-thickness skin grafts offers the best chance for cure

WIDE LOCAL EXCISION
- Experienced surgeons can undertake this definitive operation in consultation with the dermatologist and pathologist
- Diseased tissue is removed to leave disease-free tissue
- Skin grafting is required to give the best cosmetic result and reduce scarring. However, the wounds can be left to heal by secondary intention
- The patient should give full consent

Efficacy
Wide local excision gives the best chance of cure.

Risks/benefits
Benefits:
- Early surgery may prevent future relapses and complications
- Surgery is the only definitive treatment for this chronic suppurative disease, preventing multiple relapses and complications

Acceptability to patient
- The risks of surgery, including include sepsis and scarring, must be fully explained to the patient
- Consent is required from the patient, as complications may arise from surgery
- Postoperative pain may be an issue, and patients should have good postoperative care to minimize the chance of pain and sepsis occurring

Follow up plan
Careful follow up postsurgery is required as disease relapse can occur after long periods of remission.

Patient and caregiver information
- Consent is required from the patient, as complications may arise from surgery, including sepsis and scarring
- Patients should be told that surgery gives them the best hope of a cure
- Compliance with postoperative care and therapy is crucial for the success of the treatment and the skin graft
- Long-term follow up is required as disease relapse can occur after long periods of remission

Radiation therapy
RADIOTHERAPY
- Radiotherapy is a treatment option for hidradenitis suppurativa.
- This form of therapy is not used often in the treatment of hidradenitis suppurativa
- It can be very effective but has side effects
- Patients must give full consent

Efficacy
Radiotherapy can be an effective treatment for relapses of hidradenitis suppurativa.

Risks/benefits
Risk: risks of radiotherapy include burning of the skin and fibrotic scarring
Benefit: complete relief from the symptoms can be obtained with radiotherapy

Other therapies
LASER THERAPY
Carbon dioxide laser excision can be used to treat lesions of hidradenitis suppurativa.

Efficacy
Laser therapy with second-intention healing can treat lesions effectively.

Risks/benefits
Risk: complications can occur with laser therapy and the patient should give full consent.

LIFESTYLE

- Obesity, smoking, and poor hygiene are linked to disease exacerbations
- All these factors most likely exacerbate existing disease, rather than have a causal relationship to the disease itself
- All these factors should be minimized to reduce relapses of hidradenitis suppurativa
- The use of deodorants and antiperspirants should be avoided

RISKS/BENEFITS
Benefit: weight loss and cessation of smoking will be beneficial for the patient's health.

ACCEPTABILITY TO PATIENT
- Weight loss, stopping smoking, and improved hygiene may be difficult for the patient to accept
- Preventing the use of hygiene products will be difficult
- Good support and careful follow up is required

FOLLOW UP PLAN
Careful follow up to give the patient support to undertake the lifestyle changes needed to improve compliance.

PATIENT AND CAREGIVER INFORMATION
It is imperative that the patient loses weight, stops smoking, and improves hygiene to prevent relapses of this disease.

EFFICACY OF THERAPIES

- Early surgical treatment of hidradenitis suppurativa is advisable as spontaneous resolution is rare and progressive disability is the rule
- Surgical treatment is the only definitive treatment for hidradenitis suppurativa
- Medical treatment is useful for mild to moderate disease
- Medical treatment can be used to control the disease and allow for successful surgery

Review period
6 months.

PROGNOSIS

- Hidradenitis suppurativa is a chronic disabling disease
- Careful dermatological follow up is required
- Surgery offers the best chance of cure
- Long-term follow up is required as relapse can occur after long periods of remission

Clinical pearls

- Distinction from other elements of the differential diagnosis is imperative
- Patient embarrassment must be addressed to get necessary patient involvement in decision-making process

Therapeutic failure

- Referral to dermatology is required
- Surgery may be indicated

Recurrence

- Recurrence is normal for hidradenitis suppurativa
- Careful follow up by the dermatologist is required to adequately treat the skin lesions and reduce relapses and complications

Deterioration

Deterioration of hidradenitis suppurativa requires referral to a dermatologist and surgery, as both medical and surgical treatment is indicated.

COMPLICATIONS

- Abscesses, fistulas, and scarring are common complications of hidradenitis suppurativa
- Sepsis can occur, especially in immunocompromised patients
- Squamous cell carcinoma can arise in the diseased skin of hidradenitis suppurativa
- Marjolin's ulcer has been described as a complication of hidradenitis suppurativa

CONSIDER CONSULT

- If complications arise, including fistulas, abscesses, and sinuses, then referral for dermatological treatment and surgery is required

RISK FACTORS

- Cigarette smoking has been described as a triggering factor for hidradenitis suppurativa
- Obesity has been linked to hidradenitis suppurativa
- Excessive sweating, poor hygiene, and the use of antiperspirants have been associated with hidradenitis suppurativa

MODIFY RISK FACTORS
Lifestyle and wellness
TOBACCO
Cigarette smoking has been described as a triggering factor for hidradenitis suppurativa.

DIET
Weight reduction through correct diet management may prevent relapses of the disease.

PHYSICAL ACTIVITY
Exercise will help with weight reduction to prevent relapses.

DRUG HISTORY
The oral contraceptive pill has been linked to the disease and should be replaced by another method of contraception.

PREVENT RECURRENCE

- Careful follow up by the dermatologist is required as recurrences are common
- Good compliance with treatment will prevent recurrences
- Surgery gives the patient the best chance of a cure

KEY REFERENCES

- Burton J. Disorders of sweat glands. In: Essentials of Dermatology, 3rd edn. London: Churchill Livingstone, 1990
- Von der Werth, Williams HC. The natural history of hidradenitis suppurativa. J Eur Acad Dermatol Venereol 2000;14:389–92
- Boer, et al. Hidradenitis suppurativa or acne inversa. A clinicopathological study of early lesions. Br J Dermatol 1996;135:721–5
- Bedlow AJ, Mortimer PS. Dowling-Degos disease associated with hidradenitis suppurativa. Clin Exp Dermatol 1996;21:305–6
- Hamoir XL, Francois RJ, Van den Haute V, Van Campenhoudt M. Arthritis and hidradenitis suppurativa diagnosed in a 48 year man. Skeletal Radiol 1999;28:453–6
- Ortonne J. Oral isotretinoin treatment policy. Do we all agree? Dermatology 1997;195(Suppl 1):34–40
- Boer J. Long-term results of isotretinoin in the treatment of 68 patients with hidradenitis suppurativa. J Am Acad Dermatol 1999;40:658
- Fearfield L. Severe vulval apocrine acne successfully treated with prednisolone and isotretinoin. Clin Exp Dermatol 1999;24:189–92
- Herrmann A, Preusser KP, Marsch WC. Acne inversa (hidradenitis suppurativa): early detection a curative surgery. Chirurg 2000;71:1395–400
- Brown TJ, Rosen T, Orengo IF. Hidradenitis suppurativa. South Med J 1998;91:1107–14
- Lamfichekh N, Dupond AS, Destrumelle N, et al. Surgical treatment of Verneuil's disease (hidradenitis suppurativa). Ann Dermatol Venereo 2001;128:111–13
- Endo Y, Tamura A, Ishikawa O, Miyachi Y. Perianal hidradenitis suppurativa: early surgical treatment good results in chronic or recurrent cases. Br J Dermatol 1998;139:906–10
- Elwood ET, Bolitho DG.. Negative-pressure dressings in the treatment of hidradenitis suppurativa. Ann Plat Surg 2001;46: 49–51
- Ritz JP, Runkel N, Haier J, Buhr HJ. Extent of surgery and recurrence rate of hidradenitis suppurativa. Int J Colorectal Dis 1998;13:4;164–8
- Rompel R, Petres J. Long-term results of wide surgical excision in 106 patients with hidradenitis suppurativa. Dermatol Surg 2000;26:638–43
- Lorenz D. Recurrent sweat gland abscess. Langenbecks Arch Chir Suppl Kongressbd 1997;114:490–2
- Ellsworth AJ, et al. Mosby's Medical Drug Reference. Philadelphia: Mosby, 2001–2002
- Frohlich D, Baaske D, Glatzel M. Radiotherapy of hidradenitis suppurativa: still valid today. Strahlenther Onkol 2000;176:286–9
- Finley EM, Ratz JL. Treatment of hidradenitis suppurativa with carbon dioxide excision and second-intention healing. J Am Acad Dermatol 1996;34:465–9
- Lapins J, Ye W, Nyren O, Emtestam L. Incidence of cancer among patients with hidradenitis suppurativa. Arch Dermatol 2001;137:730–4
- Manolitsas T, Biankin S, Jaworski R, Wain G. Vulval squamous cell carcinoma arising in chronic hidradenitis suppurativa. Gynae Oncol 1999;75:285–8
- Lin MT, Breiner M, Fredricks S. Marjolin's ulcer occurring in hidradenitis suppurativa. Plast Reconstr Surg 1999;103:1541–3
- Konig et al. Cigarette smoking as a trigger factor of hidradenitis suppurativa. Dermatology 1999;198:261–4
- Jemec GBE. The symptomatology of hidradenitis suppuritiva and its potential precursor lesions. Br J Dermatology 1988;119:345
- Jemec GB, Heidenheim M, Nielsen NH. The prevalence of hidradenitis suppuritiva and its potential precursor lesions: J Am Acad Dermatol 1996; 35:191–4

FAQS

Question 1

How long should the antibiotic treatment continue?

ANSWER 1

Antibiotic therapy can continue for many years. If a therapeutic trial fails to achieve benefit after two months, however, it is reasonable to try alternative approaches.

Question 2
Is there a role for long-term suppressive antibiotics?

ANSWER 2
Yes, as long as they remain effective.

Question 3
Is there a role for topical antibacterial cleansers such as pHisoHex (trademark for emulsion containing hexachlorophene) or Hibiclens (trademark for a preparation of chlorhexidine gluconate)?

ANSWER 3
The bulk of the pathology is deep and therefore not amenable to topical cleansers. Such products can, however, be used to clean up superficial exudates and discharge.

Question 4
How many times should we I&D an area before recommending wider excision?

ANSWER 4
There are no set guidelines on this issue. In fact, adequate incision and drainage will resolve the specific problem first time round. The problem occurs when adjacent structures become involved and give the appearence of previously inadequate therapy. Factors to consider in determining whether or not wider excision is required include not just the frequency and severity of new lesions, but the emotional state of the patient, and his or her willingness to accept the risks of more aggressive surgery in return for the benefit of definitive curative therapy.

CONTRIBUTORS
Gordon H Baustian, MD
Seth R Stevens, MD
Douglas C Semler, MD

IMPETIGO

DESCRIPTION

- A highly communicable superficial infection of the skin
- Exists in two distinct forms: bullous impetigo, which is usually secondary to *Staphylococcus aureus* (primarily phage II, group 71, that produces an exfoliating toxin) and nonbullous impetigo, which is secondary to *Staphylococcus aureus* and/or group A beta-hemolytic streptococcal species
- Antibiotics and good hygiene are the mainstays of treatment

KEY! DON'T MISS!

Impetigo caused by *Streptococcus pyogenes* carries the sporadic risk of acute glomerulonephritis, which develops 18–21 days after cutaneous infection. Clinical lesions are no different from those in other bacterial causes of impetigo. Treatment of impetigo with antibiotics does not prevent glomerulonephritis. Specific associated strains are M groups 2, 49, 53, 55–57, and 60.

ICD9 CODE
684 Impetigo

SYNONYMS
- Superficial pyoderma
- Impetigo contagiosa

CARDINAL FEATURES
- A highly communicable superficial infection of the skin, existing in two distinct forms: bullous and nonbullous
- Nonbullous form is usually due to *Staphylococcus aureus* and/or group A beta-hemolytic streptococci and accounts for more than 70% of all cases of impetigo. Lesions start as vesicles that quickly rupture, leaving honey-colored crusts. Exposed areas such as the face and limbs are commonly afflicted
- Bullous form accounts for less than 10% of all cases of impetigo and occurs more commonly in newborns and older infants
- Bullous form usually secondary to *Staphylococcus aureus* (phage II, group 71). Lesions are vesicles that rapidly progress to bullae and contain clear or yellow fluid. Bullae rupture after 2–3 days, forming light brown crusts at the borders of erythematous erosions
- Minor traumas such as insect bites or abrasions predispose to the development of infected lesions
- Lesions remain superficial and do not ulcerate or scar
- Lesions are usually painless, but patients may complain of pruritus or burning

CAUSES
Common causes
- *Staphylococcus aureus* is currently the dominant causative micro-organism in industrialized countries
- Group A beta-hemolytic streptococcus (*Streptococcus pyogenes*) is a common cause in developing countries
- Mixed infections predominate and are due to primary infection with group A streptococcus and secondary invasion by *Staphylococcus aureus*
- Nasal carriage of *Staphylococcus aureus* by individual or close contacts
- Minor breaks in skin such as insect bites or abrasions allow impetiginization
- Pre-existing skin disease, especially atopic dermatitis

Rare causes
May be a complication of herpes simplex, pediculosis, chickenpox, thermal burns, scabies, abrasions sustained during contact sports, or any other injury to the skin's integrity.

Serious causes
Streptococcus pyogenes: may result in acute glomerulonephritis.

Contributory or predisposing factors
- Warm, humid environment or climate
- Minor trauma
- Insect bites
- Poor hygiene
- Overcrowding
- Atopic dermatitis
- Colonization of nares, axillae, or perianal area with *Staphylococcus aureus*

EPIDEMIOLOGY
Incidence and prevalence
Impetigo accounts for 10% of all skin problems in a general dermatology clinic.

FREQUENCY

Overall incidence of acute nephritis with impetigo varies between 2 and 4%.

Demographic
AGE
- Nonbullous form occurs in children of all ages, as well as adults
- Bullous form is most common in infants and preschool children

GENDER
- Among infants and children, males and females are equally commonly affected
- In adults, males are more commonly affected than females (owing to crowded living conditions such as barracks)

RACE

Affects all races.

GEOGRAPHY
- Streptococcal impetigo is more common in warm, humid environments and tropical or subtropical climates
- Impetigo caused by *Staphylococcus aureus* is more common in temperate climates
- Occurs more often in the summer months

SOCIOECONOMIC STATUS
- Common with overcrowded living conditions and/or poor hygiene
- Also occurs in healthy people with good lifestyles

DIFFERENTIAL DIAGNOSIS
Chickenpox
Chickenpox is a common illness caused by varicella-zoster virus and characterized by acute onset of vesicular rash.

FEATURES
- Predominant age is 5–10 years
- Initial lesions occur on the head or trunk as successive crops of lesions that evolve as red macules, papules, vesicles, pustules, and finally crusts. All stages can be present at one time
- Classic lesional description is 'dewdrop on a rose petal'
- Lesions spread to the extremities and are often accompanied by intense pruritus
- Crusts fall off within 5–25 days
- Other symptoms, which are usually more severe in adults, include headache, general malaise, fever, chills, backache
- Viral pneumonia and encephalitis are complications that can result in death. The risk of death is proportional to patient age

Herpes simplex virus infection
Herpes simplex is a common viral disease. Oral-facial disease is commonly caused by herpes simplex virus 1; genital disease is commonly caused by herpes simplex virus 2.

FEATURES
- Usually asymptomatic; however, constitutional symptoms can include fever, myalgias, headache, and regional lymphadenopathy, particularly during primary infection
- Recurrent lesions often preceded by a prodrome of localized pain, burning, itching, or tingling
- Grouped uniform vesicles appear, often with surrounding erythema; they frequently ulcerate or crust within 48h
- Primary oral lesions heal within 8–9 days and primary genital lesions last 2–4 weeks. Neither causes scarring, although they can scar if secondary bacterial infection supervenes
- Recurrent lesions occur in same area, but the duration of lesions and the severity of symptoms is less, and the vesicles are usually smaller

Folliculitis
Folliculitis is infection of the upper part of the hair follicle. The most common form is staphylococcal folliculitis. Predisposing factors include shaving, occlusion, topical corticosteroids, high humidity, and diabetes mellitus type 1 or type 2.

FEATURES
- Lesions are follicular papules or pustules, often surrounded by erythema and a central hair
- Usually asymptomatic, but patients may complain of pruritus or minimal tenderness
- Sycosis barbae afflicts the beard area of men who shave. It is a deep staphylococcal infection of the follicles that starts with small follicular papules or pustules that rupture, recur, and spread if not treated

Atopic dermatitis
Atopic dermatitis is often described as 'eczema' by lay public. The majority have a personal or family history of allergic rhinitis, asthma, hay fever, or atopic dermatitis.

FEATURES
- Extremely sensitive skin
- In infants, lesions are usually found on the face, neck, and trunk

- In adults, lesions are usually found on the bends (flexural) of elbows and knees, as well as on the hands
- Lesions are usually symmetric
- Primary lesions are a result of scratching caused by severe, chronic pruritus
- Acute lesions are red and edematous, sometimes with small vesicles and crusting. Chronic lesions are lichenified (accentuation of skin markings and drier) and fissured
- Constant scratching may result in hypo- or hyperpigmented areas
- People with atopic dermatitis are frequently carriers of *Staphylococcus aureus*, in which case the lesions may regularly develop into impetigo
- Eczema herpeticum is a generalized secondary infection with herpes simplex virus

Scabies

Scabies is a contagious disease caused by the *Sarcoptes scabiei* mite.

FEATURES

- Contracted by close personal contact, thus common in overcrowded living conditions, hospitals and nursing homes, and in those sleeping with an infected person
- Primary lesions result when the female mite burrows within the stratum corneum and lays eggs within the tract. The burrows end with a minute vesicle or papule from which the mite can sometimes be demonstrated
- Primary lesions are commonly found in web spaces of hand, wrists, buttocks, breasts, axillae, knees, scrotum, and penis
- Persistent pruritus, worse at night, is caused by acquired sensitivity to the mite and is usually seen 1–4 weeks after infestation
- Crusted or Norwegian scabies is characterized by widespread crusted lesions (worst on scalp and hands) that are teeming with mites in immunocompromised or institutionalized patients

Tinea corporis

Tinea corporis is a fungal infection caused by *Trichophyton* or *Microsporum* species.

FEATURES

- Most common in warm climates (because of excessive perspiration)
- Common in children with exposure to cats, dogs, horses, and cattle with the infection
- Lesions are typically annular with an advancing scaly border and may be located on the face, trunk, or extremities
- Central clearing occurs as the borders of the lesions extend outward
- Lesions may be pustular, hypopigmented, or minimally elevated

Pemphigus vulgaris

Pemphigus is an autoimmune condition (antibody production to epidermal cell membrane) that requires specialist referral.

FEATURES

- Primarily affects people between 40 and 60 years of age
- Flaccid vesicles and bullae rupture easily, leaving widespread weeping and crusted erosions
- Lesions are painful and usually present first on oral mucous membranes and may later extend to the body
- Fatal unless treated with corticosteroids or immunosuppressives

Bullous pemphigoid

Bullous pemphigoid is an autoimmune condition with antibody directed against the skin basement membrane.

FEATURES

- Primarily affects people over 60 years of age
- Tense bullae, typically affecting the legs, axillae, groin, abdomen, and flexor aspect of the arms
- Intense pruritus
- May occur initially as urticarial plaques or in association with urticarial plaques

Acute allergic contact dermatitis

An inflammatory dermatitis resulting from exposure to allergens.

FEATURES

- Acute lesions are erythematous papules and vesicles
- Chronic lesions are lichenified and scaly
- Localized to areas of contact with allergen
- Patients complain of pruritus
- Linear lesions are the classical presentation of allergic contact dermatitis caused by poison ivy

Erysipelas

A superficial cellulitis, usually found on the face, most commonly due to group A beta-hemolytic streptococci.

FEATURES

- Characterized by bright red plaques
- Well demarcated, painful, and hot
- Surface of the skin may have an orange peel appearance (*peau d'orange*) owing to dermal edema

Insect bites

Insect bites and stings tend to occur in warm weather and warm climates.

FEATURES

- Local reaction to ant, bee, or wasp sting
- Erythema followed by edema surrounding the site
- Bite may leave a punctum in the skin
- Intense pruritus usually accompanies bites or stings
- Fleas and lice cause similar lesions (small red erythematous spots)

SIGNS & SYMPTOMS
Signs

Nonbullous impetigo:

- Early lesions are vesicles or pustules
- Lesions rupture to form golden-yellow crusts
- Areas of weeping erythematous erosions
- Regional lymphadenopathy may be present
- Lesions commonly found on face or limbs

Bullous impetigo:

- Thin-walled vesicles rapidly progress to bullae containing fluid
- Honey-colored crusts bordering erosions
- Bullae commonly found on face, trunk, hands, and buttocks

Symptoms

- Pain
- Itching
- Redness
- Weeping

ASSOCIATED DISORDERS

Acute glomerulonephritis.

KEY! DON'T MISS!

Impetigo caused by *Streptococcus pyogenes* carries the sporadic risk of acute glomerulonephritis, which develops 18–21 days after cutaneous infection. Clinical lesions are no different from those in other bacterial causes of impetigo. Treatment of impetigo with antibiotics does not prevent glomerulonephritis. Specific associated strains are M groups 2, 49, 53, 55–57, and 60.

INVESTIGATION OF THE PATIENT
Direct questions to patient

Q Are you living in crowded conditions? Impetigo is a highly communicable infections and is easily spread in conditions of overcrowding.

Q What is your general standard of hygiene? Impetigo is easily spread in conditions of poor hygiene.

Q Have you recently been bitten/stung by an insect or suffered a minor skin abrasion? Insect bites/stings and minor abrasions have been implicated in impetigo.

Q Do you participate in contact sports? Minor abrasions and lacerations sustained during contact sports are easily impetiginized.

Contributory or predisposing factors

Q Do you have any other medical conditions? Conditions such as diabetes mellitus type 1 or type 2 increase risk of impetigo.

Q Do you have a history of atopic dermatitis? This condition predisposes a patient to impetigo.

Q Have you recently had chickenpox, scabies, or pediculosis? These infections cause breaks in the skin, which predispose to impetigo.

Q Are you currently living in a warm, humid environment? Spread of impetigo is facilitated by warm, humid, and overcrowded conditions.

Family history

Q Is there a family history of atopic dermatitis? There is a hereditary predisposition for atopic dermatitis, which predisposes a patient to impetigo.

Examination

- Is the patient well/unwell? Constitutional symptoms are usually absent in impetigo
- What are the lesions like? Vesicles and pustules are common in impetigo
- How widespread are the lesions? Impetigo is usually not widespread. If numerous lesions are present, consider other elements of the differential diagnosis
- What is occurring within the lesion? Lesions form vesicles that burst and form honey-colored crusts. Chickenpox may initially resemble impetigo, but all lesions are at the same stage
- Is there regional lymphadenopathy? Often present in nonbullous form of impetigo
- Is there hematuria? Acute glomerulonephritis may occur in children with impetigo; however, it usually occurs 18–21 days after impetigo

Summary of investigative tests

- Culture of exudate and Gram stain: identifies resistant organisms
- Anti-DNAase and antihyaluronidase: tests of choice to confirm prior streptococcal infection
- Urinalysis: may reveal hematuria and/or protein casts and confirm acute glomerulonephritis
- Complement tests: levels of some serum complement may be decreased in acute glomerulonephritis
- Antistreptolysin O titer: may be elevated in acute glomerulonephritis

DIAGNOSTIC DECISION

- Gram stain will confirm the presence of Gram-positive cocci, while culture will confirm whether the infecting pathogen is *Staphylococcus aureus*, *Streptococcus pyogenes*, or both
- Increased levels of anti-DNAase B and antihyaluronidase indicate preceding streptococcal infections. Anti-DNAase is the test of choice for prior skin infections
- Serologic response measured by antistreptolysin O (ASO) may be weakly positive or absent. It is elevated in acute glomerulonephritis but more closely associated with prior pharyngitis than skin infection

CLINICAL PEARL(S)

- Impetigo should be treated early because of renal implications for the patient and public health concerns due to its infectious nature
- Impetigo often occurs secondary to some primary event that impairs the skin's barrier function. These primary events are frequently trauma or insect bites, but investigation for other causes that also require medical attention (e.g. atopic dermatitis) should be performed if the cause is not obvious

THE TESTS
Body fluids
GRAM STAIN AND CULTURE
Description
Swab specimen taken from the exudate at the base of the lesion after gentle crust removal.

Advantages/Disadvantages
Advantages:
- Quick, easy, painless
- Rules out resistant bacterial strains; however, remember that many other primary dermatoses can easily develop into secondary impetigo
- Positive identification of pathogens involved, allowing the primary care physician to tailor treatment

Abnormal
- Gram-positive strains detected
- Presence of *Staphylococcus aureus* and/or *Streptococcus pyogenes*

Cause of abnormal result
Bacterial infection.

ANTI-DNAASE
Description
Blood test using serum.

Advantages/Disadvantages
Advantage: test of choice to confirm prior streptococcal skin infection.

Normal
Absent or low antibody titers.

Abnormal
Increased anti-DNAse B and antihyaluronidase.

Cause of abnormal result
Elevated titers present in 90% of patients with glomerulonephritis complicating streptococcal skin infections.

Drugs, disorders and other factors that may alter results
Previous unrelated streptococcal infection.

COMPLEMENT TESTS
Description
Blood test using serum.

Advantages/Disadvantages
Advantages:
- Sedimentation rate parallels disease activity
- Serum complement levels may indicate acute glomerulonephritis

Normal
- C3: 70–160mg/dL
- C4: 20–40mg/dL

Abnormal
- Total serum complement may be low during glomerulonephritis
- Complement C3 parallels total serum complement and may be reduced

Cause of abnormal result
- Patient may have developed acute glomerulonephritis
- Patient may have some other disease causing low complement levels (e.g. systemic lupus erythematosus)

Drugs, disorders and other factors that may alter results
Other conditions and medications can affect complement levels.

URINALYSIS
Description
Urine sample, analysis plus microscopy.

Advantages/Disadvantages
Advantages:
- Simple to perform
- Reveals hematuria in patients with acute glomerulonephritis

Normal
- No casts, blood, or protein
- No white blood cells or bacteria

Abnormal
Presence of casts, blood, protein, white blood cells, or bacteria in urine.

Cause of abnormal result
Patient may have developed acute glomerulonephritis.

Drugs, disorders and other factors that may alter results
Patients may have blood or protein in their urine as a result of many other medical or surgical conditions (e.g. urinary tract infection, renal stones, diabetes mellitus type 1 or type 2).

ANTISTREPTOLYSIN O TITER
Description
Blood sample using serum.

Advantages/Disadvantages
Advantage: Measures several streptococcal antibodies

Disadvantages:
- Moderate incidence of false-positive or false-negative results
- May be weakly positive, low, or even absent after episode of impetigo

Normal
Absent antistreptolysin O titer.

Abnormal
Antistreptolysin O titer elevated in acute glomerulonephritis

Cause of abnormal result
Patient may have developed acute glomerulonephritis or have had a prior streptococcal pharyngitis or skin infection.

Drugs, disorders and other factors that may alter results
Streptococcal pharyngitis causes the most positive titers.

TREATMENT

CONSIDER CONSULT
- Refer to nephrologist if patient develops acute glomerulonephritis due to *Streptococcus pyogenes*

IMMEDIATE ACTION
- Empiric therapy should be started before exact diagnosis is known
- Patient must avoid scratching lesions because of the risk of autoinoculation
- Good personal hygiene is important to prevent spread of infection

PATIENT AND CAREGIVER ISSUES
Patient or caregiver request
- Patient may consider washing with an antibacterial soap but may be concerned about its efficacy
- If there have been items about infections in the news recently, patients may be concerned about the outcome of their disorder

Health-seeking behavior
Has the patient waited too long? Patient may not have realized that the skin disorder is caused by bacterial infection.

MANAGEMENT ISSUES
Goals
- To eliminate skin manifestations
- To eradicate infecting organism
- To prevent spread of infection

SUMMARY OF THERAPEUTIC OPTIONS
Choices
Treatment is either topical or systemic, depending on the extent of involvement, the regional rates of bacterial resistance, and the cost of treatment.
- Topical mupirocin ointment is a safe and effective treatment, with success rates greater than 90%. Several studies have proven it to be as effective as systemic treatment with erythromycin
- In areas where erythromycin resistance is rare, patients may be treated with macrolides (erythromycin ethylsuccinate, erythromycin estolate, erythromycin base, azithromycin) or a cephalosporin (such as cephalexin)
- Alternative antibiotic treatment may be guided by culture and sensitivity results, community resistance patterns, costs, or formulary restriction
- Penicillin and amoxicillin are not recommended treatments because of increasing resistance rates
- In addition to topical or oral antibiotics, crust should be removed by soaking with wet compresses and washing involved areas with antibacterial soaps

Clinical pearl(s)
Be aggressive with treatment since impetigo is so prevalent.

Never
- Never attempt to débride lesions because this can cause permanent scarring
- Never wait to refer a patient who has failed to respond to appropriate treatment because impetigo usually responds quickly to treatment

FOLLOW UP
Plan for review
- Provide instruction on use of regular cleansing and removal of crusts
- Follow up within 7–10 days
- If impetigo is not clear within 7–10 days, repeat culture to rule out resistant organism

Information for patient or caregiver
- Regular gentle washing with antibacterial soap prevents local spread
- Avoidance of overcrowding and humid environments facilitates speed of recovery and reduces spread of infection

DRUGS AND OTHER THERAPIES: DETAILS
Drugs
MACROLIDES
- Erythromycin ethylsuccinate
- Erythromycin estolate
- Erythromycin base
- Azithromycin

Dose
- Erythromycin ethylsuccinate: children, 40mg/kg/day by mouth divided three to four times daily for 5–10 days
- Erythromycin estolate: children, 30mg/kg/day by mouth divided three to four times dally for 5–10 days (hepatotoxic in adults)
- Erythromycin base: adults, 250–500mg/day by mouth daily for 7–10 days
- Azithromycin: children, 10mg/kg by mouth up to 500mg on first day, followed by 5mg/kg by mouth up to 250mg/day to complete 5-day regimen; adults, 500mg by mouth on first day, followed by 250mg/day by mouth to complete 5-day regimen

Efficacy
Good in areas where erythromycin-resistant strains are not present.

Risks/benefits
Risks:
- Use caution in hepatic and renal impairment, and porphyria
- Avoid concomitant administration with terfenadine, astemizole, and cisapride
- Use caution with repeated or prolonged therapy

Benefits:
- Highly efficacious
- Cheap

Side effects and adverse reactions
- Gastrointestinal: anorexia, nausea, diarrhea, abdominal pain, vomiting, heartburn, hepatitis
- Cardiovascular system: dysrhythmias (uncommon)
- Skin: rashes, pruritus, vaginal candidiasis
- Ears, eyes, nose, and throat: deafness, tinnitus

Interactions (other drugs)
- Alfentanil ▪ Antiarrhythmic drugs (digoxin, disopyramide) ▪ Antihistamines (terfenadine, astemizole) ▪ Anticonvulsants (carbamazepine, valproic acid) ▪ Antiviral agents

- Benzodiazepines ■ Bromocriptine ■ Buspirone ■ Cisapride ■ Clozapine ■ Colchicine
- Cyclosporine, tacrolimus ■ Ergotamine ■ Ethanol ■ Felodipine ■ Itraconazole
- Methylprednisolone ■ Penicillin ■ Quinidine ■ Sildenafil ■ Statins ■ Theophylline
- Warfarin ■ Zopiclone

Contraindications
- Liver disease ■ Various infections (vaccinia, varicella, mycobacterial, fungal, viral)

Evidence
Erythromycin is a preferred treatment choice in terms of cost-effectiveness in the management of impetigo.
- A randomized controlled trial (RCT) compared erythromycin versus dicloxacillin in the treatment of children with impetigo. The *Staphylococcus aureus*-infected patients had similar results with both antibiotics. Erythromycin is the drug of choice in areas of low resistance because of high efficacy and relatively low cost [1] *Level P*
- A blinded RCT of children with impetigo (62% *Staphylococcus aureus*) assessed the efficacy of penicillin V, cephalexin, and erythromycin. Treatment failure occurred in 24% of patients treated with penicillin V, 4% with erythromycin, and no patients treated with cephalexin [2] *Level P*
- An RCT compared oral erythromycin with mupirocin ointment in the treatment of impetigo. Both treatment groups had a 100% bacteriologic success rate, but mupirocin had fewer side effects [3] *Level P*

There is evidence that azithromycin is effective for the treatment of skin infections.
- A controlled trial of patients with skin and soft tissue infections (most secondary to *Staphylococcus aureus*) compared azithromycin with erythromycin and cloxacillin. Clinical cure was similar between azithromycin and the other treatment groups, but azithromycin may be better tolerated [4] *Level P*
- A blinded RCT compared azithromycin (once daily for 5 days) with cephalexin (twice daily for 10 days) for patients with skin infections. The clinical and bacteriologic efficacy was similar for both medications [5] *Level P*

Acceptability to patient
High.

Follow up plan
Treatment should be for 7–10 days with erythromycin and for 5 days with azithromycin. If impetigo does not clear within this time, lesions should be cultured to identify resistant organisms.

MUPIROCIN
Dose
Topical ointment or cream 2%, applied three times daily for 7–10 days.

Efficacy
As effective and safe as erythromycin and effective against erythromycin-resistant strains.

Risks/benefits
Risks:
- Pregnancy category B: should be used during pregnancy only if clearly indicated
- Inactive against Enterobacteriaceae, *Pseudomonas aeruginosa,* and fungi

Benefits:
- Easy to use
- Pain-free
- Highly active against most frequent skin pathogens, including those resistant to other antibiotics
- Topical application allows delivery of high concentrations of drug to the site of infection

Side effects and adverse reactions
- Skin: local adverse reactions have been reported, including burning, stinging, pain, itching
- Rarely, rash, nausea, erythema, dry skin, tenderness, swelling, contact dermatitis, and increased exudate (<1%)

Interactions (other drugs)
- No drug interactions listed

Contraindications
- History of sensitivity reactions to any of its components

Evidence
Impetigo may be effectively treated with mupirocin ointment.
- An RCT compared oral erythromycin with mupirocin ointment in the treatment of impetigo. 100% bacteriologic cure was achieved in both groups. Mupirocin was found to be significantly superior in overall efficacy and safety to erythromycin when assessed by the Investigator's Global Evaluation. This was due to the low incidence of side effects [3] *Level P*

Acceptability to patient
High.

Follow up plan
- Apply mupirocin every day until lesions have cleared
- If lesions not clear within 7–10 days, culture is necessary to determine if other pathogens are present. Mupirocin is inactive against Enterobacteriaceae, *Pseudomonas aeruginosa,* and fungi

Patient and caregiver information
Night-time application also advisable.

CEPHALOSPORINS
Cephalexin.

Dose
Children: 25–50mg/kg/day orally in divided doses every 6h for 5–10 days
Adults: 250mg orally four times daily for 5–10 days

Efficacy
- More effective than erythromycin and penicillin V because of the high levels of resistance to penicillin
- Effective against staphylococcal strains

Risks/benefits
Risks:
- Use caution in patients with penicillin hypersensitivity
- Use caution in renal impairment and history of gastrointestinal disease
- Use caution in breast-feeding patients

Benefit: Broad antimicrobial coverage

Side effects and adverse reactions
- Gastrointestinal: anorexia, nausea, diarrhea, abdominal pain
- Central nervous system: headache, sleep disturbance, confusion, dizziness
- Hematologic: pancytopenia
- Skin: rashes, erythema multiforme
- Anaphylaxis

Interactions (other drugs)
- Warfarin ■ Aminoglycosides ■ Loop diuretics ■ Probenecid ■ Polymyxin B
- Vancomycin ■ Penicillins

Contraindications
- Penicillin and cephalosporin hypersensitivity ■ Children less than one month old

Evidence
There is evidence supporting the use of cephalexin in the treatment of impetigo.
- A blinded RCT of children with impetigo (62% *Staphylococcus aureus*) assessed the efficacy of penicillin V, cephalexin, and erythromycin. Treatment failure occurred in 24% of patients treated with penicillin V, 4% with erythromycin, and no patients treated with cephalexin [2] *Level P*
- An RCT compared cephalexin with dicloxacillin in the management of staphylococcal skin infections. The medications had similar efficacy, but delayed healing was more common with dicloxacillin. Twice-daily dosing of cephalexin was recommended with confidence [6] *Level P*
- A blinded RCT compared azithromycin (once daily for 5 days) with cephalexin (twice daily for 10 days) for patients with skin infections. The clinical and bacteriologic efficacy was similar for both medications [5] *Level P*

Acceptability to patient
High.

Follow up plan
Treatment should be for 7–10 days. If impetigo does not clear within this time, lesions should be re-examined and consideration given for culture to identify resistant organisms.

LIFESTYLE
Improvement in personal hygiene can be helpful.

RISKS/BENEFITS
Benefit: limits the risk of infection.

ACCEPTABILITY TO PATIENT
Medium; may not always be possible.

FOLLOW UP PLAN
Monitor patient progress and provide encouragement.

PATIENT AND CAREGIVER INFORMATION
Patients should be instructed on the use of antibacterial soaps and good hygiene.

EFFICACY OF THERAPIES

Gentle removal of crusts with wet compresses, washing with antibacterial soap, and treatment with topical mupirocin or oral antibiotics should lead to resolution of symptoms within 7–10 days.

Evidence

- *Staphylococcus aureus*-infected patients may have similar results with dicloxacillin and erythromycin. Erythromycin is the drug of choice in areas of low resistance because of high efficacy and relatively low cost [1] *Level P*
- Children with impetigo (62% *Staphylococcus aureus*) may be successfully treated with erythromycin or cephalexin [2] *Level P*
- Erythromycin and mupirocin ointment are equally effective for the treatment of impetigo, although mupirocin has fewer adverse effects [3] *Level P*
- Clinical cure for patients with skin and soft tissue infections secondary to *Staphylococcus aureus* may be similar with azithromycin, erythromycin, and cloxacillin. Azithromycin may be better tolerated [4] *Level P*
- Azithromycin and cephalexin have similar clinical and bacteriologic efficacy in the management of skin infections [5] *Level P*

Review period

Review treatment within 7–10 days.

PROGNOSIS

- Most cases of impetigo completely resolve within 7–10 days of treatment
- Both nonbullous and bullous forms heal without scarring, although scratching and prolonged infection can lead to scarring
- Acute glomerulonephritis may occur in patients with impetigo due to specific strains of group A beta-hemolytic streptococci. Systemic antibiotics cure cutaneous disease but do not prevent the development of glomerulonephritis up to 7 weeks later

Clinical pearls

In the case of recurrent impetigo, consider underlying predisposing factors and evaluate appropriately. Such causes include immunodeficiency states, such as complement, cytokine, cytokine receptor deficiencies, or atopic dermatitis, which in many ways is an immunodeficiency state confined to skin coupled with high rates of staphylococcal carriage.

Recurrence

Topical mupirocin ointment reduces *Staphylococcus aureus* carriage in the nasal passages and via the hands. Consider staphylococcal carriage by patient or close personal contacts. Reservoirs of infection are the nares, axillae, and perianal area.

Deterioration

- If impetigo has not healed within 7–10 days, lesions should be cultured to determine resistant organism
- Antibiotic treatment should be tailored to laboratory experience with local resistance patterns and culture result
- Refer to dermatologist to rule out a different diagnosis

COMPLICATIONS

- Ecthyma: similar to impetigo and caused by the same infective organisms (*Staphylococcus aureus* and/or *Streptococcus pyogenes*). Unlike impetigo, the lesions become ulcerated and are often associated with lymphadenitis

- Erysipelas: a superficial cellulitis caused by *Staphylococcus aureus* and group A beta-hemolytic streptococci
- Poststreptococcal acute glomerulonephritis: the main complication of *Streptococcus pyogenes* impetigo
- Cellulitis: deep infection of the skin
- Bacteremia
- Osteomyelitis: acute or chronic infection of bone; contiguous osteomyelitis is associated with chronic infection of skin and soft tissue
- Septic arthritis: highly destructive joint disease
- Pneumonia
- Lymphadenitis

CONSIDER CONSULT

- Refer to a dermatologist if patient does not respond to appropriate therapy or if recurrent episodes occur. Serious dermatologic diseases can present similarly to impetigo or predispose to impetigo

RISK FACTORS

- Warm, humid environment: spread of infection is facilitated by humid environments
- Tropical/subtropical climate: streptococcal impetigo is more prevalent in warmer climates
- Poor hygiene: poor personal hygiene, possibly as a result of overcrowded living conditions
- Insect bites/stings or abrasions: skin trauma provides entry point for infective organisms

MODIFY RISK FACTORS

Lifestyle and wellness
ENVIRONMENT
Avoidance of overcrowding prevents the spread of infection.

PREVENT RECURRENCE

- Patients with possible recurrent impetigo should be evaluated for colonization of themselves and close personal contacts with *Staphylococcus aureus*. Cultures should be taken of the nares, axillae, and perianal area
- Topical mupirocin ointment applied to the nares (most common site for carriage) reduces *Staphylococcus aureus* carriage
- Washing of minor trauma is effective as a preventive treatment

ASSOCIATIONS

American Academy of Dermatology
930 N. Meacham Road
Schaumburg, IL 60173
Tel: 847-330-0230
http://www.aad.org

KEY REFERENCES

- Akiyama H, Yamasaki O, Kanzaki H, et al. Streptococci isolated from various skin lesions: the interaction with *Staphylococcus aureus* strains. J Dermatol Sci 1999;19:17–22
- Baraff LJ, Fine RN, Knuston DW. Poststreptococcal acute glomerulonephritis: fact and controversy. Ann Intern Med 1979;91:76–86
- Barton LL, Friedman AD, Portilla MG. Impetigo contagiosa: a comparison of erythromycin and dicloxacillin therapy. Pediatr Dermatol 1988;5:88–91
- Birke E, Sepulveda M. Impetigo in children: etiology and response to treatment. Rev Chil Pediatr 1989;60:166–8
- Dagan R, Bar-David Y. Double blind study comparing erythromycin and mupirocin for treatment of impetigo in children: implications of a high prevalence of erythromycin-resistant staphylococcus strains. Antimicrob Agents Chemother 1992;36:287–90
- Dagan R, Bar-David Y. Comparison of amoxicillin and clavulanic acid (Augmentin) for the treatment of nonbullous impetigo. Am J Dis Child 1989;143:916–18
- Daniel R. Azithromycin, erythromycin and cloxacillin in the treatment of infections of skin and associated soft tissues. European Azithromycin Study Group. J Int Med Res 1991;19:433–45
- Darmstadt GL, Lane AT. Impetigo: an overview. Pediatr Dermatol 1994;11:293–303
- Demidovich CW, Wittler RR, Ruff ME, et al. Impetigo: current etiology and comparison of penicillin, erythromycin, and cephalexin therapies. Am J Dis Child 1990;144:1313–15
- Dillon HC Jr. Treatment of staphylococcal skin infections: a comparison of cephalexin and dicloxacillin. J Am Acad Dermatol 1983;8:177–81
- Fleisher GR, Wilmott CM, Campos JM. Amoxicillin combined with clavulanic acid for the treatment of soft tissue infections in children. Antimicrob Agents Chemother 1983;24: 679–81
- Fitzpatrick T, Freedberg IM, Eisen AZ, eds. Fitzpatrick's dermatology in general medicine, 5th edn. New York: McGraw-Hill, 1999
- Fitzpatrick T, Johnson R, Wolff K, Suurmond R. Color atlas and synopsis of clinical dermatology, 3rd edn. New York: McGraw-Hill, 1997
- Furukawa S, Okada T. A clinical evaluation of azithromycin in the treatment of pediatric infection. Jpn J Antibiot 1996;49:1013–23
- Gisby J, Bryant J. Efficacy of a new cream formulation of mupirocin: comparison with oral and topical agents in experimental skin infections. Antimicrob Agents Chemother 2000;44:255–60
- Habif TP. Clinical dermatology, 3rd edn. Philadelphia: Mosby, 1996
- Hebert A, Still JG, Reuman PD. Comparative safety and efficacy of clarithromycin and cefadroxil suspensions in the treatment of mild to moderate skin structure infections in children. Pediatr Infect Dis 1993;12:112S–117S
- Heskel NS, Siepman NC, Pichotta PJ, et al. Erythromycin versus cefadroxil in the treatment of skin infections. Int J Dermatol 1992;31:131–33
- Kakar N, Kumar V, Mehta G, et al. Clinico-bacteriological study of pyodermas in children. J Dermatol 1999;26:288–93
- Kiani R. Double-blind, double-dummy comparison of azithromycin and cephalexin in the treatment of skin and skin structure infections. Eur J Clin Microbiol Infect Dis 1991;10:88–4
- Klein GC, Jones WL. Comparison of streptozyme test with antistreptolysin O, antideoxyribonuclease B and antihyaluronidase tests. Appl Microbiol 1971;21:257–9
- Linder CW. Treatment of impetigo and ecthyma. J Fam Pract 1978;7:697–700
- McLinn S. A bacteriologically controlled, randomized study comparing the efficacy of 2% mupirocin ointment (Bactroban) with oral erythromycin in the treatment of patients with impetigo. J Am Acad Dermatol 1990;22:883–5
- Meisel C, Blenk H. The effectiveness of ciprofloxacin in bacterial skin infections. Z Hautkr 1988;63:1015–22
- Parish LC, Aten EM. Treatment of skin structure infections: a comparative study of Augmentin and cefaclor. Cutis 1984;34:567–70

■ Parish LC, Witkowski JA. Systemic management of cutaneous bacterial infections. Am J Med 1991;91:106S-110S

■ Pien FD. Double-blind comparative study of two dosage regimens of cefaclor and amoxicillin-clavulanic acid in the outpatient treatment of soft tissue infections. Antimicrob Agents Chemother 1983;24:856–9

■ Reagan DR, Doebbeling BN, Pfaller MA, et al. Elimination of coincident *Staphylococcus aureus* nasal and hand carriage with intranasal application of mupirocin calcium ointment. Ann Intern Med 1991;114:101–6

■ Sadick NS. Current aspects of bacterial infection of the skin. Dermatol Clin 1997;15:341–9

■ Schachner L, Taplin D, Scott GB, Morrison M. A therapeutic update of superficial skin infections. Pediatr Clin North Am 1983;30:397–404

■ Champion RH, Burton JL, Ebling FJG, eds. Textbook of dermatology, 6th edn. Malden, MA: Blackwell Science, 1998

■ Wortman PD. Bacterial infections of the skin. Curr Prob Dermatol 1993;5:193–228

Evidence References

1 Barton LL, Friedman AD, Portilla MGI. Impetigo contagiosa: a comparison of erythromycin and dicloxacillin therapy. Pediatr Dermatol 1988;5:88–91. Medline

2 Demidovich CW, Wittler RR, Ruff ME, et al. Impetigo. Current etiology and comparison of penicillin, erythromycin, and cephalexin therapies. Am J Dis Child 1990;144:1313–15. Medline

3 McLinn S. A bacteriologically controlled, randomized study comparing the efficacy of 2% mupirocin ointment (Bactroban) with oral erythromycin in the treatment of patients with impetigo. J Am Acad Dermatol 1990;22:883–5. Medline

4 Daniel R. Azithromycin, erythromycin and cloxacillin in the treatment of infections of skin and associated soft tissues. European Azithromycin Study Group. J Int Med Res 1991;19:433–45. Medline

5 Kiani R. Double-blind, double-dummy comparison of azithromycin and cephalexin in the treatment of skin and skin structure infections. Eur J Clin Microbiol Infect Dis 1991;10:88–4. Medline

6 Dillon HC Jr. Treatment of staphylococcal skin infections: a comparison of cephalexin and dicloxacillin. J Am Acad Dermatol 1983; 8:177–81. Medline

FAQS
Question 1
Is there any evidence to support culturing of the lesions at the initial exam?

ANSWER 1
No, treatment is typically empiric. The decision to culture infections should be based on local patterns of resistance, which should be checked with local microbiology laboratories. The local emergence of significant resistance should prompt a lower threshold to culture rather than to initiate empiric therapy.

Question 2
What is the risk of developing methicillin-resistant *Staphylococcus aureus* (MRSA)?

ANSWER 2
Adequate and complete therapy should minimize the development of MRSA. The likelihood of initial infection with MRSA in impetigo in most areas remains low; however, local variation is possible and likely over time. Communication with microbiology laboratories is helpful in choosing appropriate antibiotics.

Question 3
Is there a role for treatment of close contacts in recurrent cases?

ANSWER 3
Close contact of recurrent cases should be first cultured prior to treatment. Because asymptomatic carriers are reasonably common, treating such carriers can be helpful in reducing recurrence.

Question 4
How long does a child need to be kept home from school?

ANSWER 4
Only one day of therapy prior to return to school is necessary.

CONTRIBUTORS
Gordon H Baustian, MD
Seth R Stevens, MD
Andrea Trowers, MD

INGROWN NAIL

SUMMARY INFORMATION

DESCRIPTION

■ Common condition in shoe-wearing people
■ Mainly affects great toe
■ Defect is due to the nail pushing into the soft tissue with consequent pressure necrosis, edema, infection, and granulation tissue
■ Treatment is initially conservative, then operative

URGENT ACTION

■ Exclude osteomyelitis – institute antistaphylococcal antibiotic and refer to emergency room if suspected
■ If critical limb ischemia present (peripheral vascular disease), refer immediately

KEY! DON'T MISS!

■ Do not miss a sinus track which may indicate osteomyelitis
■ Never miss a possible neoplastic lesion

BACKGROUND

ICD9 CODE

- 703.0 Ingrowing nail (unguis incarnatus)
- 703.9 Diseases of nail

SYNONYMS

- Onychocryptosis
- Unguis incarnatus

CARDINAL FEATURES

- Signs of inflammation (e.g. pain, redness, swelling) in affected toe (usually great toe)
- Suppuration from inflamed nail fold

CAUSES
Common causes

- Soft tissue abnormalities: a soft lax pulp as occurs in debilitating disease and hyperhidrosis (soft tissue rolls over the nail plate edge); ill-fitting shoes causing an overcrowded foot (extrinsic pressure of soft tissue onto nail edge)
- Nail abnormalities: improper cutting of nail (short and curved); congenitally hypercurved nail; acquired hypercurved nail (occurs in peripheral vascular disease, pulmonary disease, and old age)
- Bone abnormalities: subungual exostosis; upward tilt of tip of distal phalanx
- Other causes: trauma; infection (e.g. in diabetics); drugs (e.g. indinavir)

Rare causes

Tumors of the soft tissue or bone causing changes in the relationship of the nail to the soft tissue, e.g. subungual melanoma, osteosarcoma.

Serious causes

Tumors of the soft tissue or bone causing changes in the relationship of the nail to the soft tissue, e.g. subungual melanoma, osteosarcoma.

Contributory or predisposing factors

- Shoes (ill-fitting): ingrown nail is rare in people who do not wear shoes
- Debility: infection and poor vascular supply contribute to the condition
- Poor foot care: a nail cut short and curved is most likely to cut into the soft tissue under extrinsic pressure from a shoe

EPIDEMIOLOGY
Incidence and prevalence
FREQUENCY
Common condition.

Demographics
AGE

- Common in the elderly because of associated disorders, e.g. peripheral vascular disease, diabetes
- Common in children and adolescents because of foot growth and tendency to wear ill-fitting footwear

GEOGRAPHY
Tends not to occur in populations where shoes are not worn.

SOCIOECONOMIC STATUS

May occur more commonly in poorer socioeconomic groups due to shoes being ill-fitting or passed down through families.

DIFFERENTIAL DIAGNOSIS
Overgrown nail
An ingrowing nail needs to be distinguished from an overgrown nail.

FEATURES
- Excess growth of the nail plate
- Generally thickened, lengthened, piled-up nail
- Nail is often discolored
- No soft tissue involvement

Soft tissue pulp infection
Infection of the distal phalanx pulp may involve the nail folds and be difficult to distinguish from an ingrown nail.

FEATURES
- Tense swelling of the whole pulp
- Increased local skin temperature
- Possible foreign body entry wound

Osteomyelitis
Osteomyelitis is a serious infection of the bone which is difficult to distinguish clinically, but must be treated promptly.

FEATURES
- Definitive diagnosis is radiologic
- Patient may be systemically unwell
- May be a discharging sinus rather than localized pus from inflamed nail fold tissue
- Localized inflammation often accompanied by proximal spread
- Bone pain (unremitting, gnawing character)
- Fever and lethargy may be present

Paronychia
Paronychia is an infection of the nail fold which may be acute or chronic.

FEATURES
- No sign of nail impingement
- Red, warm, tender nail fold (acute)
- Boggy, swollen, inflamed nail fold (chronic)
- Often follows an injury to a nail fold
- Chronic lesions often occur in people who have wet-work jobs

SIGNS & SYMPTOMS
Signs
- Inflamed toe around the nail fold
- Granulation tissue or frank pus often present
- Nail plate appears normal in consistency
- Tenderness of nail fold to palpation
- May affect medial and/or lateral aspects of toenail, and may be bilateral

There are three recognized stages of ingrown toenail.

Stage 1:
- Mild erythema, swelling, and tenderness along the nail fold

Stage 2:
- Increased erythema, hyperhidrosis, and tenderness
- Nail fold bulges over the nail plate edge and drainage occurs
- Initially serous discharge, which rapidly becomes infected
- Walking becomes difficult and wearing a shoe almost impossible

Stage 3:
- Granulation covers the lateral nail fold and inhibits free drainage
- Untreated, the epithelium will creep over the edge of the granulation tissue
- Condition becomes chronic, with recurrent acute inflammatory episodes

Symptoms
- Painful toe, especially when walking in shoes
- Red toe often with discharge (pus or serous fluid)

KEY! DON'T MISS!
- Do not miss a sinus track which may indicate osteomyelitis
- Never miss a possible neoplastic lesion

CONSIDER CONSULT
- Referral is mandatory if suspicion of neoplastic lesion, exostosis identified, or osteomyelitis

INVESTIGATION OF THE PATIENT
Direct questions to patient
General history:

Q **Have you suffered from any medical problems, either now or in the past?** Especially consider diabetes or other debilitating disease. Concurrent illness may affect the nature of the disease and treatment.

Q **Are you taking indinavir?** Indinavir is associated with an increased risk for developing ingrown nail.

Q **Have you suffered with any chest or leg cramps on walking?** May indicate presence of peripheral vascular disease.

Foot history:

Q **When did the toenail problem first occur and how did it progress?** For example, was it related to trauma or a new pair of shoes.

Q **Have you had previous problems or infections in your feet?** Determines if it is a recurrent problem, and likely cause.

Q **Have you had previous surgery to your feet?** This may indicate severity of previous similar episodes and determine future surgery.

Q **What self-treatments have you tried?** May indicate a problem with foot care methods used.

Contributory or predisposing factors

Q **How do you buy your shoes, and how often?** Ill-fitting shoes are a major predisposing cause of ingrown nails.

Q **What is your regular foot care method?** Poor foot hygiene and nail care are very important factors.

Examination

- **Are there any signs of debilitating disease?** General examination for signs such as pallor, lymphadenopathy
- **Are there any obvious skeletal malformations of the spine or lower limbs? Is the patient's gait normal?** This may indicate unusual pressures being applied to the foot
- **Are there any obvious structural abnormalities of the foot? Is there any unusual pattern of wear on the footwear?** This may indicate unusual pressures being applied to the foot
- **Is there any sign of vascular or nervous impairment to the foot?** Poor blood supply to the foot predisposes to infection and a neuropathic foot is more likely to incur injury
- **Is the nail normal?** Is it, for example, curved, misshapen
- **Is the nail fold normal?** Signs of infection/granulation tissue
- **Is there any other sign of dermatologic disease?** May indicate complicating factors or alternative diagnosis

Summary of investigative tests

- There are no routine tests for uncomplicated ingrown nail
- Microbial culture and sensitivity: not routinely necessary, but may be of value in persistent or secondary infection
- Plain radiograph of affected toe: not useful in ingrown nail, but necessary if diagnosis of osteomyelitis or exostosis suspected, and therefore normally performed by a specialist

DIAGNOSTIC DECISION

Diagnosis is based on clinical grounds.

Guidelines

Ingrown toenails. Philadelphia (PA): Academy of Ambulatory Foot and Ankle Surgery; 2000. [1]

CLINICAL PEARLS

Dyspigmentation of the adjacent skin or nail plate may suggest otherwise unapparent acral melanoma.

THE TESTS
Body fluids
MICROBIAL CULTURE AND SENSITIVITY
Description
Frank pus may be swabbed and cultured for bacteria if the physician believes antibiotic treatment may be warranted.

Advantages/Disadvantages
Advantage: not necessary in most cases, but provides targeted antibacterial treatment if done
Disadvantage: may be difficult to differentiate inflammation from infection

Normal
No culture of pathologic bacteria.

Abnormal
Significant pathologic bacteria present.

Cause of abnormal result
Bacterial infection.

Drugs, disorders and other factors that may alter results
Previous antibiotic therapy may distort result.

Imaging
PLAIN RADIOGRAPH OF AFFECTED TOE
Advantages/Disadvantages
Advantages:
- Toe X-ray presents no radiologic safety issue (minuscule exposure)
- Useful for identifying underlying bony abnormalities
- Necessary for specialist diagnosis of osteomyelitis or malignant bone tumor

Disadvantage: Definitive reporting should be done by radiologist

Normal
No significant bony abnormality (radiologist report).

Abnormal
Radiologic findings suggestive of pathology.

Cause of abnormal result
- Bony abnormalities (benign tumors, malignant tumors, fractures, mineral/collagen deficit, or infection)
- Soft tissue abnormalities (tumors, infection)
- Foreign body

TREATMENT

CONSIDER CONSULT

- Structural nail or toe deformities which may need formal surgery
- Ascending infection represents possible escalation to systemic infection; intravenous antibiotics may be required
- Complications (impaired circulation or increased infection risk such as diabetes)
- When procedure under local anesthetic would not be tolerated (mental impairment, children, allergy to local anesthetics, severe anxiety)

IMMEDIATE ACTION

Treat any serious infection present with broad-spectrum antibiotic with antistaphylococcal activity.

PATIENT AND CAREGIVER ISSUES
Patient or caregiver request

- **Is the procedure curative?** Usually – recurrence rates vary
- **How long is it likely to be before I can wear shoes again?** One week, or when pain and dressing allow
- **Is my toenail going to look normal?** Depends on procedure, but often there is a noticeable difference
- **Is an operation necessary?** Yes, if condition is not amenable/responsive to conservative measures
- **What aftercare do I need?** Postoperative nursing plan is necessary

Health-seeking behavior

- How does patient decide if their footwear is a good fit?
- How does patient cut their nails?
- How has patient been treating foot problem?

MANAGEMENT ISSUES
Goals

- Relief of pain
- Resolution of the condition, allowing return to normal activity level
- Prevention of recurrence

Management in special circumstances
COEXISTING DISEASE

- Diabetic patients must have their glycemic control optimized, need strict aseptic procedures and prophylactic antibiotics, and may require antibiotic support at an earlier stage of ingrown nail
- Other debilitated patients may benefit from early antibiotic use
- Patients with anxiety disorders may be most easily treated in hospital

COEXISTING MEDICATION

Over-the-counter and alternative therapies should normally be discontinued once definitive management has been agreed.

SPECIAL PATIENT GROUPS

- Elderly patients may prefer conservative management, including referral to a podiatrist
- Anxious young adults may prefer a general anesthetic

PATIENT SATISFACTION/LIFESTYLE PRIORITIES

■ Normal footwear is not normally worn for one week after surgery
■ Pressure in the foot may continue to cause pain for up to 3 weeks; therefore, those with jobs involving walking or foot pedal pressure may need a period of absence from work

SUMMARY OF THERAPEUTIC OPTIONS
Choices

Stage 1 ingrown nail (nonoperative treatment):

■ Involves lifting the lateral edge of the nail plate from its embedded position in the dermis of the nail fold
■ Nonabsorbent cotton wool or acrylic mesh is passed beneath the corner of the nail
■ As the lesion is painful, the patient may need a few days of intermittent warm soaks, a cutout shoe and reduced physical activity before inflammation subsides enough to allow this procedure to occur
■ Treatment (self administered) is continued daily and the patient returns weekly for inspection
■ Resolution usually takes 2–3 weeks

Stage 2 ingrown nail (nonoperative treatment):

■ All pressure must be removed from the toe (including hosiery)
■ Toe is soaked in warm water for 10–15min four or five times a day
■ Drainage is cultured and the sensitivities determined
■ Broad-spectrum antibiotic (cloxacillin, erythromycin) is prescribed
■ Once swelling recedes and drainage stops, use of material under the distal nail corner can occur as in stage 1
■ Nail splinting by flexible tube enables resolution without permanent nail matrix damage for stage 2 and 3

Stage 2 ingrown nail (operative treatment):

■ Surgical intervention may be preferred at this stage
■ Choice is between definitive surgery such as partial matricectomy or the lesser procedure of nail avulsion (complete or partial) which carries a high recurrence rate

Stage 3 ingrown nail (surgical intervention):

■ Surgical intervention is the treatment of choice
■ There are many surgical procedures described for ingrown nail. It is advised that the one most familiar to the physician is used. Chemical partial matricectomy is suitable for performance in an office

Lifestyle measures such as proper foot care, particularly correct trimming of nails, or podiatry input for those who are less dextrous, may also be beneficial.

Guidelines

Ingrown toenails. Philadelphia (PA): Academy of Ambulatory Foot and Ankle Surgery; 2000. [1]

Never

Never use local anesthetic containing epinephrine for digital ring-block anesthesia.

FOLLOW UP

■ Nonoperative treatment: treatment (self-administered) is continued daily and the patient returns weekly for inspection; resolution usually takes 2–3 weeks
■ Surgical treatment by chemical partial matricectomy: wound inspection and dressing renewal 24h after surgery are recommended, with further inspection at weekly intervals until toe has healed

Plan for review
- It is usual to see the patient within the first week of treatment to check for any complications
- Review following this can usually take place weekly (often with the nurse alone) until healing is complete

DRUGS AND OTHER THERAPIES: DETAILS
Drugs
CLOXACILLIN

Cloxacillin is the penicillin of choice for its antistaphylococcal action.

Dose
Cloxacillin adult dose usually 250–500mg four times a day for 5 days.

Efficacy
Highly effective against staphylococcal infection.

Risks/benefits
Risks:
- Use caution in penicillin hypersensitivity
- Do not administer for prolonged or repeated doses

Benefit: Reduces local nail fold infection and minimizes risk of spread

Side effects and adverse reactions
- Gastrointestinal: nausea, vomiting, diarrhea, abdominal pain, colitis, gastritis, anorexia
- Central nervous system: headache, fever, depression, anxiety, seizures
- Skin: rashes
- Hematologic: bone marrow depression, hemolytic anemia
- Genitourinary: impotence, proteinuria, hematuria, vaginitis

Interactions (other drugs)
- Aminoglycosides - Anticoagulants - Chloramphenicol - Erythromycin

Contraindications
- No known contraindications

Acceptability to patient
Cloxacillin is generally highly acceptable as it is available in either capsule or suspension form.

Follow up plan
Review after completion of course.

Patient and caregiver information
The prescribed course should always be completed.

ERYTHROMYCIN
Dose
Erythromycin 500mg twice daily or 250mg four times daily for 5–10 days.

Risks/benefits
Risks:
- Caution in hepatic and renal impairment, porphyria
- Avoid concomitant administration with terfenadine, astemizole, and cisapride

- Use caution with repeated or prolonged therapy
- Potential risk of superinfection with resistant bacteria

Side effects and adverse reactions
- Cardiovascular system: dysrhythmias (uncommon)
- Eyes, ears, nose, and throat: deafness, tinnitus
- Gastrointestinal: anorexia, nausea, diarrhea, abdominal pain, vomiting, heartburn, hepatitis
- Genitourinary: moliniasis, vaginitis
- Skin: rashes, pruritus, vaginal candidiasis

Interactions (other drugs)
- Alfentanil ■ Antiarrhythmic drugs (digoxin, disopyramide) ■ Antihistamines (astemizole) ■ Anticonvulsants (carbemazepine, valproic acid) ■ Antiviral agents ■ Benzodiazepines ■ Bromocriptine ■ Buspirone ■ Cisapride ■ Clozapine ■ Colchicine ■ Cyclosporine, tacrolimus ■ Ergotamine ■ Ethanol ■ Felodipine ■ Itraconazole ■ Methylprednisolone ■ Penicillin ■ Quinidine ■ Sildenafil ■ Statins ■ Theophylline ■ Warfarin ■ Zopiclone

Contraindications
- Liver disease ■ Various infections (vaccinia, varicella, mycobacterial, fungal, viral)

Acceptability to patient
Erythromycin is available in several presentations.

Follow up plan
Review after completion of course.

Patient and caregiver information
The prescribed course should always be completed.

Surgical therapy
CHEMICAL PARTIAL MATRICECTOMY
- Surgical treatment for ingrown toenail should be individualized; the physician may find it necessary during the procedure to modify the technique being used
- Partial matricectomy (partial nail plate removal and matrix destruction) is the most commonly used operative procedure for ingrown toenail
- Matricectomy can be accomplished either surgically or with a locally cytotoxic chemical (described here); all matricectomy techniques should be aseptic procedures

Regional anesthesia is achieved using a ring-block technique:
- 1% local anesthetic sterile solution (lidocaine or mepivacaine) without epinephrine is introduced with a small-gauge needle 1cm distal to the first web space
- Ensure that both plantar digital nerves and dorsal sensory branches of the superficial peroneal nerve are well anesthetized by injecting up to 5mL in an inverted 'U' fashion around the base of the toe
- Allow full anesthesia to develop over 20min before undertaking the surgical procedure
- Use of a light rubber tourniquet is traditionally said to prolong useful anesthetic time (but there is no evidence for this)

Estimate how much nail plate border will need to be removed:
- Decide on the line of nail excision that will prevent future impinging on the nail fold in its uninflamed state

- Use a flat sterile dissector (e.g. a MacDonald) to lift the nail plate away from the nailbed lateral to this line by blunt dissection
- Straight scissors or a scalpel can be used to divide the nail along this line from distal to proximal, ensuring complete division through the growth plate (it may be necessary to dissect or reflect the eponychium)
- Nail fragment is carefully avulsed making sure its proximal subeponychial portion is completely removed
- Brief pressure may be necessary to achieve hemostasis

Debride any severely infected/inflamed nail fold tissue as necessary:
- Use of a curette (e.g. Volkmann spoon) is preferred to a scalpel
- Apply liquid phenol to cotton bud (thinned in bulk if necessary); avoid unnecessary contact of phenol with surrounding tissues
- Push phenol-soaked cotton bud into space left by excised nail portion, as deeply under the eponychium as it will go
- Maintain phenol application for a minimum of 90s before removing and irrigating with saline
- Apply sterile nonadherent dressing (containing antiseptic if local infection present) and bandage securely

Efficacy
Good outcome with only a small recurrence rate.

Risks/benefits
Risk: small risk of recurrence and a very small risk of postoperative infection or hemorrhage
Benefit: primarily a rapid resolution over 2–3 weeks of a painful chronic condition

Evidence
- A systematic review found that simple nail avulsion combined with the use of phenol is more effective for the prevention of symptomatic recurrence of ingrown toenails than surgical excision without phenol [2] *Level M*
- Symptomatic recurrence rate is dramatically reduced with the addition of phenol when performing simple nail avulsion; however, this is achieved at the expense of significantly increased postoperative infection rates [2] *Level M*

Acceptability to patient
- Operative procedure is usually acceptable to a patient whose discomfort has become intolerable with conservative treatment
- Cosmetic result is usually acceptable

Follow up plan
- Usual to see patient within 24–48h to check for any complications and to change the dressing
- Review following this can take place (often with the nurse) weekly until healing is complete

Patient and caregiver information
- Extremity should be elevated for 48h
- Dressing is then removed by the nurse
- Soaks are begun for 10min several times a day and the wound is covered with only an adhesive bandage
- No shoe or hosiery should be worn for 5–7 days; it is acceptable to wear a postoperative wooden-soled shoe that has no toe box in this period
- After a week it is usually comfortable to wear a wide-toed shoe

Other therapies

NAIL SPLINTING BY FLEXIBLE TUBE

- This novel technique offers the prospect of enabling resolution of stage 2 or 3 ingrown nail without permanent nail matrix damage
- Involves lifting the lateral edge of the nail plate from its embedded position in the dermis of the nail fold
- A small flexible plastic tube (e.g. a sterile drainage tube), split lengthways to form a gutter, is then pushed along the 'ingrowing' nail plate edge as far proximally as it will go, under local anesthesia

Efficacy
First reports suggest promising results.

Risks/benefits
Risk: recurrence rates may be higher
Benefit: less invasive procedure, may reduce complications

Acceptability to patient
Likely to be highly acceptable.

Follow up plan
Similar to conventional nonsurgical method.

Patient and caregiver information
Similar to conventional nonsurgical method.

LIFESTYLE

- Proper foot care, particularly correct trimming of nails
- Podiatry input may benefit those who are less dextrous

RISKS/BENEFITS

Benefit: nails cut in a noncurved fashion are less likely to impinge on the nail fold.

ACCEPTABILITY TO PATIENT

- May be difficult to self-manage
- May be expensive to use regular podiatry

FOLLOW UP PLAN

- No routine follow up
- Report new problems or recurrences promptly

PATIENT AND CAREGIVER INFORMATION

This is potentially a lifelong problem and requires constant awareness of preventive measures and the need for prompt treatment of exacerbations.

EFFICACY OF THERAPIES

- Stage 1 and some stage 2 ingrown nails can be expected to respond to nonsurgical management, although resolution may take several weeks
- Stage 3 and some stage 2 ingrown nails can be expected to resolve with surgical treatment within 2–3 weeks

Evidence

- A systematic review found that simple nail avulsion combined with the use of phenol is more effective for the prevention of symptomatic recurrence of ingrown toenails than surgical excision without phenol [2] *Level M*
- Symptomatic recurrence rate is dramatically reduced with the addition of phenol when performing simple nail avulsion; however, this is achieved at the expense of significantly increased postoperative infection rates [2] *Level M*

Review period

- Nonoperative treatment: treatment (self-administered) is continued daily and the patient returns weekly for inspection; resolution usually takes 2–3 weeks
- Surgical treatment by chemical partial matricectomy: wound inspection and dressing renewal 24h after surgery are recommended, with further inspection at weekly intervals until toe has healed

PROGNOSIS

- While resolution of the presenting condition can usually be attained without much difficulty, it must be recognized that ingrown nail has a significant recurrence rate
- Patient education on foot care and definitive surgical intervention lessen the recurrence rate

Clinical pearls

For many patients, wide-toe box shoes will prevent recurrence.

Therapeutic failure

- Failure of nonsurgical management usually leads to consideration of surgical treatment
- Failure of surgical treatment in the office warrants specialist referral for consideration of more complex definitive procedures

Recurrence

- There is a wide range of further procedures for recurrent ingrown nail – laser surgery, cryotherapy, negative galvanic therapy, trephine, and onychotripsy; these have not been critically evaluated in controlled trials
- Most require referral to a surgical specialist

Deterioration

- Deterioration after surgical treatment may be due to infection which may respond to a broad-spectrum antibiotic
- Any other deterioration may necessitate specialist referral

COMPLICATIONS

- Ascending infection is rare, but represents the possible escalation to systemic infection
- Complications due to impaired circulation necessitate consideration of degree of vascular compromise and its management as well as the ingrown nail
- Increased infection risk in diabetes requires consideration of additional anti-infective measures such as broad-spectrum antibiotics, and the effect such infection has on glycemic control

CONSIDER CONSULT

- Failure of surgical treatment in the office warrants specialist referral for consideration of more complex definitive procedures, unless the PCP is confident undertaking revision surgery on the toenail

- Ingrown nail is rare in people who do not wear shoes
- Poor foot hygiene and nail care are very important factors

RISK FACTORS

- **Wearing shoes:** ingrown nail is commoner in people who wear shoes; avoidance of ill-fitting footwear helps prevent the condition
- **Nail cut short and curved:** this is more likely to cut into the soft tissue under extrinsic pressure from a shoe; education in correct nail-cutting technique helps prevent progression to ingrown nail or its complications

MODIFY RISK FACTORS

SCREENING

Selective screening is only of value in patients with diabetes because of their increased risk of infection and complications.

REGULAR FOOT INSPECTION

Diabetic foot care is an essential screening tool to maintain health and prevent a number of foot complications, including ingrown nail.

Cost/efficacy

Annual foot inspection by a trained podiatrist or diabetic specialist nurse is highly cost effective in the diabetic population.

PREVENT RECURRENCE

Once an ingrown nail has been resolved successfully with either nonoperative or surgical treatment, the patient must be instructed to take precautions against recurrence by care in choice of footwear and proper technique for cutting nails.

KEY REFERENCES

- Mori H. A comparison of the nail matrix phenolization method with the elevation of the nail bed-periosteal flap procedure. J Dermatol 1998;25:1–4
- Schulte KW, Neumann NJ, Ruzicka T. Surgical pearl: nail splinting by flexible tube: a new noninvasive treatment for ingrown toenails. J Am Acad Dermatol 1998;39:629–30
- Canale ST. Ingrown toenail (onychocryptosis, unguis incarnatus). In: Campbell's operative orthopedics. 9th edn. St Louis (MO): Mosby , 1998

Evidence references and guidelines

1. Ingrown toenails. Philadelphia (PA): Academy of Ambulatory Foot and Ankle Surgery; 2000. Available at the National Guidelines Clearinghouse
2. Rounding C, Bloomfield S. Surgical treatments for ingrowing toenails (Cochrane Review. In: The Cochrane Library, 1, 2002. Oxford: Update Software

CONTRIBUTORS

Joseph E Scherger, MD, MPH
Seth R Stevens, MD
Rolland P Gyulai, MD, PhD

LICHEN PLANUS

DESCRIPTION

- A papular skin eruption
- Occurs on flexor surfaces of limbs, mucous membranes, and genitalia
- Cutaneous rash is typically itchy, violaceous
- Exhibits fine, white, reticulate pattern
- Self-limiting

ICD9 CODE
697.0 Lichen planus

SYNONYMS
- Lichen
- Lichen planus et atrophicus

CARDINAL FEATURES
- Lichen planus is a papulosquamous skin disorder characterized by the six 'P's: pruritus, polygonal shape, planar, purple color, papules, and plaques
- Symmetrical lesions
- Common on flexor aspects of extremities, e.g. wrists
- Shows fine, white, reticulate pattern (Wickham's striae)
- Exhibits Koebner's phenomenon
- Mucosal involvement, especially oral, is common

CAUSES
Common causes
- Unknown
- Mainly thought to be an autoimmune disorder as there is a lymphocytic infiltrate in the dermis
- Some familial tendency with an association to human leukocyte antigen (HLA)-B7 genotype

Contributory or predisposing factors
- May be found in association with other autoimmune disorders such as ulcerative colitis, dermatomyositis, myasthenia gravis, alopecia areata, lichen sclerosis
- Drug-induced: tetracyclines, chloroquine, penicillamine, gold, thiazide diuretics, beta-blockers, and NSAIDs
- There is an association with hepatitis C infection. The reason for this is not known

EPIDEMIOLOGY
Incidence and prevalence
No accurate figures are available. There may be a higher incidence in December and January.

INCIDENCE
- 10/1000 new patients seen in US dermatology clinics
- 20–40/1000 new patients seen in European dermatology clinics

PREVALENCE
4.4/1000 population.

Demographics
AGE
- Mainly occurs in middle-aged people 30–60 years of age
- Uncommon in children

GENDER
No significant gender difference.

RACE
No good evidence but lichen planus may be more common in Europe and Asia than in Australia and the US.

GENETICS

There is an increased prevalence in three HLA types: HLA-B7, -DR1, and -DR10. The extent of this association is not known.

GEOGRAPHY

No good evidence but lichen planus may be more common in Europe and Asia.

SOCIOECONOMIC STATUS

There is no known association.

DIFFERENTIAL DIAGNOSIS
Drug eruptions
Idiopathic or allergic reaction to medication.

FEATURES
- Positive drug history
- Rash is usually more generalized and not specifically on flexor surfaces

Psoriasis
Psoriasis is a chronic, papulosquamous, inflammatory skin disease. A positive family history is common.

FEATURES
- Affects extensor rather than flexor surfaces
- Scale present plus Auspitz sign
- Nail changes are more common
- No involvement of oral mucosa
- Not as itchy as lichen planus

Lichenified eczema
Can appear in areas of chronic eczema. Infection may also be present.

FEATURES
- Lesions poorly demarcated
- Exhibits crusting and edema
- No mucosal involvement
- No nail changes
- No flat-topped, shiny papules

Pityriasis rosea
Pityriasis rosea is a self-limiting condition that may be of viral origin. Disease shows seasonal variation.

FEATURES
- Begins with pink, solitary, scaly lesion called a 'Herald' patch
- Typically on the chest
- Fine scale present
- Not specifically the flexor surfaces, no mucosal involvement, pink rather than violaceous, no lichenification, itch is less a feature

Leukoplakia
Associated with immune deficiency and usually involves oral or genital mucosa. This condition can be premalignant.

FEATURES
- Lesions typically on the tongue rather than mucosa
- White patches
- Fissuring is common

Systemic lupus erythematosus
Systemic lupus erythematosus is an autoimmune disease characterized by antinuclear antibodies and vasculitis. Most commonly affects women.

FEATURES

■ Fewer lesions
■ Affects palms and face (malar butterfly rash)
■ Less itchy than lichen planus
■ Sun sensitive

Oral candidiasis

Oral candidiasis is a fungal overgrowth that is usually opportunistic, though may indicate immunocompromise.

FEATURES

■ Lesions appear in the mouth
■ White mucosal flecks, surrounded by erythema, which can be scraped off
■ Lacks the fine, reticulate pattern of lichen planus
■ Responds to antifungal therapy

Secondary syphilis

Secondary syphilis is a sexually transmitted disease where *Treponema pallidum* enters via skin abrasion. Skin manifestations occur 4–8 weeks after primary chancre.

FEATURES

■ May affect trunk, palms, and soles
■ There may be associated systemic effects

Seborrheic dermatitis

Seborrheic dermatitis is a scaly, greasy rash typically in the hairline or areas with many sebaceous glands.

FEATURES

■ Crusting and scaling often present
■ Different distribution of rash

Lichen simplex

Also known as neurodermatitis.

FEATURES

■ Localized
■ Itchy
■ Light-purple exaggerations of skin creases
■ Occurs in scratch areas, such as calves in men and nape of neck in females

SIGNS & SYMPTOMS
Signs

■ Clinical signs vary depending on the location of affected sites, including the limbs, scalp, nails, mucous membranes, and genitalia
■ Mucous membranes are commonly affected and may be sole site of involvement. White streaks in a linear or reticular pattern may be present on the buccal mucosa or tongue (must be distinguished from 'bite-line'). Lesions may be reticular, plaque-like, atrophic, erosive, papular, or bullous. The background may be red or violaceous. Ulcerated oral lesions may have a tendency to malignant transformation but the evidence for this is not strong
■ Genital involvement is common amongst men. Papules, in a ring formation, may be present on the glans penis. Women may have white striae, papules, or erosions on the vulva and/or vagina

- Nail changes can be present in patients with lichen planus. The nails develop longitudinal ridges and grooves, subungual hyperkeratosis, pterygium, and hyperpigmentation. There may be onycholysis, thinning, and atrophy
- The scalp may have scaly, pruritic, violaceous papules. Scarring alopecia can result. Nail and mucosal involvement are commonly associated
- Cutaneous rash may be present. Lichen planus has several forms, i.e. hypertrophic, atrophic, annular, linear, follicular, erosive, vesicular, guttate, and actinic. Violaceous, shiny papules may present. Scarring and residual pigmentation are common

Symptoms

- Slow onset is usual, with maximal spread within 1–4 months
- Initial lesions on flexor aspects of limbs
- Maximal spread within 1–4 months
- Itch, especially hypertrophic lesions
- Oral lesions are painful or burning, but can be asymptomatic
- Bald patches in the scalp
- Dyspareunia, pruritus, or burning can present in genital lesions

ASSOCIATED DISORDERS

- Chronic, host-versus-graft disease
- Ulcerative colitis
- Alopecia areata
- Myasthenia gravis
- Hepatitis C infection
- Dermatomyositis
- Vitiligo
- Lichen sclerosis

CONSIDER CONSULT

- When diagnosis is in doubt

INVESTIGATION OF THE PATIENT

Direct questions to patient

Q **Where did the rash start?** Lichen planus usually starts on the flexor surface of wrists or lower legs.

Q **For how long have you noticed the lesions?** Typically, the appearance is insidious over 1–4 months.

Q **Is the rash itchy?** Lichen planus is usually itchy, especially hypertrophic lesions.

Q **Are there any lesions or white patches in the mouth?** Lichen planus involves the mouth in 50% of cases.

Q **Is there any rash or lesion on the genitalia?** Genital involvement is also common. Also, question women regarding symptoms of dyspareunia or burning.

Q **Have you noticed any bald patches on the scalp?** Lichen planus can give rise to irreversible alopecia.

Q **Are there any nail changes?** There are nail changes in 10% of cases.

Contributory or predisposing factors

Q **Is there any history of infection/exposure to hepatitis C?** There is an association between hepatitis C and lichen planus. The reason for this is not known.

Q **Are you taking medication?** Lichen planus is associated with many drugs, including tetracyclines, gold, thiazides, beta-blockers, and NSAIDs. There is uncertainty whether ACE inhibitors are implicated.

Family history

Q Is there a family history of lichen planus? Some patients have a positive family history. This is probably an association with human leukocyte antigen (HLA)-B7, DR1, and DR10.

Q Is there a personal or family history of autoimmune disease, including ulcerative colitis, dermatomyositis, myasthenia gravis, alopecia areata, lichen sclerosis, or vitiligo? There is an increased incidence of lichen planus in autoimmune disorders.

Examination

- **Where is the rash?** Lichen planus is typically found on the limb flexor surfaces, mouth, scalp, and genitalia
- **What is the morphology of the rash?** The typical rash of lichen planus is violaceous, pruritic, flat-topped, and shiny. The papules are usually between 1mm and 1cm in size. Wickham's striae may be present. These fine, white, reticulate patterns on individual lesions are common, particularly in the mouth
- **Does the rash exhibit the Koebner effect?** The lesions often appear along the line of scratch or trauma to the skin. Linear lesions may appear similar to herpes zoster
- **Are there any areas of atrophy?** Atrophy may result from healing hypertrophic or annular lesions
- **Are there any erosive lesions?** Erosive lichen planus is most common on mucosal surfaces
- **Is there altered pigmentation?** Actinic lesions are annular with a hypopigmented area surrounding a hyperpigmented center. These lesions usually affect exposed areas and spare the scalp, nails, and mucous membranes. Actinic form of lichen planus is more common in India, Africa, and the Middle East
- **Are the nails involved?** There is nail involvement in 10% of cases. Changes include longitudinal ridges and grooves, subungual hyperkeratosis, pterygium, hyperpigmentation, onycholysis, thinning, and atrophy

Summary of investigative tests

- Investigations are not usually necessary as the diagnosis is made on clinical appearance
- If there is diagnostic doubt, a biopsy of skin taken from the lesion and examined histologically will confirm diagnosis; however, there is the possibility of patient discomfort or scarring, and some areas, e.g. genitalia, are difficult to biopsy. Abnormal results present as a band-like infiltrate of lymphocytes at the epidermal/dermal junction with basal cell layer damage, and hypergranulosis and acanthosis in the epidermis. This procedure is normally performed by a specialist

DIAGNOSTIC DECISION

The diagnosis is clinical and depends on recognition of the sites and types of lesions. The typical lesions of lichen planus are summarized by the six 'P's:

- Pruritus
- Purple color
- Polygonal
- Planar
- Papules
- Plaques

CLINICAL PEARLS

Evaluation for lichen planus should include examination of the volar wrists (common location), the scalp (follicular hyperkeratosis), and oral cavity (buccal streaking to ulceration may present). Nail dystrophy may also present.

PATIENT AND CAREGIVER ISSUES
Impact on career, dependants, family, friends
As with all skin disease, the social stigma of abnormal skin may be great or perceived as great by the patient. Appropriate attention must be paid to the psychosocial aspects of skin disease. Pruritus may interfere with the ability to focus and may reduce effectiveness at work or school.

Patient or caregiver request
- **What causes lichen planus?** The cause is unknown. A few cases are associated with specific medications
- **Is it infectious?** No, there is no infectious agent that could be passed on
- **Is it a form of cancer?** No, it is not a malignant condition
- **Is it inherited?** Lichen planus is not inherited, although there are some genetic types in which it is more common
- **What areas of my body can be affected?** Lichen planus can involve the skin, mouth, nails, scalp, and genitalia
- **Does it need treating?** Not always. It is usually self-limiting and if it is not itchy or painful, it can be left alone
- **Will it get worse?** After about 4 months the rashes are stable and will not extend
- **Will it leave any marks?** As the papules fade, they can leave a brown discoloration. These may eventually fade
- **Will I get it again?** About one in 6 people get another attack
- **Is there a cure?** There is no known cure. Treatment aims to stop itching and improve appearance until it goes on its own
- **How long will it take to go away?** In 50% of cases it has gone by 6 months. By 18 months, 85% of cases have cleared
- **Is there a risk of developing cancer?** Not in most forms. There may be an increased risk of mouth cancer if you have lichen planus in the mouth, especially under the tongue. The evidence for this is not strong but regular check-ups are advised

Health-seeking behavior
- **Have you taken any medications, prescribed or not?** Lichen planus is associated with many medications
- **Have any creams already been tried?** Lichen planus is treated with topical steroid creams

MANAGEMENT ISSUES
Goals
- Aim to relieve itching
- Aim to improve appearance
- Aim to follow up oral lesions until possible spontaneous resolution

Management in special circumstances
COEXISTING DISEASE
If the patient is already being treated for an autoimmune disease they may already be taking oral steroids or immunosuppressants. This would restrict treatment choices to topical therapies.

COEXISTING MEDICATION
If the patient is taking a drug known to be associated with lichen planus, the drug should be stopped and an alternative found.

SPECIAL PATIENT GROUPS

Although rare in children, the response to treatment and the course of the disease is similar to that of adults.

PATIENT SATISFACTION/LIFESTYLE PRIORITIES

- Some patients will be affected by the physical appearance of the rash more than others will. This may influence whether or not to treat
- Long-term use of potent topical steroids and oral steroids should be avoided

SUMMARY OF THERAPEUTIC OPTIONS
Choices

- In mild or localized disease, the first-choice therapy is a potent, topical steroid
- Topical retinoids may be used as second-line therapy, especially for oral lichen planus
- If the itch is severe, an oral antihistamine can be used
- Systemic steroids, such as prednisolone, may be used if there is poor symptom control or no improvement with the use of creams. Usually, this is for more severe disease and the evidence of efficacy is poor
- Oral retinoids can be used for severe cases. They are usually prescribed by a specialist due to the possible side effects
- Psoralen plus ultraviolet A (PUVA) has been used, but the evidence on efficacy is poor. Usually prescribed by a specialist after failure of other treatments
- Topical tacrolimus or cyclosporines have been used, but the evidence for efficacy is poor. Usually used by a specialist only as a last resort if all other treatment has failed

Clinical pearls

Lichen planus can be surprisingly difficult to treat, and occasionally requires more aggressive therapy than initially believed.

Never

Never use oral retinoids in women of childbearing years without ensuring effective contraception. This is due to the risk of teratogenicity.

FOLLOW UP

Most cases resolve spontaneously with no need for follow up.

Plan for review

- Check for adequate symptom control
- Check for any new sites of disease
- If on active treatment, review at 1–2 monthly intervals is reasonable
- Oral lichen planus should be followed-up until resolved. This is due to the small risk of developing squamous carcinoma

Information for patient or caregiver

A useful patient information site is The British Association of Dermatologists or American Academy of Dermatology.

DRUGS AND OTHER THERAPIES: DETAILS
Drugs
TOPICAL STEROIDS

Examples include:

- Fluocinonide cream or ointment 0.05%
- Triamcinolone acetonide cream or ointment 0.1%
- Clobetasol propionate cream or ointment 0.05%

Dose
- Apply a thin layer twice daily to the lesions
- Occlusion may be used in severe cases
- Generally, use for maximum of 4 weeks
- Clobetasol is a strong topical steroid; total dosage should not exceed 50g/week, use for a maximum of 2 weeks, not recommended for use in children under 12

Efficacy
Widely used, but no proven efficacy in lichen planus.

Risks/benefits
Risks:
- The potential for systemic absorption must be considered
- Use with caution in children

Benefits:
- Inexpensive
- First-line choice for oral lichen planus is fluocinonide in an adhesive or gel base
- Intradermal triamcinolone can be used for thick, hyperkeratotic lesions. The evidence for this is anecdotal only

Side effects and adverse reactions
- Skin: rash
- Dermatitis
- Pruritus
- Atrophy
- Hypopigmentation
- Striae
- Xerosis
- Burning
- Stinging upon application
- Alopecia
- Conjunctivitis

Interactions (other drugs)
- No known interactions with topical betamethasone

Contraindications
- Do not use on face, axilla, or groin

Acceptability to patient
- Use of topical preparations is inconvenient for some patients
- Ointments can be messy and stain clothing

Follow up plan
Avoid use after lesions have healed.

Patient and caregiver information
- Apply sparingly to the affected area only
- Use for short courses and apply regularly
- If skin becomes irritated, stop using it and see the doctor

TOPICAL RETINOIDS

Examples include:

- Tretinoin cream, gel, solution, or lotion 0.025%
- Isotretinoin gel 0.05%

Dose

Apply thinly once daily.

Efficacy

- Not proven by clinical trials
- Anecdotal evidence only

Risks/benefits

Risks:

- Side effects may be worse than no treatment in some cases
- Increased sensitivity to UVB light and sunlight
- Use caution with broken or sunburnt skin
- Use caution in renal and hepatic impairment
- Avoid UV light

Benefit: May provide symptom relief

Side effects and adverse reactions

- Gastrointestinal: nausea, vomiting, diarrhea, constipation
- Skin: irritation, rash, pruritus, alopecia, changes in pigmentation, sweating, dryness, erythema, burning, photosensitivity, peeling, blistering
- Ears, eyes, nose, and throat: visual disturbances
- Central nervous system: fever, headache, dizziness
- Cardiovascular system: hypertension, dysrhythmias

Interactions (other drugs)

- Soaps ■ Salicylic acid ■ Benzoyl peroxide ■ Sulfur ■ Resorcinol

Contraindications

- Pregnancy and breastfeeding ■ Cutaneous epithelioma

Acceptability to patient

- Dependent on the degree of side effects
- Women of childbearing age may find the risk or teratogenicity unacceptable

Follow up plan

Cease use after lesions have healed.

Patient and caregiver information

- Apply sparingly to the affected area only
- Use for short courses and apply regularly
- If skin becomes irritated, stop using it and see the doctor
- Women of childbearing age should take adequate contraceptive precautions

ANTIHISTAMINES
Promethazine can be used.

Dose
Promethazine: 12.5–25mg orally at night, increasing to twice daily if required.

Efficacy
Efficacious in treating pruritus.

Risks/benefits
Risks:
- Use caution in acute asthma or COPD
- Use caution in bladder neck and intestinal obstruction, cardiovascular disease, hypertension, prostatic hypertrophy, urinary retention, history of peptic ulcer, hepatic disease
- Use caution in children and the elderly
- Sedation may be unacceptable to some patients

Benefit: May provide symptomatic relief

Side effects and adverse reactions
- Gastrointestinal: anorexia, constipation, diarrhea, dry mouth, nausea and vomiting, jaundice, cholestasis
- Genitourinary: urination difficulties, impotence, galactorrhea, menstrual irregularities, ejaculation difficulties
- Central nervous system: drowsiness, excitation in children, restlessness, extrapyramidal symptoms, tardive dyskinesia, neuroleptic malignant syndrome
- Hematologic: blood cell dyscrasias
- Cardiovascular system: orthostatic hypotension, palpitations, tachycardia
- Eyes, ears, nose, and throat: blurred vision, dry nose and throat, retinopathy, corneal opacification
- Skin: rash, skin hyperpigmentation, photosensitivity

Interactions (other drugs)
- Amantidine ▪ Aminolevulinic acid ▪ Amoxipine ▪ Antidiabetics ▪ Antimuscarinics (e.g. phenothiazines, H_1 blockers, tricyclic antidepressants) ▪ Antipsychotics ▪ Antithyorid agents ▪ Bromocriptine ▪ Cabergoline ▪ Central nervous system depressants ▪ Clozapine ▪ Cyclobenzaprine ▪ Disopyramide ▪ Epinephrine ▪ Levodopa ▪ MAOIs ▪ Methoxsalen ▪ Metoclopramide ▪ Vitamin A analogs

Contraindications
- Glaucoma ▪ Seizure disorders or those receiving anticonvulsants ▪ Pregnancy or breastfeeding ▪ Propylthiouracil

Acceptability to patient
- Usually highly acceptable due to availability of newer, nonsedating antihistamines
- Some people may find risk of drowsiness unacceptable, e.g. machine operators

Follow up plan
Check for adequate symptom control.

Patient and caregiver information
- Use as required
- If taking sedating antihistamine, suggest using it at night

PREDNISOLONE
Oral steroid.

Dose
- Adult: 5–60mg once daily for 4–6 weeks, tapering over the following 4–6 weeks
- Dose reduction is required in children

Efficacy
No good scientific evidence available, particularly on effect on duration of disease.

Risks/benefits
Risks:
- Overwhelming septicemia if patient has an infection
- Loss of control of blood glucose in those with diabetes
- Prolonged use causes adrenal suppression
- Use caution in elderly due to risk of diabetes and osteoporosis
- Use caution in patients with psychosis, seizure disorders, or myasthenia gravis
- Use caution in congestive heart failure, hypertension
- Use caution in ulcerative colitis, peptic ulcer, or esophagitis

Side effects and adverse reactions
- Side effects are minimized by short duration of therapy
- Cardiovascular system: hypertension, thromboembolism
- Central nervous system: insomnia, euphoria, depression, psychosis
- Endocrine: adrenal suppression, impaired glucose tolerance, growth suppression in children
- Eyes, ears, nose, and throat: cataract, glaucoma, blurred vision
- Gastrointestinal: dyspepsia, peptic ulceration, oesophagitis, oral candidiasis
- Musculoskeletal: proximal myopathy, osteoporosis
- Skin: delayed healing, acne, striae

Interactions (other drugs)
- Aminoglutethamide ▪ Barbiturates ▪ Cholestyramine ▪ Clarithromycin, erythromycin ▪ Colestipol ▪ Isoniazid ▪ Ketoconazole ▪ NSAIDs ▪ Oral contraceptives ▪ Rifampin ▪ Salicylates ▪ Troleandomycin ▪ Warfarin

Contraindications
- Systemic infection ▪ Avoid live virus vaccines in those receiving immunosuppressive doses

Acceptability to patient
- Many possible side effects may limit use
- Offers speedy relief from itching

Follow up plan
- Avoid long-term therapy
- Monitor blood sugar, potassium, blood pressure, and growth in those at risk

Patient and caregiver information
- Take single dose in the morning
- Report symptoms of anorexia, weakness, vomiting, and diarrhea
- Avoid stopping therapy abruptly
- Long or repeated courses to be avoided

ORAL RETINOID
- Example is acitretin
- Mechanism of action is unknown, but may inhibit abnormal keratinization

Dose
- Initially 25–30mg daily for 2–4 weeks, then adjust dose according to response; usual dose required 25–50mg/day; treatment should be discontinued once lesions have resolved (or if there is no significant response)
- Pediatric dose not established

Efficacy
Has been shown in controlled trials to improve remission and symptoms.

Risks/benefits
Risks:
- Side effects can be significant
- Women of childbearing age should use contraception; should be used during and for 3 years after therapy
- Use caution in renal insufficiency, liver disease, hyperlipidemia, pancreatitis

Benefit: An effective therapy taken for brief duration

Side effects and adverse reactions
- Cardiovascular system: flushing, edema
- Central nervous system: dizziness, fatigue, headache, hot flashes
- Eyes, ears, nose, and throat: cheilitis, dry eyes and nose, conjunctivitis, xerostomia
- Gastrointestinal: anorexia, increased appetite
- Metabolism: abnormal liver function tests, hypertriglyceridemia, hyperglycemia
- Musculoskeletal: arthralgia, myalgia
- Skin: alopecia, dry skin

Interactions (other drugs)
- **Methotrexate toxicity** ■ **Alcohol** ■ **Tetracyclines** ■ **Progesterone**

Contraindications
- **Pregnancy and breastfeeding** ■ **Alcohol** ■ **Use of vitamin A**

Acceptability to patient
- Severe risk of teratogenicity may make this medication unacceptable to women of childbearing age. Women need to use effective contraception for 3 years post-therapy
- Many side effects can also limit use

Follow up plan
- Transaminase levels pretreatment and monthly thereafter
- Lipid levels pretreatment and monthly thereafter

Patient and caregiver information

- Avoid low-dose progestin contraception
- Women of childbearing years to use effective contraception during therapy and for 3 years after therapy
- Avoid alcohol
- Should not donate blood for at least one year after last dose

EFFICACY OF THERAPIES

Good, randomized controlled trials to support the use and effectiveness of most treatments for lichen planus are lacking. Many treatments are based on anecdote. It is appropriate to remember that the natural course is spontaneous resolution within one year.

PROGNOSIS

■ 65% of cases clear within 12–18 months
■ 10–20% of cases will recur
■ Oral lichen planus or nail involvement can persist for years

Clinical pearls

Lichen planus can be difficult to treat and, often, spontaneous remission occurs prior to satisfactory treatment.

Recurrence

■ 10–20% of cases will have recurrences
■ First-line treatments remain the same
■ In resistant cases, psoralen plus ultraviolet A (PUVA) or immunosuppressants, e.g. cyclosporine or topical tacrolimus, have been tried. These require specialist supervision and there is little scientific evidence for their use or efficacy

COMPLICATIONS

■ Malignant transformation has been reported in ulcerative oral lesions in men. There are confounding factors that make this evidence insecure
■ Alopecia is of the scarring variety and can be permanent
■ Hypertrophic lesions can leave hyperpigmentation
■ Lichen planus has been linked to hepatitis C infection. The manner in which hepatitis C virus (HCV) predisposes patients to lichen planus is not known. It is argued that it may be appropriate to screen patients with lichen planus for HCV infection
■ Vulvar lesions can be painful

CONSIDER CONSULT

■ If treatment with retinoids or PUVA or immunosuppressants is needed
■ If oral lichen planus is persistent or painful

PREVENTION

RISK FACTORS

Hepatitis C infection is epidemiologically associated with lichen planus. The etiology remains unclear.

ASSOCIATIONS
American Academy of Dermatology
930 N Meacham Road
PO Box 4014
Schaumburg, IL 60168-4014
Tel: (847) 330-0230
Fax: (847) 330-0050
http://www.aad.org

British Association of Dermatologists
19 Fitzroy Square
London W1T 6EH
United Kingdom
Tel: 0044 20 7383 0266
Fax: 0044 20 7388 5263
E-mail: admin@bad.org.uk
http://www.bad.org.uk

American Academy of Family Physicians
11400 Tomahawk Creek Parkway
Leawood, KS 66211-2672
Tel: (913) 906-6000
E-mail: fp@aafp.org
http://www.aafp.org

KEY REFERENCES
- Chan ES-Y, Thornhill M, Zakrzewska J. Interventions for treating oral lichen planus (Cochrane Review). In: The Cochrane Library, 1, 2002. Oxford: Update Software
- American Family Physician. Katta R. Lichen planus
- Sharma R, Maheshwari V. Childhood lichen planus: a report of fifty cases. Pediatr Dermatol 1999;16(5):345–8
- Cribier B, Frances C, Chosidow O. Treatment of lichen planus. An evidence-based medicine analysis of efficacy. Arch Dermatol 1998;(12):1521–30
- Laurberg G, Geiger JM, Hjorth N, et al. Treatment of lichen planus with acitretin. A double blind, placebo-controlled study in 65 patients. J Am Acad Dermatol 1991;24(3):434–7
- Nasr IS. Topical tacrolimus in dermatology. Clin Exp Dermatol 2000;25(3):250–4

FAQS
Question 1
Could you speculate on the pathogenesis?

ANSWER 1
A variety of findings suggest immune system abnormality. Clearly, some cases relate to infectious agents such as hepatitis C, while others to drug eruptions, and others suggest autoimmune phenomenon. Thus, while we correctly state in this file that the pathogenesis is unknown, the vast majority of evidence incriminates an immune pathogenesis.

Question 2
Should other sequelae be considered?

ANSWER 2
Persistent injury to the epidermis by lichen planus can lead to exposure of neoantigens to the immune system. This can give rise to secondary, rather than causative, autoimmune phenomena. Therefore, in long-standing and particularly severe disease, a secondary skin disease may develop.

Question 3
Do variants exist?

ANSWER 3
Yes, a number of variants exist. An actinic variant occurs classically in those of west Asian descent (e.g. Afghanistan) which is photoexacerbated. Lichenoid drug eruptions occur as a drug eruption that can be very difficult to treat and may persist for over one year after the discontinuation of the offending agent. Lichen planopilaris presents predominantly as an alopecia. Twenty nail dystrophy is, as the name implies, an abnormality of all nails and may present without other abnormality.

CONTRIBUTORS
Fred F Ferri, MD, FACP
Seth R Stevens, MD
Richard Averitte, MD

MELANOMA

SUMMARY INFORMATION

DESCRIPTION

- Skin neoplasm resulting from malignant degeneration of melanocytes caused most commonly by overexposure to the sun
- The common clinical classifications include superficial spreading melanoma, nodular melanoma, lentigo maligna melanoma, acral lentiginous melanoma, mucosal lentiginous melanoma, and unclassified melanoma
- Diagnosis is based on the clinical features, reinforced by pathologic examination of a biopsy sample
- Warning signs include (A) asymmetric appearance (color and/or shape), (B) irregular borders, (C) variable colors (tan, brown, blue, red, white, pink, or gray), (D) large diameters (>6mm), and (E) elevation above the skin surface
- Treatments include surgical removal of the tumor, lymph node dissection in cases of nodal metastasis, isolated limb perfusion, chemotherapy, immunotherapy, radiation therapy
- Patient self-examination and screening are critical for early detection, successful treatment, and positive response

URGENT ACTION

Patients who have suspicious lesions should be referred for additional diagnostic procedures or undergo biopsy.

KEY! DON'T MISS!

Any suspicious lesion should result in a referral for the patient or an immediate excisional biopsy.

ICD9 CODE
172.9 Melanoma of the skin, site unspecified.

SYNONYMS
Malignant melanoma.

CARDINAL FEATURES
- Characteristic history is of a changing existing mole or a newly appearing pigmented skin or mucosal lesion, often in a patient with a history of chronic sun exposure or a family history of skin cancer
- Typical characteristics include variegated colors, irregular borders, raised surfaces, and ulcerations
- Most commonly found on the legs in women and on the back in men
- Superficial spreading melanoma occurs in women more than men; it is the most common growth pattern and progresses from a flat lesion to a glossy, lacy (notched and indented), darkly colored, deep lesion
- Nodular melanoma occurs more in men than women; it is found mainly on the trunk, head, and neck, is the second most common growth pattern, and quickly progresses to a small lesion (1–2cm) of uniform color (blue-black) with greater vertical growth than horizontal growth and irregular borders
- Lentigo maligna melanoma is usually located on the face and is frequently large (at least 3cm), flat, speckled (tan, black, and white), and accompanied by other changes in the skin that result from sun exposure
- Acral lentiginous melanoma occurs in dark-skinned people more than light-skinned people and is a stain-like lesion of variegated color
- Subungual melanoma (a type of acral lentiginous melanoma) occurs in dark-skinned people more often than in light-skinned people and usually presents as dark discolorations under the nail bed, usually on a thumb or big toe

CAUSES
Common causes
There are no direct causes associated with the development of melanoma.

Contributory or predisposing factors
- Skin that sunburns easily
- Poor tanning response
- Light-colored skin
- History of several severe sunburns
- Exposure to ultraviolet-B light
- Numerous nevi, especially atypical nevi
- Tendency for freckling
- History of skin cancer
- Genetic predisposition and familial history of melanoma
- Use of tanning salon
- Previous melanoma

EPIDEMIOLOGY
Incidence and prevalence
Incidence and prevalence rates rose steeply during the 1980s and 1990s, although the rates of increase have slowed recently.

INCIDENCE
In the US:

- 0.19 new cases per 1000 males/year
- 0.14 new cases per 1000 females/year

Rates are higher in Australia, where the population has more sun exposure:

- 0.37 new cases per 1000 males/year
- 0.28 new cases per 1000 females/year

PREVALENCE
13 cases per 1000 Caucasian Americans.

Demographics
AGE

- Median age at diagnosis is 53 years; however, melanoma occurs most commonly in young adults
- Superficial spreading melanoma is more common in young adults who take part in sun-exposing activities and is more commonly reported in women than in men
- Nodular melanoma usually occurs during middle age and is more commonly reported in men than in women
- Lentigo maligna melanoma occurs most commonly in older Caucasian women
- Acral lentiginous melanoma occurs most commonly in older people

GENDER
The lifetime risk of being diagnosed with melanoma is significantly higher for men (1.91%) than for women (1.37%).

RACE

- Caucasians are more likely to develop melanoma than other people in the US
- Dark-skinned people are more likely to develop acral lentiginous melanoma and subungual melanoma than light-skinned people

GENETICS
Familial history of melanoma increases the risk of melanoma.

GEOGRAPHY
A higher frequency rate of melanoma is reported among people who live near the equator.

SOCIOECONOMIC STATUS
The highest frequency of melanoma is reported among educated, professional, urban people who participate in sun-exposing activities on an irregular basis.

DIFFERENTIAL DIAGNOSIS
Dysplastic nevus
FEATURES
- Tan or brown lesions are the most common, but lesions may be red, pink, or black
- Larger than 5mm in diameter
- Usually appear on the back, chest, buttocks, or scalp
- Potentially malignant
- Perform skin biopsy to confirm diagnosis

Solar lentigo
FEATURES
- Spot on face or other exposed skin surface
- Tan or brown lesion
- Caused by sun exposure
- No treatment is required

Blue nevus
FEATURES
- Skin nodule of 2–7mm diameter
- Steel-blue color
- Usually found on face or arms
- Grows slowly but may change characteristics and require immediate medical attention

Basal cell carcinoma
It is usually only pigmented basal cell carcinoma that poses differential diagnostic problems with melanoma. Amelanotic melanomas may look like basal cell carcinoma.

FEATURES
- Caused by the proliferation of basal keratinocytes
- Usually occurs on sun-exposed skin
- Locally aggressive tumor
- Rarely metastasizes
- Diameter can range from a few millimeters to a few centimeters

Seborrheic keratosis
FEATURES
- Slightly raised greasy bump that may itch
- Tan or black
- Usually on the face, neck, chest, or upper back
- Has a more 'stuck-on' appearance and frequently has a pitted surface

Spitz nevus
Also known as benign juvenile melanoma.

FEATURES
- Most commonly seen in children, although it does occur in adults
- Usually appears suddenly
- Hairless, red-brown, dome-shaped papules or nodules
- Smooth or warty surface
- Lesions vary in size from a few millimeters to 1–2cm
- Lesions sometimes bleed after trauma

SIGNS & SYMPTOMS
Signs
Warning signs that a lesion may be a melanoma can be summarized as 'ABCDE':

- A: asymmetry
- B: border irregularity
- C: color variegation
- D: diameter enlargement (>6mm)
- E: elevation

Specific types of melanoma have their own pattern:

- Superficial spreading melanoma occurs in women more than in men; is the most common growth pattern; and progresses from a flat lesion to a glossy, lacy (notched and indented), darkly colored, deep lesion
- Nodular melanoma occurs in men more than in women; is found mainly on the trunk, head, and neck; is the second most common growth pattern; and quickly progresses to a small lesion (1–2cm) of uniform color (blue-black) with greater vertical growth than horizontal growth and irregular borders
- Lentigo maligna melanoma is usually located on the face and is usually large (at least 3cm), flat, speckled (tan, black, and white), and accompanied by other changes in the skin that result from sun exposure
- Acral lentiginous melanoma occurs in dark-skinned people more often than in light-skinned people and is a stain-like lesion of variegated color
- Subungual melanoma (a type of acral lentiginous melanoma) occurs in dark-skinned people more often than in light-skinned people and usually presents as dark discolorations under the nail bed, usually on a thumb or big toe

Symptoms
- Lesions reported by patient, often on the lower body extremities in women and on the back in men
- Itch (occasional)
- Bleeding (rare)

ASSOCIATED DISORDERS
- Melanoma-associated retinopathy and melanoma-associated vitiligo are thought to be the result of autoimmune reactions induced by melanoma antigens targeting retinal or melanocyte proteins. They are usually associated with more favorable prognosis
- Paraneoplastic syndromes, such as paraneoplastic pemphigus, can be associated with malignant melanoma
- Other nonspecific, associated disorders can develop as the direct or indirect consequences of therapy (e.g. immunosuppression, hair loss, radiation ulcers)

KEY! DON'T MISS!
Any suspicious lesion should result in a referral for the patient or an immediate excisional biopsy.

CONSIDER CONSULT
- Refer to dermatology if uncomfortable distinguishing melanoma from other elements of the differential diagnosis
- Any suspicious lesion should result in referral to a dermatologist or an immediate excisional biopsy for diagnostic testing

INVESTIGATION OF THE PATIENT
Direct questions to patient
Q **How much sun exposure have you had?** Sun exposure is the main cause of melanoma.

Q **Have you ever had a melanoma?** Potential for current lesion being malignant increases. Also, potential for recurrence increases.

Q **Has this mole changed? If so, how?** Changing moles are the primary warning sign of melanoma.

Q **Do you have any other unusual skin problems or lumps or bumps?** The patient may have noticed lymph nodes or other lesions (e.g. intransit metastases) apart from the presenting lesion.

Contributory or predisposing factors
Q **Do you have a history of severe sunburns?** This is an important risk factor for melanoma.

Q **Do you find it difficult to tan?** People who do not tan are at increased risk of melanoma.

Family history
Q **Do you have a family history of melanoma?** This is an important risk factor.

Examination
- **Physical examination of the suspect lesion.** Check for typical characteristics and growth patterns – use the 'ABCDE' rules
- **Perform complete skin examination.** Examination should include the mucous membranes, looking for other suspicious lesions
- **Check the lymph nodes for lymphadenopathy and the abdomen for hepatosplenomegaly.** These findings may indicate metastatic spread

Summary of investigative tests
- Perform a diagnostic biopsy of the suspicious lesion (or refer the patient to a specialist for the biopsy); have the diagnosis confirmed by histology; and assess tumor thickness (by the Breslow staging method), tumor invasion (by the Clark staging method), and ulceration
- The presence or absence of regional lymph node metastases should be assessed by sentinel lymph node biopsy – recommended for all patients with melanomas with a Breslow's thickness (depth) of >1mm
- Distant visceral or lymph node metastases should be assessed by imaging methods (chest X-ray, computed tomography, or positron electron tomography). Imaging studies should be performed on patients with melanomas of Breslow's thickness >4mm and are optional for patients with melanomas of <4mm
- Routine laboratory tests (complete blood count, urea, creatinine, and electrolytes, and lactate dehydrogenase) should be performed
- Excisional biopsies are preferable for smaller (<1.5cm in diameter) lesions
- Incisional biopsy procedures are acceptable for large melanomas or when the melanoma is on the face, hands, or feet, and the amount of skin obtained is critical. It is no longer believed that incisional biopsy increases risk of metastasis
- Punch biopsies are acceptable, but only when the entire melanoma is able to be removed
- Whichever biopsy procedure is used, it is imperative that the biopsy be full-thickness and include the subcutaneous layer
- Shave or curette biopsies are contraindicated if the entire depth of the lesion cannot be assessed with certainty

DIAGNOSTIC DECISION

- Characteristic clinical features suggest the diagnosis of melanoma and prompt biopsy of the suspicious lesion
- Absolute diagnosis is dependent on the histopathologic evaluation of the biopsy sample
- Tumor thickness (assessed by the Breslow staging method) and ulceration are the most powerful characteristics and are critical for determining the potential for nodal involvement, systemic metastases, and the prognosis. Recent multicenter analysis demonstrated that the level of invasion, assessed by the Clark staging method, has a significant impact only within the group of thin melanomas (up to 1mm Breslow's thickness)
- In patients with melanomas thicker than 1mm, the presence or absence of regional lymph node metastases should be assessed by sentinel lymphadenectomy
- Distant visceral or lymph node metastases should be assessed by imaging methods

Guidelines

- Guidelines of care for primary cutaneous melanoma. The American Academy of Dermatology Melanoma Guidelines [1]
- Final version of the American Joint Committee on Cancer staging system for cutaneous melanoma [2]

CLINICAL PEARLS

- For patients with numerous atypical moles, biopsy of the most abnormal-appearing will help establish the histologic correlates of the clinical lesions and provide guidance on the approach to other lesions
- Do not discount pigmented lesions on dark-skinned patients. While acral lentiginous melanomas are most common, other sorts of melanoma can occur in these populations
- Comfort with the diagnosis of seborrheic keratoses should be developed in those wishing to perform biopsy of pigmented lesions. These extremely common pigmented lesions, described above, can meet all the ABCDE features of melanoma yet be obviously benign
- In melanomas that are candidates for sentinel lymph node biopsy, the biopsy should be performed before wide local excision in order to identify the sentinel lymph node better
- If a patient insists that a mole needs to be removed, it should be biopsied

THE TESTS
Body fluids
COMPLETE BLOOD COUNT
Description
Venous blood sample.

Advantages/Disadvantages
Advantages:
- Easy, inexpensive, and readily available test
- Provides baseline measurement

Disadvantage: Very nonspecific

Normal
- Hemoglobin (adult male): 13.5–18.0g/dL
- Hemoglobin (adult female): 12.5–16.0g/dL
- Hematocrit (adult male): 42–52%
- Hematocrit (adult female): 37–47%
- White blood cell count (adult): 4.0–10.5x1000/mm^3

- Red blood cell count (adult male): 4.7–6.0x10^6/mm^3
- Red blood cell count (adult female): 4.2–5.4x10^6/mm^3
- Mean corpuscular volume (adult): 78–100fL
- Mean corpuscular hemoglobin (adult): 27–31pg
- Mean corpuscular hemoglobin concentration: 32–36g/dL
- Platelet count: 150,000–450,000/mm^3

Abnormal
- Values outside the normal ranges
- Keep in mind the possibility of a falsely abnormal result
- Abnormal results are usually associated with advanced disease or caused by treatment

Cause of abnormal result
Advanced disease or aggressive treatment.

UREA, CREATININE, AND ELECTROLYTES
Description
Venous blood sample.

Advantages/Disadvantages
Advantages:
- Easy, inexpensive, and readily available test
- Provides baseline measurements

Disadvantage: Very nonspecific

Normal
- Blood urea nitrogen: 3.3–6.7mmol/L (8–25mg/dL)
- Creatinine: 60–120mcmol/L (0.6–1.6mg/dL)
- Sodium: 135–147mmol/L
- Potassium: 3.8–5.0mmol/L

Abnormal
- Values outside the normal ranges
- Keep in mind the possibility of a falsely abnormal result
- Abnormal results are usually associated with advanced disease or caused by treatment

Cause of abnormal result
Advanced disease or aggressive treatment.

LACTATE DEHYDROGENASE
Description
Two or more venous blood samples obtained more than 24h apart.

Advantages/Disadvantages
Advantages:
- Easy and inexpensive test
- One of the most predictive independent factors of diminished survival. Patients with distant metastases and elevated lactate dehydrogenase levels are assigned to the worst prognostic group regardless of the site of the distant metastases

Normal
50–150U/L.

Abnormal
>150U/L.

Cause of abnormal result
Increased lactate dehydrogenase levels are presumably associated with the growing and disintegration of the tumor mass.

Drugs, disorders and other factors that may alter results
Hemolysis.

Biopsy
BRESLOW'S MICROSTAGING METHOD
Description
- Histologic determination of the thickness of the melanoma in the biopsy sample
- Measured at the thickest part of the tumor (tumor invasion associated with skin appendages is excluded)
- Expressed as the distance of the deepest melanoma cell from the top of the epidermis in millimeters
- Thresholds are: T1, 0–1.00mm; T2, 1.01–2.00mm; T3, 2.01–4.00mm; T4, >4.00mm

Advantages/Disadvantages
Advantages:
- Primary category for the T classification of melanoma
- Strongest predictor of survival and disease outcome

Disadvantage: Should be assessed by a specialist

CLARK'S MICROSTAGING METHOD
Description
- Histologic assessment of the level of melanoma invasion into the skin in the biopsy sample
- Measured at the thickest part of the tumor (tumor invasion associated with skin appendages is excluded)
- Expressed as the skin level at the deepest melanoma cell
- Thresholds are: I, epidermis; II, papillary dermis; III, lower papillary dermis; IV, reticular dermis; V, subcutis

Advantages/Disadvantages
Advantage: Significant predictor of disease outcome and survival within the subgroup of thin melanomas (up to 1mm Breslow's thickness)

Disadvantages:
- Less predictive of survival outcome for melanomas >1mm Breslow's thickness
- Should be assessed by a specialist

SENTINEL LYMPHADENECTOMY
Description
- Surgical removal and histologic evaluation of the first-draining regional lymph nodes of the affected skin area
- Sentinel lymph node is detected by the combination of lymphatic mapping, dye detection, and radioactive probes
- Recommended for all patients with melanomas >1mm Breslow's thickness

Advantages/Disadvantages
Advantages:
- Very significant predictor of disease outcome and survival
- Relatively well tolerated by the patients, and complications are rare and usually mild
- Good indicator of lymphatic spread, and positive results should prompt regional lymphadenectomy

Disadvantage: Requires skilled surgical personnel

Imaging
CHEST X-RAY
Advantages/Disadvantages
Advantages:
- Readily available
- Can help to rule out metastases to the chest

Disadvantage: Exposes patient to ionizing radiation

Abnormal
Evidence of metastases in the chest.

Cause of abnormal result
Secondary spread to the chest.

COMPUTED TOMOGRAPHY SCAN
Advantages/Disadvantages
Advantages:
- Reasonably readily available
- Can help to rule out or diagnose metastases to the chest, abdomen, or brain

Abnormal
Evidence of metastases in the chest, abdomen, or brain.

Cause of abnormal result
Secondary spread to the chest, abdomen, or brain.

POSITRON ELECTRON TOMOGRAPHY
Advantages/Disadvantages
Advantages:
- May be more sensitive than radiography or computed tomography scanning at detecting metastatic spread
- Provides full body images

Disadvantages:

- Positive results often require further evaluation with other diagnostic methods
- Expensive
- Not readily available in all medical centers

Abnormal
Evidence of metastases.

Cause of abnormal result
Secondary spread to the affected body area.

CONSIDER CONSULT

- After biopsy, if the diagnosis is confirmed by histology, patients should be referred to a surgical specialist for sentinel lymphadenectomy and wide re-excision
- Refer to a multidisciplinary melanoma program, which provides better outcomes at lower cost
- Refer to a dermatologic, surgical, or medical oncologist for adjunctive therapy in appropriate patients

IMMEDIATE ACTION

Patients who present with suspicious lesions should undergo immediate excisional biopsy for diagnostic testing.

PATIENT AND CAREGIVER ISSUES
Patient or caregiver request

- **How much sun exposure is too much?** There is no exact amount below which the risk of melanoma is eliminated. Epidemiologic data consistently show that blistering sunburns during childhood increase the risk of subsequent melanoma; therefore these should be avoided
- **How can I protect myself?** Reduce exposure to sunlight by limiting outdoor activity in the middle of the day (10am–3pm). Photoprotective clothing, hats, and sunscreens can supplement behavioral approaches. Avoid tanning salons
- **Is sunscreen a protection or a hindrance?** Patients may have heard that using sunscreen protects them from only one type of ultraviolet light. There has been recent controversy regarding sunscreen use and subsequent melanoma risk. In particular, the question has been, do sunscreens protect against sunburn (redness, pain, blistering) to a greater extent than against carcinogenesis, thereby removing the natural signal to get out of the sun and so causing increased exposure to sunlight and enhanced melanoma risk? The issue is greatly clouded by the evolution in sunscreen formulations over the past few decades, including the former use in Europe of psoralens as sunscreens, which form DNA adducts and are clearly mutagenic. More recently, broad-spectrum sunscreens have been and are being developed that protect against ultraviolet-A (the so-called tanning rays) as well as ultraviolet-B (the so-called burning rays). Currently, opinion leaders believe that broad-spectrum, high-factor sunscreens are protective
- **Are sun protection factors greater than 15 superfluous?** The sun protection factor (SPF) of a sunscreen formulation is determined experimentally by exposing human subjects with and without sunscreen protection to simulated sunlight. The SPF is the amount of light that induces redness (usually measured in seconds) in sunscreen-protected skin divided by the amount of light that induces redness in unprotected skin. SPF is predominantly a measure of ultraviolet-B protection. Thus a sunscreen with an SPF of 15 will delay the onset of sunburn in an person who would otherwise burn in 10min so that burning does not start until 150min (2.5h). This sort of exposure is not uncommon. Additionally, inadequate application of the sunscreen, inadequate reapplication (should be at least every 2h), and the variability of SPF between people have all led to the recommendation that high-SPF, broad-spectrum sunscreens be used

MANAGEMENT ISSUES
Goals

- Identify and remove early melanomas
- Remove malignant tumor successfully
- Prevent recurrence of malignant melanoma

Management in special circumstances

Melanoma in childhood:

- Melanoma is rare in children and often poses differential diagnostic difficulty (pigmented Spitz nevus) – excision biopsy is usually warranted
- If melanoma is diagnosed, a second histopathology opinion should be sought to confirm the diagnosis
- The recommended treatment of melanoma in children is the same as that for adults

Melanoma during pregnancy:

- Pregnancy does not seem to affect the clinical course or prognosis of melanoma
- Melanoma has been reported to cross the placenta, but this appears to occur only in mothers with highly advanced melanoma
- Pregnancy is not advisable for at least 2 years after the excision of a clinically significant melanoma (>1.5mm) and for at least 5 years with melanoma in the lymph nodes
- The treatment of primary melanoma does not usually differ because a woman is pregnant

COEXISTING DISEASE

- Multiple primary melanoma is relatively common: at least 5% of patients with a previous melanoma subsequently develop a new primary melanoma
- Multiple primary melanomas are more common in patients with multiple atypical nevi
- The treatment for multiple primary melanomas is based entirely on the tumor thickness of each specific melanoma

COEXISTING MEDICATION

Neither hormone replacement therapy nor the use of the contraceptives seem to play any role in the natural history of melanoma.

SPECIAL PATIENT GROUPS

- Pregnant women with melanoma should be immediately referred to specialist for a complete evaluation and recommendations
- Evaluation and final treatment recommendations for a pregnant patient with melanoma is individualized, depending on the stage of the tumor and the pregnancy status
- Regardless of the gestational age, each pregnant patient should undergo excisional biopsy for any suspicious lesions

PATIENT SATISFACTION/LIFESTYLE PRIORITIES

The following may cause compliance problems:

- Significant change in outdoor activities, including amount of sun exposure, change in attire for protection against the sun, and use of sunscreens
- The critical need for diligent self-examination of the skin

SUMMARY OF THERAPEUTIC OPTIONS
Choices

- The first step in treatment of a primary melanoma is to perform a biopsy (excisional preferred) in order to remove the melanoma and to determine the clinical nature of the lesion, the potential for metastasis, and the prognosis for recurrence and survival
- For a primary melanoma, perform wide local excision of the tumor based on Breslow's thickness and ulceration, determined by the biopsy; sentinel lymph node dissection is recommended for patients with melanomas thicker than 1mm
- Therapeutic lymph node dissection – in cases of positive sentinel lymphadenectomy or clinically detectable lymphadenopathy, surgical excision of the affected nodes is advised
- Local recurrence – options in order of preference include surgical excision, isolated limb perfusion combined with chemotherapy and hyperthermia, or radiation therapy

- Intransit metastases – options include surgical excision, regional lymph node dissection, isolated limb perfusion, regional chemotherapy infusion, radiation therapy, intralesional immunotherapy, systemic chemotherapy, and electroporation
- High-risk or recurrent stage II or III melanoma – adjuvant therapy involving therapeutic dissection, radiotherapy, or systemic therapy
- Stage IV metastatic melanoma – because cure is not expected, options for treatment include no treatment, palliative surgical excision, radiation therapy, systemic chemotherapy including investigational studies, single-agent chemotherapy, biologic agents – immunotherapy, monoclonal antibodies, tumor vaccines, gene therapy, intralesional therapy, or combinations of any of these treatments
- Interferon-alfa may be used as adjuvant to surgery in patients at high risk of recurrence (specialist advice must be sought)

Guidelines
- Guidelines of care for primary cutaneous melanoma. The American Academy of Dermatology Melanoma Guidelines [1]

Clinical pearls
Congenital nevi are associated with increased risk of malignant transformation. Guidelines for therapy are frequently changing, though excision at an age when the child is able to co-operate with surgery under local anesthesia is appropriate for many such patients.

Never
- Never use shave or curette biopsies in cases of melanoma – they are contraindicated
- Never ignore a suspicious lesion because a patient is in a low-risk group (e.g. a patient with a darkly pigmented skin type or a child)

FOLLOW UP
Plan for review
- Skin examinations must be performed regularly to detect any recurrence
- Laboratory and radiographic examinations are not very helpful in the follow up care for melanoma

The following signs and symptoms should be looked for:
- Constitutional – weight loss, malaise, decreased appetite, weakness, fatigue, fever
- Respiratory – cough, hemoptysis, pneumonia, pleurisy, chest pain, dyspnea
- Gastrointestinal – cramping, abdominal pain, bleeding, nausea, anorexia, vomiting, constipation, jaundice
- Neurologic – headache, memory disturbance, depression, focal neurologic symptoms, visual disturbances, seizures, balance problems, blackouts, numbness, local weakness, paralysis, mood swings
- Skin/lymphatics – color change, swollen glands, nonhealing/bleeding skin lesion, lumps, new pigmented skin lesion, easy bruising
- Musculoskeletal – bone pain

Information for patient or caregiver
- Adjustments for specific lifestyle issues (sun exposure, clothing for outside activities, sunscreen, periodic skin examinations) can reduce the potential of recurrence of melanoma
- Educate patient how to perform proper self-examination
- Advise patient that first-degree family members are at increased risk of melanoma

DRUGS AND OTHER THERAPIES: DETAILS
Surgical therapy
SURGICAL EXCISION

- Early and complete excision of melanoma with appropriate clinical margins is the hallmark of melanoma treatment
- Use a wide local excision and adjust margin of normal skin obtained, depending on tumor thickness and presence or absence of ulceration
- Suggested margins for wide local re-excision (based on the 2001 guidelines of the American Academy of Dermatology): melanoma in situ, 0.5cm; melanoma <2mm thick, 1cm; melanoma >2mm thick, 2cm
- Preferably perform surgical excision of all easily accessible (e.g. skin, lymph node) metastases
- Primary closure of surgical wound is usually possible, but sometimes skin transplantation, flaps, or other methods are required
- Surgical excision is limited in patients with poor prognosis to cases where the lesion is accessible and involves a 'safe' number and size of lesions

Efficacy
- For melanomas up to 2mm thick, a 1cm margin provides local control and survival rates similar to those observed with a 3cm margin (frequency of local recurrence is approximately 2% with a 1cm excision)
- For melanomas of 1–4mm thick, a 2cm margin of resection provides local control and survival rates that are as good as a 4cm margin (frequency of local recurrence is approximately 2% with a 2cm excision)
- Surgical excision in patients with poor prognosis is purely palliative

Risks/benefits
Risks:
- Skin transplantation, flaps, or other methods of surgical wound closure may cause cosmetically less acceptable results
- Surgical excision used in patients with a poor prognosis may prolong life for a short time only

Benefit: Early and complete excision of melanoma with appropriate clinical margins is the hallmark of melanoma treatment

Evidence
There is evidence that less radical surgery is effective in the management of melanoma:
- The recommended clinical excision margin is 0.5cm for melanoma in situ, 1cm for lesions <2mm, and 2cm for lesions up to 2mm [1] *Level C*
- Wide surgical margins (3–5cm) have not been shown in randomized controlled trials (RCTs) to improve survival or local recurrence rates [3] *Level P*
- An RCT of patients with melanomas up to 2mm thick compared wide and narrow excision. A 1cm excision margin was compared with 3cm. No significant difference was noted in the occurrence of metastatic disease between the groups. Disease-free and overall survival rates were similar. Three of 305 patients in the narrow resection group had local recurrence of disease as first relapse [4] *Level P*
- An RCT compared 2cm with 4cm excision margins for melanomas of 1–4mm thickness. At follow up, there was no significant difference in local recurrence, intransit metastases, or overall survival between the groups. The narrow excision group had less need for skin grafting and a shorter hospital stay [5] *Level P*

Acceptability to patient
- Acceptable, since surgery is the definitive treatment
- Cosmetic result is usually acceptable

Follow up plan
- Routine follow up Is required, at least annually, where a full history and examination should be performed
- Patients with thicker tumors or lymph node involvement require more regular follow up
- Low-risk melanoma patients are generally examined 6-monthly for 2 years and then annually. Patients with melanomas >1mm are seen 3-monthly for the first year, then 4-monthly for 2 years, and then 6-monthly for 2 years. Annual visits commence at 5 years. Patients should be followed for 10 years
- Full skin examination, inspection of the primary surgical site, and examination for metastasis are important
- Clinical information is a better indication of recurrence than laboratory and imaging investigations
- Lactate dehydrogenase measurements and chest X-rays may be indicated

Patient and caregiver information
- Patients should be educated on skin and lymph node self-examination and sun protection
- Information on early warning signs of melanoma should be given

LYMPH NODE DISSECTION
- Sentinel lymphadenectomy is recommended for all melanoma patients with >1mm tumor thickness
- In patients who have a positive sentinel lymphadenectomy or clinically evident lymph node metastases, total lymph node dissection should be performed

Efficacy
- Patients with lymph node metastases have a less favorable disease outcome than patients with only skin-limited disease
- The number of positive nodes is the most effective predictor of survival. Treatment recommendations are based on the thresholds: one positive lymph node; two or three positive lymph nodes; four or more positive lymph nodes
- Ulceration of the primary tumor and metastatic burden of lymph nodes (micro- or macrometastasis) are the second most significant determinants of disease outcome for patients with lymph node metastases
- 5-year survival rates range from 88% (one positive node, no ulceration of primary melanoma) to <50% (four or more nodes, with ulceration)
- Efficacy for axillary node dissection is dependent on complete removal versus partial removal
- Overall, the prognosis after lymphadenectomy is good, especially when only one node is involved

Risks/benefits
Risks:
- Complications after ilioinguinal lymph node dissection include leg edema, seroma, functional deficits, persistent severe lymphedema, and residual edema
- Complications after complete axillary node dissection include seroma, infection, nerve dysfunction, pain, hemorrhage, and arm edema
- Complications after neck dissection include seroma, pain, skin slough, neck pain, functional deficit, and chylous leak
- Risks of parotidectomy include facial nerve injury, temporary facial paralysis, and gustatory sweating

Evidence
There is no evidence for the benefit of elective lymph node dissection; however, it may provide benefit for certain patients.

- Patients with cutaneous melanoma and no clinical evidence of lymph node involvement were randomized to receive elective lymph node dissection or surgery at the time of clinical recurrence. No significant survival benefit was noted for elective lymph node dissection in four RCTs. In a retrospective analysis, there was a trend towards benefit for elective dissection for certain patients [3] *Level P*
- Sentinel node biopsy is appropriate for patients with melanoma thickness greater than 1mm, lesions that are 1mm or less with histologic ulceration, or Clark level 4 or higher [6] *Level C*

Acceptability to patient
Possible complications and the risk/benefit aspects of lymph node dissection should be carefully discussed with the patient before surgery.

Follow up plan
- Patients with thicker tumors or lymph node involvement require more regular follow up
- Low-risk melanoma patients are generally examined 6-monthly for 2 years and then annually. Patients with melanomas >1mm are seen 3-monthly for the first year, then 4-monthly for 2 years, and then 6-monthly for 2 years. Annual visits commence at 5 years. Patients should be followed for 10 years
- Full skin examination, inspection of the primary surgical sites, and examination for metastasis are important
- Clinical information is a better indication of recurrence than laboratory and imaging investigations
- Lactate dehydrogenase measurements and chest X-rays may be indicated

Patient and caregiver information
- Patients should be educated on how to perform periodic skin self-examination
- Sun protection education is essential
- Lymphedema and edema secondary to lymph node dissection is a possible complication

Radiation therapy
LOCAL RADIATION THERAPY
- Radiation therapy should be used when surgical excision is not possible in patients with local recurrence or intransit metastases
- Radiation therapy may be used alone or in combination with hyperthermia

Risks/benefits
Risk: Acute or chronic radiation side effects (inflammation, ulcer, tumor)
Benefit: Can provide palliation

Acceptability to patient
Usually well tolerated.

Follow up plan
Attention should be paid to long-term radiation side effects.

ADJUVANT RADIATION THERAPY
Use in combination with surgery in patients with nodal involvement.

Efficacy
Local response has been reported as >85%.

Risks/benefits
Risk: Acute or chronic radiation side effects (inflammation, ulcer, tumor)
Benefit: Can provide palliation

Acceptability to patient
Usually well tolerated.

Follow up plan
Attention should be paid to long-term radiation side effects.

Chemotherapy
REGIONAL CHEMOTHERAPY INFUSION
Intra-arterial infusion therapy with dacarbazine or cisplatin is used to treat patients with intransit metastases who have failed isolated limb perfusion.

Efficacy
Partial and transient responses of 40–50% have been reported.

Risks/benefits
Benefit: Regional chemotherapy appears to offer a better chance of improvement than systemic chemotherapy in cases of intransit metastases.

Acceptability to patient
Possible side effects may discourage patients from undergoing therapy.

Follow up plan
- Specialist follow up is required
- Blood workup to check for possible side effects
- Discontinue therapy if disease is progressing despite treatment

SYSTEMIC CHEMOTHERAPY
- Use single-agent or combination chemotherapies to treat recurrent melanoma or when surgical methods have failed
- Many systemic chemotherapy regimens are still in the investigational stage, but patients who have poor prognosis for survival should be encouraged to participate in clinical studies
- Use in patients with isolated metastases to visceral organs
- Dacarbazine is the most active agent against melanoma: 850–1000mg/m^2 intravenously for one day every 3–4 weeks, 250mg/m^2 per day intravenously for 5 days every 3 weeks, or 4.5mg/kg per day intravenously for 10 days every 4 weeks
- Clinical studies with nitrosoureas, cisplatin, carboplatin, vinca alkaloids, taxol, and other agents have shown some response but still remain investigatory

Efficacy
- Systemic chemotherapy regimens with dacarbazine have resulted in response rates of 20% among patients with skin, subcutaneous tissue, and nodal involvement, with 2% achieving complete responses for at least 6 years
- Duration of response is usually 5–6 months

Risks/benefits
Risk: Effects of dacarbazine therapy include nausea, vomiting, pain at injection site, neutropenia, thrombocytopenia, flu-like symptoms, photosensitivity, and liver failure.

Evidence
Combination chemotherapy and dacarbazine have been compared with placebo in RCTs. No survival advantage was noted in patients receiving chemotherapy [3] *Level P*

Acceptability to patient
Possible side effects (nausea, vomiting, pain at injection site, neutropenia, thrombocytopenia, flu-like symptoms, photosensitivity, and liver failure) may discourage patients from undergoing therapy.

Follow up plan
- Perform regular blood workup to check for possible side effects
- Discontinue therapy if disease is progressing despite treatment

Patient and caregiver information
Possible side effects (nausea, vomiting, pain at injection site, neutropenia, thrombocytopenia, flu-like symptoms, photosensitivity, and liver failure) and the risk/benefit aspects of the treatment should be discussed with the patient.

INTERFERON-ALFA
Interferon-alfa is a frequently utilized adjunctive modality.

Efficacy
Increases disease-free survival. Best evidence is that interferon is particularly beneficial in stage IIB or III patients in whom relapse-free survival is increased from 26% to 36% and 5-year survival is increased from 37% to 46%.

Risks/benefits
Risks:
- Flu-like symptoms (e.g. fever, chills, malaise, anorexia, myalgia)
- Renal, hepatic, and cardiac toxicities

Benefit: Prolonged disease-free and overall survival in appropriately selected patients

Evidence
There is some evidence for the use of alpha-2b interferon in the treatment of certain patients with melanoma.
- The use of alpha-2b interferon may be appropriate for patients with melanoma tumor depth >4mm or for patients with known lymph node metastases or metastasis intransit. Use is uncertain in cases of ulcerated tumors 2.01–4mm deep [6] *Level C*
- An RCT compared high-dose alpha-2b interferon with observation in patients with melanoma (>4mm or resectable stage III tumor). The treatment group was found to have an improved disease-free and overall survival at follow up [7] *Level P*
- Early results from a large RCT comparing alpha-2b interferon with placebo have not shown any benefit for the treatment group [8] *Level P*
- Low-dose alpha-2b interferon was compared with observation only in two RCTs of patients with stage II melanoma. A trend towards survival advantage was noted in the treatment groups of one trial, and there was an increase in the period before relapse in both trials [3] *Level P*

Acceptability to patient
- May be administered intravenously or intramuscularly, both of which can be unpleasant
- Toxicities are usually bothersome to some extent and may be dose limiting

Follow up plan
Administration and follow up should be by those who are expert in the use of this drug for melanoma patients.

Patient and caregiver information
Significant side effects may occur.

Other therapies
ISOLATED LIMB PERFUSION
- Isolated limb perfusion is combined with regional chemotherapy and hyperthermia in patients who have experienced multiple recurrences and have a poor prognosis
- Isolated limb perfusion is performed for intransit metastatic disease in an extremity when there is no suggestion of systemic disease
- Isolated limb perfusion may be combined with melphalan, tumor necrosis factor, and interferon-gamma to improve response rate of intransit metastatic disease

Efficacy
Overall complete response rates of 91% have been reported when limb perfusion methods are combined with melphalan, interferon, and tumor necrosis factor; response rates may be increased to 100% in cases of intransit metastases.

Risks/benefits
Risks:
- Requires general anesthetic and an operative procedure
- More than one administration is difficult
- Regional toxicity

Benefit: Allows for dose escalation, since the high concentration of agents is not metabolized or excreted

Acceptability to patient
Regional toxicity may make the therapy less acceptable.

Follow up plan
Specialist follow up is required.

LIFESTYLE
- Avoidance of sun exposure
- Use of sunscreen

RISKS/BENEFITS
Benefit: Decreased potential for melanoma.

ACCEPTABILITY TO PATIENT
Although these lifestyle changes seem simple in themselves, overall compliance may be a problem.

FOLLOW UP PLAN
Patients should:
- Perform self-examination of the skin periodically
- Undergo medical skin examination every 6 months

PATIENT AND CAREGIVER INFORMATION
- Educate patients about protection measures, including limiting sun exposure, use of sunscreen, and wearing of suitable clothing
- Educate patients about proper methods for self-examination

OUTCOMES

EFFICACY OF THERAPIES

- Overall recurrence rates after treatment of primary melanoma are very low (3.2%) and appear to be associated with prognostic parameters, including metastases, thickness, ulceration, and anatomic location of the melanoma
- Local recurrences are usually indicative of higher risk of metastatic disease
- Prognosis for recurrence and survival depend on factors such as thickness of the tumor, number and type of lymph nodes involved, presence of ulceration in the melanoma, and anatomic location of the melanoma

Evidence

- Wide surgical margins have not been shown to improve survival or local recurrence rates. Narrow margins are effective and reduce the need for skin grafting [3] *Level P*
- No significant survival benefit was noted for elective lymph node dissection (in patients with no clinical evidence of metastases) in four RCTs. In a retrospective analysis, there was a trend towards benefit for elective dissection for certain patients [3] *Level P*
- Combination chemotherapy and dacarbazine have been compared with placebo in RCTs. No survival advantage was noted in patients receiving chemotherapy [3] *Level P*
- Increased disease-free and overall survival have been found with high-dose interferon-alfa-2b, and there is evidence of increased time before relapse [3] *Level P*

Review period

Perform skin examination every 6 months, and have patient perform diligent self-examinations.

PROGNOSIS

- Nodal involvement and number of metastatic sites are the most important prognostic factors for survival (survival rates are directly correlated with the number of nodes and metastatic sites involved)
- 5-year survival rates have been reported as 88% for one metastatic node and <50% for four or more metastatic nodes
- 5-year survival rates have been reported as 37% or less with visceral or distant lymph node metastases
- Local recurrence is usually associated with poor prognosis and systemic metastases (10-year survival rate with local recurrence is 20%)
- The fewer the number of intransit metastases the better the prognosis for survival; however, intransit metastases are associated with regional nodal involvement, which are associated with lower survival rates as previously indicated
- Thick melanomas (>4mm diameter) are associated with an increased risk of regional nodal metastases, which are associated with lower survival rates
- Distant metastasis is associated with survival times of 9 months or less
- Systemic metastasis is associated with survival times of about 6 months

Clinical pearls

- When detected early (<1mm), there is a remarkably high chance of cure (>95%). Primary care physicians should screen for melanoma and have suspicious lesions examined by a dermatologist. Overuse of biopsies on benign lesions should be discouraged; however, underuse of biopsy and excision may lead to a missed opportunity to cure a fatal malignancy
- Extracutaneous melanoma exists. Examination by an ophthalmologist is appropriate for those at increased risk of melanoma

Therapeutic failure

- If recurrence of the primary melanoma occurs, several options are available, including additional surgical excision, amputation (toes, fingers, ears), isolated limb perfusion combined with regional chemotherapy and hyperthermia, and radiation therapy
- If regional metastasis from the primary tumor occurs, treatment options include surgical excision and node dissection
- If regional metastasis occurs from an unknown primary tumor, treatment options include surgical excision and lymphadenectomy
- If intransit metastasis occurs, treatment options include surgical excision; isolated limb perfusion; regional chemotherapy infusion with dacarbazine; radiation therapy; intralesional immunotherapy with bacille Calmette-Guèrin (BCG), vaccinia virus, or dinitrochlorobenzene; systemic chemotherapy with dacarbazine; or electroporation

Other treatments for metastatic disease include elective lymph node dissection, clinical trial participation with investigational agents, adjuvant therapies, biologic therapies, immunotherapy, monoclonal antibodies, tumor vaccines, gene therapy, and no treatment

Recurrence

Patients with stage I or II melanoma have been found to have recurrence rates of 13% when the thickness is >4mm, 11.5% when ulceration is present, and between 5 and 12% when the melanoma is located on the face, scalp, foot, or hand.

COMPLICATIONS

- Pathologic fracture of bony metastases
- Seizure disorder or other neurologic impairment due to brain metastasis

PREVENTION

- Limit exposure to the sun
- Avoid tanning booths
- Use sunscreen whenever sun exposure is anticipated
- Wear proper protective clothing (e.g. hat, sunglasses, long-sleeved shirts) as necessary
- Perform self-examination of the skin
- Undergo skin examination by medical personnel periodically

RISK FACTORS

- Sun exposure; this is the main cause of melanoma
- Multiple raised nevi on the arms (predisposing factor)
- Previous history of melanoma increases the risk of melanoma
- Familial history of melanoma increases the risk of melanoma
- History of multiple severe sunburns and poor ability to suntan
- Fair complexion and light skin tone increases the risk of melanoma

MODIFY RISK FACTORS

The most important modification is to limit sun exposure and to wear sunscreen and protective clothing.

Lifestyle and wellness

PHYSICAL ACTIVITY
Adhere to protection methods when participating in outside activities (sunscreen, proper clothing for sun protection, sun avoidance).

ENVIRONMENT
- Limit activities with sun exposure
- Adhere to protection methods (sunscreen, sun avoidance, proper protective clothing)

FAMILY HISTORY
Patients should be aware of any familial history of melanoma and adhere to protective methods (sunscreen, sun avoidance, proper clothing during outside activities).

SCREENING

- Screening and removal of suspicious lesions are extremely important preventive methods and decrease the risk of and development of melanoma
- Self-screening increases the chance of finding suspicious lesions in the early stages of disease and decreases the chance of melanoma, metastatic disease, and recurrence
- Physical examination by a medical provider decreases the risk of metastatic disease and recurrence
- Public screening programs provide patient education materials, brief skin examinations, and referrals for patients with suspicious lesions

EYE EXAMINATION
Eye examinations are important for diagnosing intraocular melanoma.

PREVENT RECURRENCE

- Diligent self-screening and periodic physical examination by medical personnel are two very effective methods for prevention of recurrence
- Use of sunscreen and other protective methods (clothing, hats, sunglasses) are extremely important preventive measures

ASSOCIATIONS
American Academy of Dermatology
930 N. Meacham Road
PO Box 4014
Schaumburg, IL 60168–4014
Tel: 847–330–0230
Fax: 847–330–0050
http://www.aad.org

KEY REFERENCES

- Abeloff MD, Armitage JO, Lichter AS, Niederhuber JE. Clinical oncology, 2nd edn. Chapter 55, Skin: Malignant melanoma. London: Churchill Livingstone, 2000
- Balch CM, Urist MM, Karakousis CP et al. Efficacy of 2cm surgical margins for intermediate-thickness melanomas (1 to 4mm). Results of a multi-institutional randomized surgical trial. Ann Surg 1993;218:262–7. Medline
- DeVita VT, Jr. Cancer: Principles and practice of oncology, 5th edn. Philadelphia: Lippincott-Raven Publishers, 1997, p1935–1989
- Goroll AH. Primary care medicine, 3rd edn. Philadelphia: Lippincott-Raven, 1995, p880–886
- Habif TP. Clinical dermatology, 3rd edn. Philadelphia: Mosby, 1996, p700–719

Evidence references and guidelines

1 Guidelines of care for primary cutaneous melanoma. The American Academy of Dermatology Melanoma Guidelines Development Task Force, and Guidelines/Outcomes Committee. J Am Acad Dermatol 2001;45:579–86. Available at the National Guideline Clearinghouse
2 Balch CM, Buzaid AC, Soong SJ et al. Final version of the American Joint Committee on Cancer staging system for cutaneous melanoma. J Clin Oncol 2001;19:3635–3648. Medline
3 Crosby T, Mason M, Crosby D. Malignant melanoma: non-metastatic. Skin disorders. In: Clinical Evidence 2001,5:1175–1182. London: BMJ Publishing Group
4 Veronesi U, Cascinelli N, Adamus J et al. Thin stage I primary cutaneous malignant melanoma. Comparison of excision with margins of 1 or 3cm. N Engl J Med 1988;318:1159–62. Medline
5 Balch CM, Soong SJ, Gershenwald JE et al. Prognostic factors analysis of 17,600 melanoma patients: Validation of the American Joint Committee on Cancer melanoma staging system. J Clin Oncol 2001;16:3622–3634
6 Dubois RW, Swetter SM, Atkins M et al. Developing indications for the use of sentinel node biopsy and adjuvant high-dose interferon alfa-2b in melanoma. Arch Dermatol 2001;137:1217–24. Medline
7 Cole BF, Gelber RD, Kirkwood JM et al. Quality-of-life-adjusted survival analysis of high risk resected cutaneous melanoma: the Eastern Co-operative Oncology Study Group. J Clin Oncol 1996;14:2666–2673. Reviewed in Clinical Evidence 2001,5:1175–1182
8 Kirkwood JM, Ibrahim J, Sondak V, et al. Preliminary analysis of the E1690/S9111/C9190 intergroup postoperative adjuvant trial of high- and low-dose IFN-2b in high risk primary of lymph node metastatic melanoma. Proc ASCO 1999;18. Reviewed in Clinical Evidence 2001;5:1175–1182

FAQS
Question 1
Does sunscreen use increase the risk of melanoma?

ANSWER 1
There has been recent controversy regarding sunscreen use and subsequent melanoma risk. In particular, the question has been, do sunscreens protect against sunburn (redness, pain, blistering) to a greater extent than against carcinogenesis, thereby removing the natural signal to get out of the sun, causing increased exposure to sunlight-enhancing melanoma risk? The issue is greatly clouded by the evolution in sunscreen formulations over the past few decades, including the former use in Europe of psoralens as sunscreens, which form DNA adducts and are clearly mutagenic. More recently, broad-spectrum sunscreens have been and are being developed that protect against ultraviolet-A (the so-called tanning rays) as well as ultraviolet-B (the so-called burning rays). Currently, opinion leaders believe that broad-spectrum, high-SPF sunscreens are protective.

Question 2
What is SPF?
ANSWER 2
SPF (sun protection factor) is determined experimentally for sunscreens by exposing human subjects to simulated sunlight with and without sunscreen protection. The amount of light that induces redness (usually measured in seconds) in sunscreen-protected skin, divided by the amount of light that induces redness in unprotected skin, is the SPF. SPF is predominantly a measure of ultraviolet-B protection. Thus a sunscreen with SPF of 15 will delay the onset of sunburn in an individual who would otherwise burn in 10min, to burn in 150min (2.5h). This sort of exposure is not uncommon.

Question 3
Is melanoma universally fatal?
ANSWER 3
No. Early (<1mm deep, nonulcerated) melanomas without lymph node involvement are usually curable by excision (5-year survival of about 95%). In contrast, involvement of lymph nodes or deeper tumors is associated with a much worse prognosis. These data highlight the need for early detection and excision.

Question 4
Should all 'changing moles' be removed?
ANSWER 4
If suspicion for melanoma exists, yes. Seborrheic keratoses often fulfill all the 'ABCDE' signs of melanoma and grow. They often have a 'stuck-on' appearance and have a pitted surface.

CONTRIBUTORS
Martin Kabongo, MD, PhD
Seth R Stevens, MD
Rolland P Gyulai, MD, PhD

ONYCHOMYCOSIS

DESCRIPTION

- Chronic fungal infection of the nail affecting up to 3% of the population
- Dermatophtye organisms are the usual causal agents
- Distal and lateral margins of the nail are infected – distal and lateral subungual onychomycosis
- Onycholysis (splitting of the nail plate from the nail bed) is the primary event
- Nail becomes thickened and discolored, and splits
- Toenail infection is more common than fingernail infection
- Can be a painful condition leading to functional impairment
- Generally difficult to treat and reinfection is common

ICD9 CODE
110.1 Onychomycosis

SYNONYMS
- Tinea unguium
- Ringworm of the nails
- Dermatophyte infection of the nail
- Distal subungual onychomycosis
- Lateral subungual onychomycosis

CARDINAL FEATURES
- Chronic fungal infection of the nail affecting up to 3% of the population
- Dermatophtye organisms are the usual causal agents (>90% of cases)
- Distal and lateral margins of the nail are infected – distal and lateral subungual onychomycosis
- Onycholysis (splitting of the nail plate from the nail bed) is the primary event
- Initially there is a distal yellow or white patch of discoloration that extends and darkens with time; then the nail becomes thickened, crumbly, and splits
- Toenail infection is more common than fingernail infection and often all toenails become infected
- Can be a painful condition leading to functional impairment
- Adjacent skin is usually infected
- Difficult to treat and reinfection is common

CAUSES
Common causes
- Dermatophyte organisms are the most common cause (>90% of cases)
- *Trichophyton rubrum* is the most common cause
- *Trichophyton interdigitale* is less common and affects the great toenail
- *Trichophyton mentagrophyte* can infect the nail plates
- *Candida albicans* is responsible for 5% of cases

Rare causes
- Yeasts and nondermatophyte infections
- *Aspergillus niger*
- *Scopulariopsis brevicaulis*

Contributory or predisposing factors
- Local warmth and humidity favor the presence of fungus
- Exercise: dermatophyte fungi live on the nail plate and repeated minor trauma permits the fungal organism to invade the nail plate and become established
- Tight occlusive footwear causes crowding of the toes, promoting fungal infection
- Communal showers, where untreated fungal organisms can spread rapidly
- Occupations requiring constant hand washing
- Diseases that influence local and systemic immunity can predispose to onychomycosis, including diabetes mellitus, AIDS, and peripheral ischemia

EPIDEMIOLOGY
Incidence and prevalence
INCIDENCE
20–100/1000.

PREVALENCE
3% of the population.

Demographics

AGE
- Peak incidence is between 40 and 60 years
- Incidence increases with increasing age
- Rare before puberty

GENDER
More males than females are affected.

GEOGRAPHY
Rare in rural undeveloped countries (e.g. in Zaire the incidence is 1%) compared to urban areas in developed countries (13%).

SOCIOECONOMIC STATUS
- Developed countries have a greater incidence
- Communal showers in health clubs are fertile ground for onychomycosis

DIFFERENTIAL DIAGNOSIS
Psoriasis
Psoriasis is a chronic skin condition due to excessive keratinocyte proliferation. Nail changes occur in 10–40%.

FEATURES
- Symmetrical involvement of the nails
- Nail plate is affected from the proximal end
- Pinpoint pitting of nail bed
- Air, debris, and exudate accumulate between nail plate and nail bed, and results in loss of the pink hue
- Onycholysis (removal of the nail plate from the nail bed) results in the 'spot of oil' appearance and usually develops from the free edge and proceeds proximally
- Transverse ridging of the dorsal surface of the nail plates
- Splinter hemorrhages are common
- Subungual hyperkeratosis (thickening of the skin of the nail bed)
- Presence of a psoriatic rash and terminal interphalangeal joint arthritis simplifies diagnosis

Eczema
Eczema of any etiology can affect nail folds, disturb matrix function, and result in nail plate abnormalities.

FEATURES
- Nail plate becomes pitted
- Transverse ridges can form even when there is no rash on the nail fold
- Subungual hyperkeratosis may occur, causing onycholysis (nail plate lifting off nail bed)
- Onycholysis may be painful and cause functional impairment

Lichen planus
Lichen planus can affect the skin and nail matrix.

FEATURES
- Lichen planus thins the nail matrix
- Onycholysis (separation of the nail plate from the nail bed)
- Nail becomes brittle and longitudinal ridges become prominent
- Whole nail may be shed and inflammation may be intense
- Skin of flexor surfaces of the wrists may have papules that itch intensely and spread to the trunk and shins
- Scarring alopecia can occur
- Oral involvement includes fine white Wickham striae and ulceration
- Can be triggered by viral, drug, or neoplastic processes
- Histology reveals a lymphocytic infiltrate at the epidermis with a saw-tooth pattern of the lower border and patchy degeneration of the basal layer

Subungual exostosis
Phalanx bony overgrowth underneath the nail bed which is often mistaken for onychomycosis.

FEATURES
- Reddish brown discoloration of nail plate
- Lesion is tender on pressure
- X-ray of the phalanx is diagnostic

Paronychia

Paronychia is a localized infection (most commonly *Candida albicans* or *Staphylococcus aureus*) or abscess of the lateral and proximal nail fold that is acute or chronic in nature.

FEATURES
- Loss of the natural seal between nail plate and nail bed leads to bacterial and fungal invasion
- Nail fold becomes red, tender, and swollen
- Gentle pressure can lead to release of pus
- Chronic paronychia occurs with loss of the nail cuticle allowing for colonization with *Candida* and bacterial pathogens
- Nail plate becomes discolored (brown or bluish-black)
- Predisposing factors include digital ischemia and frequent immersion of hands in water; paronychia is an occupational hazard of nurses, bakers, cleaners, and restaurant staff

Yellow nail syndrome

Due to defective lymphatic drainage in the lungs.

FEATURES
- Nails appear small and curved
- Nail plate is thick, yellow/green, and slow-growing
- Patient may be predisposed to pulmonary infections and pleural effusions

SIGNS & SYMPTOMS
Signs
- Onychomycosis is classified according to its clinical pattern
- Infected distal and lateral margins of the nail (distal and lateral subungual onychomycosis (DLSO)) is the most common clinical pattern; superficial and proximal subungual onychomycosis are less common clinical patterns
- Onycholysis (splitting of the nail plate from the nail bed) is the primary event
- Initially there is a distal yellow or white patch of discoloration that extends and darkens with time
- Nail becomes thickened, crumbly, and splits
- Eventually the nail plate loosens, separates from the nail bed, and falls off
- Can be painful and lead to functional impairment
- Toenail infection is more common than fingernail infection and all toenails can become infected
- Adjacent skin is usually infected

Symptoms
- Early fungal infection is usually asymptomatic
- Nail discoloration leads to a poor cosmetic appearance and can be distressing
- May be painful
- Patient may complain of loss of the nail in more advanced disease

ASSOCIATED DISORDERS

Tinea pedis often coexists with onychomycosis.

CONSIDER CONSULT
- Refer to a dermatologist if another diagnosis is being considered (e.g. psoriasis)

INVESTIGATION OF THE PATIENT
Direct questions to patient
Q For how long have you noticed discoloration of the nail? Often the fungal nail infection has been present for months.

Q Have you tried any treatment? The patient may have tried to self-treat the nail infection.

Q Is the condition painful? Pain suggests that the fungal infection is advanced.

Contributory or predisposing factors

Q Do you suffer from athlete's foot? Fungal infection of the skin predisposes the person to infection of the nail.

Q What is your occupation? Those in occupations that require frequent immersion of the hands in water (e.g. nurses, caterers, restaurant staff, cleaners) are predisposed to fungal infection.

Q Has the infected nail been damaged? Nail damage can predispose the person to onychomycosis.

Q Do you do any exercise? Use of training equipment and communal showers, and mechanical trauma to the nails predispose a person to onychomycosis.

Q Do you suffer from diabetes, peripheral ischemia, or any immunosuppressive disease including AIDS? All of these diseases are associated with onychomycosis.

Family history

Q Do members of your family suffer from fungal skin or nail infections? Fungal infections cross-infect members of the same household.

Examination

▪ What is the pattern of the nail bed infection? Fungal nail infection is classified by its infection pattern, including distal and lateral subungual onychomycosis, and superficial and proximal subungual onychomycosis

▪ Which nails are involved? Fungal nail infection usually starts asymmetrically but can progress to affect all nails. Toenails are affected far more commonly than fingernails

▪ What color is the infected nail? Fungal nail infection causes the nail to turn yellow to brown in color

▪ What is the appearance of the nail infection? The infected nail is thickened, brittle, hard, and distorted

▪ Is onycholysis (separation of the nail plate form the nail bed) present? Onycholysis occurs early in fungal nail infection

▪ Is the nail plate loose? Later stages of the disease cause the nail plate to loosen, separate form the nail bed, and fall off

▪ Is the adjacent skin infected? This is common with fungal nail infections

Summary of investigative tests

As treatment for onychomycosis is prolonged and expensive, fungal nail infection should always be confirmed by:

▪ Direct microscopy, using KOH to dissolve the keratin and then looking for fungal elements, including hyphae (microscopy can also be used to check on treatment compliance and to verify eradication of the condition)

▪ A fungal culture, which can be done by sending nail clippings and subungual debris for laboratory analysis using Sabouraud medium

DIAGNOSTIC DECISION

Diagnosis is based on clinical appearance of the nails in the context of the differential diagnosis. Nail dystrophy is commonly caused by psoriasis or trauma. Demonstrating the organism is confirmatory.

Guidelines:
The American Academy of Dermatology. [1]

CLINICAL PEARLS
Onychomycosis usually does not have associated pits.

THE TESTS
Biopsy
DIRECT MICROSCOPY
Description
- Use a good pair of pincer-type nail clippers to take clippings from the discolored, thickened part of the nail
- Take clippings from the whole thickness of the nail and remove the scales beneath the nail as well
- Cut the nail back as far as possible – the most important tissue to obtain is the keratin debris from under the nail plate
- If the sample is to be sent to a laboratory, it must be put into a suitable mycology transport pack that includes the patient's name, clinical details, and a description of previous treatment
- Place clippings in KOH for up to one hour to soften the keratinized cells
- Specific staining of the solution is helpful to demonstrate organism
- Direct microscopy will reveal fungal elements including hyphae

Advantages/Disadvantages
Advantages:
- Easy to obtain specimen
- Can be performed in the examining room
- Relatively inexpensive
- Diagnostic for fungal elements, which leads to appropriate antifungal therapy
- Can be used for diagnosis and during and after treatment to assess compliance with treatment and eradication of the condition

Disadvantages:
- Not all infected nail clippings will reveal fungal elements
- Experienced microscopist required to reduce false-positive rates

Abnormal
Fungal elements seen under microscopy.

Cause of abnormal result
Fungal infection of the nail – onychomycosis.

FUNGAL CULTURE
Description
- Use a good pair of pincer-type nail clippers to take clippings from the discolored thickened part of the nail
- Take clippings from the whole thickness of the nail and remove the scales beneath the nail as well
- Cut the nail as far back as possible – the most important tissue to obtain is the keratin debris from under the nail plate
- Collect the sample in a suitable mycology transport pack and include the patient's name, clinical details, and a description of previous treatment
- Clippings are then prepared and cultured on Sabouraud medium

Advantages/Disadvantages
Advantages:
- Easy to obtain sample
- Identifies the fungal organism causing the infection so appropriate antifungal therapy can be started

Disadvantages:
- Laboratory culture on Sabouraud medium needed
- Failure to grow fungi is common with nail clippings
- For a successful result, it is important to obtain material as near the proximal edge of the nail as possible
- Dermatophyte identification usually occurs within 14 days, but may take up to 30 days

Abnormal
Fungal growth on the Sabouraud medium.

Cause of abnormal result
Fungal infection – onychomycosis.

CONSIDER CONSULT

- If the patient is diabetic, refer to a podiatrist for advice on footwear, foot hygiene, nail debridement, and surgical removal of the toenail

PATIENT AND CAREGIVER ISSUES
Patient or caregiver request

- **For how long will I need to treat the nails?** Onychomycosis is a chronic condition requiring prolonged treatment of up to 6 months
- **When will I see the treatment working?** No discernable benefit will be seen for months and compliance is important
- **For how long will it take my nails to recover?** Normally, it takes 3–6 months for the fingernail plate and 9–12 months for the toenail plate to grow 1cm
- **Is the condition infectious?** Fungal nail infections are contagious so hygiene precautions, such as using separate towels, will help prevent cross-infection in the household

Health-seeking behavior

- **Have you tried self-treatment of the nail?** Often the patient will have tried a topical steroid, which has exacerbated the onychomycosis
- **Have you complied with previous treatment?** Treatment regimens can be up to 6 months and often patients stop using the medication as no discernable benefit is seen for months

MANAGEMENT ISSUES
Goals

- Treat diagnosed onychomycosis appropriately with specific antifungal drugs
- Clear the fungal nail infection completely
- Maximize compliance with the treatment regimen
- Prevent reinfection and infection of other household members

Management in special circumstances
COEXISTING DISEASE

- Diseases that influence local and systemic immunity, including diabetes mellitus, AIDS, and peripheral ischemia, must be treated appropriately to clear the fungal infection and prevent recurrence of onychomycosis
- Diabetic patients should be referred to a podiatrist for advice on footwear, foot hygiene, nail debridement, and for surgical removal of the toenail
- Treat tinea pedis appropriately to prevent reservoir of fungal infection

COEXISTING MEDICATION

- Certain antifungal treatments cannot be used with certain medications, with most of the problems relating to drugs metabolized by the cytochrome P450 system. Before starting any oral antifungal agent in patients who take other medication, drug-drug interaction must be excluded or appropriately managed
- A full drug history is needed to prevent drug interactions

SPECIAL PATIENT GROUPS

- Newer oral antifungal agents cannot be used in children; griseofulvin is the only drug licensed in this age group
- Oral antifungal therapies should not be initiated in pregnancy

PATIENT SATISFACTION/LIFESTYLE PRIORITIES
Prolonged treatment up to 6 months can cause problems with patient compliance.

SUMMARY OF THERAPEUTIC OPTIONS
Choices
- Spontaneous remission of onychomycosis is rare and, therefore, treatment using systemic antifungal agents is required
- Terbinafine and itraconazole are the therapeutic choices for adults; griseofulvin is the first-line therapeutic choice for children (only antifungal agent licensed for children)
- Careful monitoring of these agents will permit eradication rates of up to 80–90% for dermatophyte onychomycosis
- Periodic monitoring of liver function is required with oral antifungal agents
- These drugs are incorporated into the nail and are effective after treatment ends
- Continuous oral terbinafine therapy is the most effective against dermatophytes
- Intermittent dosing with itraconazole is as safe and effective as short-term continuous dosing but is more economical, convenient, and carries fewer risks
- Griseofulvin is seldom used in adults because it has a high risk of side effects and low efficacy compared to newer antifungal therapies
- Candidal onychomycosis should be treated with itraconazole because terbinafine is ineffective
- Fluconazole has not been labeled for use in onychomycosis by the US FDA
- Superficial or distal onychomycosis cases can be treated using topical treatments – clotrimazole 1% cream
- Nail debridement or removal may be necessary for advanced disease and refractory onychomycosis
- Lifestyle changes may be useful in preventing reinfection

Guidelines:
- The American Academy of Dermatology. [1]
- The Infectious Diseases Society of America. [2]
- The American Academy of Family Physicians [3]

Clinical pearls
- Itraconazole requires close monitoring of blood and has several drug-drug interactions. These risks can be reduced by pulse dosing
- Terbinafine is easy to use and may be preferred for more complex patients
- Topical agents and griseofulvin are not usually effective for onychomycosis and should be prescribed accordingly. Griseofulvin, however, is less costly, thus may be an appropriate choice

Never
Never use topical steroids in onychomycosis as proliferation of the fungal infection occurs.

FOLLOW UP
- Careful follow up is needed to check on treatment compliance
- Direct microscopy of nail clippings will verify compliance and eradication
- Nail changes are not always discernable during treatment as it may take several months for the new nail to completely replace the diseased nail
- Periodic liver monitoring is required for patients taking oral antifungal agents

Plan for review

- Periodic follow up reviews should be initiated while the patient is taking oral antifungal therapy
- Direct microscopy can be performed to verify eradication after treatment regimen has been completed

Information for patient or caregiver

- Patient must be motivated to complete the treatment regimen
- Patient must not be pregnant when taking oral antifungal agents
- Patient must undergo liver function monitoring while on oral antifungal agents

DRUGS AND OTHER THERAPIES: DETAILS
Drugs
TERBINAFINE

- Systemic and topical antifungal agent
- Topical treatment is only for early superficial onychomycosis
- Inhibits fungal sterol biosynthesis
- Synthetic allylamine
- First-line oral antifungal for dermatophyte infection
- Only for patients over 12 years

Dose

- Topical treatment: apply twice daily for 6 weeks for fingernail onychomycosis; apply twice daily for 12 weeks for toenail onychomycosis
- Oral treatment: 250mg once daily for 6 weeks for fingernail onychomycosis; 250mg once daily for 12 weeks for toenail onychomycosis

Efficacy

- First-line oral antifungal for dermatophyte infection – eradication rates of 70–90%
- Ineffective against *Candida* spp.

Risks/benefits
Risks:

- Long-term treatment with good patient compliance required
- Contact with the eyes should be avoided

Benefits:

- Effective against dermatophyte species
- Once-daily oral regimen for better compliance

Side effects and adverse reactions

- Central nervous system: headache, taste disturbance
- Gastrointestinal: abdominal discomfort, nausea, diarrhea, liver toxicity
- Skin: rash, urticaria

Interactions (other drugs)

- Caffeine (decreased clearance of caffeine) ■ Cyclosporine (increased clearance of cyclosporine) ■ Rifampin (increased clearance of terbinafine) ■ Cimetidine (decreased clearance of terbinafine) ■ Terfenadine (increased exposure/area under the curve (AUC) of terbinafine)

Contraindications

- Children under 12 years of age ■ Pregnancy and breast-feeding

Evidence

Oral terbinafine is effective for the treatment of onychomycosis secondary to dermatophyte infection:

- Oral terbinafine or itraconazole are effective treatments for onychomycosis. For the treatment of onychomycosis secondary to *Candida* infection, terbinafine has limited and unpredictable in vitro activity, and does not have consistent clinically proven efficacy [2] *Level C*
- An RCT compared 12 weeks treatment with oral terbinafine vs griseofulvin in patients with fingernail dermatophytosis. Significantly more patients receiving terbinafine achieved complete cure at 48 weeks [4] *Level P*
- Terbinafine (for 16 weeks) and griseofulvin (for 52 weeks) were compared in another RCT in patients with toenail onychomycosis. Terbinafine was significantly more effective than griseofulvin, in terms of total cure and mycological cure [5] *Level P*
- An RCT compared terbinafine (daily treatment for 12 or 16 weeks) vs itraconazole (daily for one week every month; for 3 or 4 months) in patients with fungal toenail infections. The continuous regimens of terbinafine were significantly more effective than either intermittent regimen of itraconazole, in terms of clinical and microbiological care rates at 1.5 years [6] *Level P*

Acceptability to patient

- Expensive
- Willingness of the patient to comply with treatment is necessary as twice-daily application is required (if topical treatment is chosen)

Follow up plan

- Liver function and complete blood count monitoring are needed while taking oral terbinafine
- Terbinafine should be stopped if liver function is abnormal

Patient and caregiver information

- Full clinical benefit may not be apparent until several months after terbinafine treatment has stopped
- Antifungal agent is incorporated into the nail matrix and is effective after the treatment has finished

ITRACONAZOLE

- Oral antifungal triazole derivative
- Inhibits the cytochrome P450-dependent synthesis of ergosterol, a vital component of fungal cell membranes
- Therapeutic choice for *Candida* onychomycosis and second choice for dermatophyte infections

Dose

- Adult, toenails (with or without fingernail involvement): 200mg four times daily for 3 months
- Adult, fingernails only: two treatment pulses, each consisting of 200mg twice daily for one week, separated by 3 weeks without itraconazole

Efficacy

Very effective antifungal agent against both dermatophyte and *Candida* spp.

Risks/benefits

Risks:

- Use caution in hepatic and renal disease
- Discontinue use if peripheral neuropathy occurs

Side effects and adverse reactions
- Cardiovascular system: edema, hypertension
- Central nervous system: depression, dizziness, headache, fever, fatigue
- Gastrointestinal: vomiting, nausea, diarrhea, hepatitis, altered liver function, abdominal pain
- Genitourinary: sexual dysfunction
- Metabolic: hypokalemia
- Skin: rashes, pruritus

Interactions (other drugs)
- Antiulcer drugs (cimetidine, famotidine, lansoprazole, nizatidine, omeprazole, sucralfate)
- Antivirals (amprenavir, didanosine, indinavir, nelfinavir, ritonavir, saquinavir) Antacids
- Astemizole Atevirdine Benzodiazepines Buspirone Chlordiazepoxide
- Cyclosporine Digoxin Ethanol Felodipine Macrolide antibiotics Methadone
- Methylprednisolone Oral anticoagulants Phenytoin Pimozide Quinidine
- Rifampin Statins Tacrolimus Terfenadine Tolbutamide

Contraindications
- Nursing mothers Pregnancy Not recommend in children or the elderly
- Do not administer with pimozide, quinidine, triazolam, oral midazolam, or statins

Evidence
- Oral terbinafine or itraconazole are effective treatments for onychomycosis. Itraconazole appears to be effective for the treatment of onychomycosis secondary to *Candida* infection [2] *Level C*
- An RCT compared terbinafine (daily treatment for 12 or 16 weeks) vs itraconazole (daily for one week every month; for 3 or 4 months) in patients with fungal toenail infections. The continuous regimens of terbinafine were significantly more effective than either intermittent regimen of itraconazole, in terms of clinical and microbiological care rates at 1.5 years [6] *Level P*

Acceptability to patient
- Expensive
- Compliance can be problematic in pulsed therapy and clear instructions should be given

Follow up plan
Liver function must be monitored while patients are taking this oral antifungal agent.

Patient and caregiver information
- Full clinical benefit may not be apparent for several months after itraconazole treatment has stopped
- Antifungal agent is incorporated into thc nail matrix and is effective after the treatment has finished
- Treatment should be taken with food to ensure maximal absorption
- Avoid antacids within 2h of administration

GRISEOFULVIN
- Binds to keratin of nail and prevents fungal invasion
- Active against dermatophytes
- Inexpensive
- Only oral antifungal agent licensed for children
- Protracted administration time

Dose
- Adult: 1g orally four times daily for a minimum of 4 months for fingernails and a minimum of 6 months for toenails
- Child: 10–15mg/kg orally four times for a minimum of 4 months for fingernails and a minimum of 6 months for toenails

Efficacy
- Cure rate of up to 60% for fingernail infection and 30% for toenails if the correct treatment is taken
- Protracted administration and poor cure rates make newer antifungal agents more attractive

Risks/benefits
Risks:
- Causes side effects in 20% of patients
- Use caution with known penicillin allergy

Side effects and adverse reactions
- Central nervous system: headache, fatigue, insomnia, confusion, dizziness
- Gastrointestinal: diarrhea, nausea, vomiting, gastrointestinal bleeding, hepatoxicity
- Hematologic: leukopenia, agranulocytosis
- Hypersensitivity: rashes, photosensitivity

Interactions (other drugs)
- Aspirin ■ Cyclosporine ■ Oral contraceptives ■ Phenobarbital ■ Tacrolimus ■ Warfarin

Contraindications
- Lupus erythematosus ■ Porphyria ■ Pregnancy ■ Severe liver disease

Evidence
- An RCT compared 12 weeks treatment with oral terbinafine vs griseofulvin in patients with fingernail dermatophytosis. Significantly more patients receiving terbinafine achieved complete cure at 48 weeks [4] *Level P*
- Terbinafine (for 16 weeks) and griseofulvin (for 52 weeks) were compared in another RCT in patients with toenail onychomycosis. Terbinafine was significantly more effective than griseofulvin, in terms of total cure and mycological cure [5] *Level P*

Acceptability to patient
Side effects of griseofulvin are common and cause poor compliance with the treatment regimen.

Follow up plan
Liver, renal, and hematopoietic function need to be monitored.

Patient and caregiver information
- Full clinical benefit may not be apparent for several months after griseofulvin treatment has started; complete entire treatment course
- Avoid prolonged exposure to sunlight or sunlamps
- Seek medical attention if sore throat or skin rash occurs

CLOTRIMAZOLE
- Topical antifungal treatment used for superficial onychomycosis
- Broad-spectrum, inhibiting growth of dermatophytes, yeasts, *Candida*, and other fungal species
- Fungistatic and fungicidal activity as it interferes with fungal DNA replication by binding sterols in fungal cell membrane, which increases permeability and leaks cell nutrients

Dose
Topical dose: 1% twice daily to infected nail.

Efficacy
Only effective for superficial infection.

Risks/benefits
Risk: None listed

Benefits:
- Inexpensive
- No blood tests required during treatment

Side effects and adverse reactions
- Gastrointestinal: nausea, abdominal pain (oral administration)
- Genitourinary: dyspareunia, urinary frequency
- Skin: burning, rash, urticaria, stinging

Interactions (other drugs)
- Cyclosporine ▪ Tacrolimus

Contraindications
- Hypersensitivity to clotrimaxole

Acceptability to patient
- Topical treatment has few side effects
- Twice-daily application can be demanding on a patient's time

Follow up plan
- Careful follow up to check on onychomycosis eradication
- Oral antifungal agents may be needed if onychomycosis persists

Patient and caregiver information
Patients must be told to comply with the treatment regimen to eradicate the fungal infection.

Surgical therapy
NAIL REMOVAL
- Nail debridement or removal may be necessary for advanced disease and refractory onychomycosis
- Primary care physicians, dermatologists, or podiatrists can perform this minor operation
- Relapse rate is high

Efficacy
Eradicates fungal infection with nail removal.

Risks/benefits
Risks:
- Potentially painful procedure
- Secondary infection may occur
- Nail regrowth may be uneven
- Nail regrowth may be reinfected with the causal fungal agent

Acceptability to patient
- Cosmetic results may be distressing
- Removal of the diseased nail prevents the need for further antifungal agents

Follow up plan
Careful follow up is necessary to check for secondary infection and reinfection of onychomycosis.

Patient and caregiver information
Full consent for this procedure is necessary.

LIFESTYLE

Reinfection can be prevented if the patient:
- Wears properly fitting shoes to reduce repeated trauma to toenails
- Avoids communal showers, where fungal infections spread easily
- Keeps feet and nails clean and dry

After successful treatment, new shoes should be worn as old shoes will serve as a reservoir for spores that may reinfect the nails.

ACCEPTABILITY TO PATIENT

Minimal changes in footwear and hygiene patterns can prevent reinfection and the need for prolonged treatment regimens.

EFFICACY OF THERAPIES

- Oral terbinafine is the therapeutic choice for dermatophyte onychomycosis
- Oral itraconazole is the therapeutic choice for candidal onychomycosis
- Topical antifungal agents are the therapeutic choice for superficial onychomycosis

Evidence

- A systematic review found insufficient evidence to draw conclusions on the efficacy of topical antifungals for the treatment of nail infections [7] *Level M*
- Terbinafine is more effective than griseofulvin for the treatment of patients with dermatophyte onychomycosis [4,5] *Level P*
- Continuous terbinafine was found to be more effective than intermittent itraconazole in patients with fungal toenail infections in one RCT [6] *Level P*

Review period

One year.

PROGNOSIS

A long-term disease-free toenail occurs in 25–50% of patients treated with the oral antifungal agents.

Clinical pearls

- Shoes serve as a reservoir of fungal elements. After successful therapy, new shoes should be worn to reduce the risk of relapse
- Protective footwear should be advised for those using communal shower facilities, particularly with history of previous fungal infection or athlete's foot

Therapeutic failure

- Refractory onychomycosis may require nail removal, although relapse rates are high
- A dermatology referral may be indicated if the original diagnosis is uncertain

Recurrence

- Recurrence is common
- Removal of the nail may be indicated
- Dermatology referral is indicated if the management is uncertain

Deterioration

Referral to a dermatologist is indicated.

COMPLICATIONS

- Nail removal due to the nail plate lifting from the nail bed can occur in severe infection
- Secondary infection can occur

CONSIDER CONSULT

- Refer if the fungal nail infection is not responding to treatment

Prevention, early identification, and treatment will minimize severity of disease and risk of functional impairment.

RISK FACTORS
- **Poor hygiene** standards: use of communal showers leads to fungal infection
- **Ill-fitting footwear:** increases microtrauma to the nail plate
- **Nail damage**
- **Poor foot care** for patients at risk (e.g. those with diabetes mellitus, AIDS, and peripheral ischemia)
- **Tinea pedis**

MODIFY RISK FACTORS
- Improve hygiene standards
- Modify footwear
- Prevent nail damage
- Improve foot care for patients at risk
- Treat tinea pedis appropriately to prevent reservoir of infection

Lifestyle and wellness
PHYSICAL ACTIVITY
- Sports shoes that fit well will reduce microtrauma to the nail plate
- Using communal showers leads to fungal infection

FAMILY HISTORY
Care with hygiene is needed to reduce cross-infection between family members.

PREVENT RECURRENCE
Improve hygiene standards, modify footwear, and prevent nail damage. The fungi that cause onychomycosis are ubiquitous; thus, while meticulous hygiene will reduce the rate of recurrence, it may not prevent recurrence.

Reassess coexisting disease
- Improve foot care for patients at risk (e.g. those with diabetes mellitus, AIDS, and peripheral ischemia)
- Treat tinea pedis appropriately to prevent reservoir of fungal infection

RESOURCES

ASSOCIATIONS
Mycology Center
Department of Dermatology
University Hospitals of Cleveland
11100 Euclid Avenue
Lakeside 1400
Cleveland, OH 44106–5028
Tel: (216) 844-3177
Fax: (216) 844-8993
http://www.uhri.org/divinfojsp?GroupID=38deptd=28path=1

KEY REFERENCES
- Berker D. Nails. Medicine 1997;25:14–16
- Mirza B, Ashton R. Recognising nail conditions: a guide. Practitioner 2000;244:873–83
- Fungal toenail infections; definitions and results. Bandolier 1999 Oct;68–8
- Gupta AK, Sauder DN, Shear NH. Antifungal treatment: an overview. Part II. J Am Acad Dermatol 1994;30:911–33

Evidence references and guidelines
1 The American Academy of Dermatology. Guidelines of care for superficial mycotic infections of the skin: onychomycosis. J Am Acad Dermatol 1996;34:116–21
2 The Infectious Diseases Society of America. Practice guidelines for the treatment of candidiasis. Clin Infect Dis 2000;30:662–78. Available at the National Guideline Clearinghouse
3 The American Academy of Family Physicians has published the following information: Rodgers P, Bassler M. Treating onychomycosis. Am Fam Physician 2001;63:663–72, 677–8
4 Haneke E, Tausch I, Brautigam M, et al. Short-duration treatment of fingernail dermatophytosis: a randomized, double-blind study with terbinafine and griseofulvin. LAGOS III Study Group. J Am Acad Dermatol 1995;32:72–7. Medline
5 Faergemann J, Anderson C, Hersle K, et al. Double-blind, parallel-group comparison of terbinafine and griseofulvin in the treatment of toenail onychomycosis. J Am Acad Dermatol 1995;32:750–3. Medline
6 Evans EG, Sigurgeirsson B. Double blind, randomised study of continuous terbinafine compared with intermittent itraconazole in treatment of toenail onychomycosis. The LION Study Group. BMJ 1999;318:1031–5. Medline
7 Crawford F, Hart R, Bell-Syer S, et al. Topical treatments for fungal infections of the skin and nails of the foot (Cochrane Review). In: The Cochrane Library, Issue 2, 2002. Oxford: Update Software. Reviewed in: Clinical Evidence 2001;6:1261–1265

FAQS
Question 1
With no guarantee that oral therapy will work, is it worth the inconvenience, expense, and many-month observation trial involved?

ANSWER 1
Oral therapy is effective at one year in about one-half of its users. Considering the pain, deformity, shoe-wear and toenail difficulties sufferers experience, along with the unattractive cosmetic appearance, patients are often urged to attempt a trial of therapy.

Question 2
What are the potential liver problems the patient may experience while on oral therapy?

ANSWER 2
In a rare patient, the oral antifungal agents may cause liver enzyme elevation to a degree that necessitates discontinuation of the medication. Typically, there are no symptoms of liver problems. A blood test is advised to screen for this.

Question 3
Are the oral antifungal medications safe when used concomitantly with other medications?

ANSWER 3
Itraconazole and to a lesser extent terbinafine are metabolized through the cytochrome P450 enzyme system of the liver. This system is responsible for metabolizing a number of other commonly used medications. If the enzyme system gets 'overloaded', blood levels of some of the medications may either increase or decrease to dangerous or nontherapeutic levels. All of the patient's medications should be reviewed to ensure addition of the antifungal drugs is safe.

Question 4
If the patient has fungal toenails, is the infection likely to spread to the digits of the hands?

ANSWER 4
Theoretically, the infection can spread. However, the hands are much less likely to become infected than the feet and this problem is rarely encountered.

Question 5
If the fungal toenails are successfully treated, will the infection come back? If they become reinfected, can they be retreated?

ANSWER 5
There is no guarantee of a permanent cure. Preventive measures may be helpful in preventing recurrence. Nails can be retreated so long as the medication is well tolerated.

CONTRIBUTORS
Kathleen M O'Hanlon, MD
Seth R Stevens, MD
Douglas C Semler, MD

PARONYCHIA

DESCRIPTION

- Acute or chronic localized, superficial infection of periungual tissues on fingers or toes (much more common on fingers)
- Associated with hangnail, ingrown nail, trauma to nail fold, or chronic irritation
- Acute infection typically staphylococcal
- Chronic infection typically caused by *Candida albicans* or fungi; seen in people whose occupations require prolonged water contact, such as dishwashers
- May need incision and drainage

URGENT ACTION

- Empiric antibiotic therapy may be necessary before causative organism is determined, especially if osteomyelitis is suspected
- Incision and drainage may be required

KEY! DON'T MISS!

- Be sure to differentiate paronychia from herpetic whitlow: incision and drainage is appropriate treatment for paronychia but contraindicated in herpes infection
- Never miss a neoplastic lesion!

ICD9 CODE
- 681.02 Paronychia
- 112.30 Candidiasis of skin and nails

CARDINAL FEATURES
- Superficial infection and inflammation of perionychium
- Infection typically follows nail margin and may extend beneath nail
- Acute infection may be associated with trauma such as a cut hangnail, ingrown nail, or nail-biting
- Chronic infection may be associated with repeated irritation such as exposure to water and detergents
- A break in the epidermis allows organisms to enter
- Begins as cellulitis, but frank abscess can result
- May be seen in children as a result of finger-sucking and nail-biting

CAUSES
Common causes
Acute:
- *Staphylococcus aureus*; less commonly *Streptococcus* or *Pseudomonas* species
- Mixed flora may be present in people with diabetes

Chronic:
- *Candida albicans*; less commonly other fungi

Contributory or predisposing factors
- Trauma to perionychium or ingrown nails, resulting in a break in the epidermis
- Chronic exposure of hands to water and detergent
- Immunocompromise, particularly people taking antiviral drug therapy (indinavir and lamivudine)
- Diabetes mellitis

EPIDEMIOLOGY
Incidence and prevalence
FREQUENCY
Most common hand infection in the US.

Demographics
AGE
Adults and children.

GENDER
Female > male (3:1).

GENETICS
No link known.

SOCIOECONOMIC STATUS
Chronic paronychia is more common in people whose occupations expose their hands to water and irritants (detergent): dishwashers, bartenders, healthcare workers.

DIFFERENTIAL DIAGNOSIS
Ingrown nail
Ingrown nail is caused by the nail pushing into adjacent soft tissue with consequent pressure necrosis, edema, infection, and granulation tissue development.

FEATURES
- Relatively common
- Mainly affects great toe
- Signs of inflammation (pain, redness, swelling) in affected toe
- Suppuration from inflamed nail fold
- Treatment is initially conservative, then operative

Contact dermatitis
Contact dermatitis is caused by either an irritative or allergic reaction to chemicals.

FEATURES
- After contact with the chemical, skin becomes red, itchy, oozing, and subsequently lichenified (chronic form)
- Can become superinfected by bacteria or fungi
- Requires anti-inflammatory (topical steroid) treatment and elimination of causative agent

Felon
Felon is a painful abscess on the palmar aspect of a fingertip.

FEATURES
- Infection of the pulp of the fingertip, not necessarily localized around the nail folds as in paronychia
- Paronychia is more superficial than felon; paronychia may progress to felon if untreated
- Edema in closed pulp space, resulting in intense, throbbing pain
- Underlying bone, joint, or tendons may be affected
- Most commonly seen in thumb and index finger

Tumors of distal phalanx
Benign or malignant proliferation originating from tissues of distal phalanx (e.g. basal cell carcinoma, squamous cell carcinoma, melanoma, osteoblastoma).

FEATURES
- Excess mass of tissue, usually without signs of inflammation
- Ulceration and bleeding are not uncommon in malignant neoplasms
- Bacterial superinfection may occur
- Definitive diagnosis depends on histology
- Treatment is usually surgical

Herpetic whitlow
Herpetic whitlow results from herpes simplex infection of the finger.

FEATURES
- Most common in healthcare workers
- Swollen, painful, erythematous lesion on fingertip (self-limited) rather than an inflammation and infection based in the nail fold
- Vesicles are often present

- Systemic features such as fever, malaise, and axillary lymphadenopathy are more common in herpetic whitlow than paronychia
- Important to differentiate since treatment of paronychia is incision and drainage; this procedure is contraindicated for herpetic lesions

Psoriasis

Psoriasis is a chronic proliferative disease of the skin.

FEATURES

- Varies from few localized lesions to widespread disease
- May be associated with arthritis, unlike paronychia
- Pitting of nails, onycholysis, and splinter hemorrhages may be seen (in paronychia, nails are typically unaffected in this way)
- Silvery scales on skin are pathognomonic

Osteomyelitis

Osteomyelitis is a serious infection of bone, which can affect the distal phalanx. Can be difficult to diagnose clinically.

FEATURES

- Inflammation is often accompanied by proximal spread
- Development of discharging sinus is not uncommon
- Bone pain (unremitting, gnawing character)
- Fever and malaise may be present
- Definitive diagnosis is with pathologic evaluation of bone biopsy
- Prompt antibiotic treatment is required

SIGNS & SYMPTOMS
Signs

Acute phase:

- Erythematous, warm swelling of skin around nail initially
- Suppurative infection with fluctuance develops
- Usually associated with regional lymph node enlargement
- Nail fold may separate from nail plate

Chronic phase:

- Signs of inflammation (tenderness, redness) are less prominent
- Green nail discoloration that may be due to *Pseudomonas* infection
- Chronic infection may result in boggy nail folds (not present in acute infection)

Symptoms

Painful area around nail, particularly skin along lateral nail fold.

ASSOCIATED DISORDERS

- Paronychia has been reported in association with malignant lesions
- If skin is pigmented or irregular in appearance, or if there is a history of malignancy, the patient should be referred for a biopsy

KEY! DON'T MISS!

- Be sure to differentiate paronychia from herpetic whitlow: incision and drainage is appropriate treatment for paronychia but contraindicated in herpes infection
- Never miss a neoplastic lesion!

CONSIDER CONSULT

- Patients with diabetes and ingrown toenail associated with paronychia may require referral to a podiatrist

INVESTIGATION OF THE PATIENT
Direct questions to patient

Q **Why did you seek care?** Patients with paronychia typically seek care for acute onset of a red, swollen, painful finger that may or may not express pus around the nail. Chronic paronychia is more insidious, and patients may not immediately seek care for chronic inflammation and infection.

Q **When did you notice this change in your finger?** The sooner the patient seeks care for symptoms, the less risk there is of extension of the infection into the deeper tissues. If treatment is sought in the early cellulitis phase, incision and drainage is usually not required.

Q **Have you tried any treatments yourself?** Patients who use topical over-the-counter antibiotic ointments may not be candidates for culture of any purulent drainage.

Q **Do you bite your nails/suck on your fingers? Have you had a hangnail recently? Have you had a break in the skin on your finger before this swelling and redness started?** Trauma to skin around the nails can allow organisms to enter, resulting in paronychia.

Contributory or predisposing factors

Q **Does your occupation or daily routine require you to have your hands in water?** Chronic paronychia is associated with jobs that require frequent immersion of hands in water, such as dishwashing, bartending, and healthcare work.

Q **Are you a healthcare worker?** This helps identify risk of exposure to herpes virus while considering the differential diagnosis of herpetic whitlow.

Q **Have you or your current sexual partner been diagnosed with herpes virus infection?** Helps exclude differential diagnosis of herpetic whitlow.

Q **Do you have artificial nails?** Perionychial trauma caused by filing during placement (or removal) of artificial nails can create a port of entry for organisms into perionychial tissue. Some salons' poor hygiene practices increase risk of contamination from equipment resulting in infection.

Q **Do you have regular manicures that include cuticle trimming?** Trauma from cuticle trimming can lead to paronychia.

Q **Do you have diabetes?** Diabetes increases risk for finger and toe infections.

Q **Do you use your hands a lot in your work?** Repetitive finger trauma such as typing, other keyboard work, or piano playing can increase risk for infection.

Examination

- **Inspect the affected area for erythema and swelling.** Green discoloration of nails may be present with *Pseudomonas* infection
- **Palpate the affected area for tenderness** along the nail folds and for separation of the nail from the nail plate
- **Palpate the affected area for fluctuance**
- **Look for evidence of herpetic whitlow,** such as vesicles
- **Look for evidence of malignancy,** such as proliferation of tissue
- **Look for silvery scales** in the presence of nail pitting and onycholysis, which suggest psoriasis
- **Palpate regional lymph nodes for enlargement**

Summary of investigative tests

In uncomplicated acute paronychia, laboratory tests are not indicated; treatment can be empiric based on the high likelihood of staphylococcal infection.

Tests that may be ordered in acute paronychia include:
- Gram stain of exudate from nail fold
- Bacterial culture and sensitivity tests of exudate from nail fold

Tests that may be ordered in chronic paronychia include:
- Potassium hydroxide (KOH) test of smear from nail fold
- Fungal culture of exudate from nail fold
- Radiology and histology should be considered in selected cases to rule out osteomyelitis and malignancy, respectively. Investigations are normally performed by a specialist

DIAGNOSTIC DECISION
- Diagnosis of paronychia is based on clinical findings
- Laboratory investigations may confirm infection with organisms in unclear or complicated cases

Guidelines:
The American Academy of Family Physicians has produced the following: Acute and chronic paronychia. [1]

CLINICAL PEARLS
- The diagnosis of paronychia is usually straightforward
- Atypical presentations prompt one to think more broadly about differential diagnosis

THE TESTS
Body fluids
GRAM STAIN

Description
Swab of purulent discharge from perionychium fixed onto glass slide and stained with Gram stain.

Advantages/Disadvantages
Advantages:
- Useful if there is reasonable suspicion infection is not staphylococcal or if antibacterial therapy is ineffective
- Simple test
- Reasonably fast results

Normal
No/few bacteria seen.

Abnormal
- Bacteria present in considerable numbers and characteristics identified: Gram-positive or Gram-negative
- Fungal elements, if present, may be identified
- Keep in mind the possibility of a false-positive or false-negative result

Cause of abnormal result
Bacterial infection.

Drugs, disorders and other factors that may alter results
- If patient has self-treated with topical antibiotic ointment, Gram stain may be negative despite infection
- Laboratory technique may affect results

CULTURE FOR PATHOGENS AND SENSITIVITY TO ANTIBIOTICS
Description
Swab of purulent discharge from perionychium is collected; exudate is inoculated onto culture medium and then incubated to support growth of organisms.

Advantages/Disadvantages
Advantages:
- Useful if there is reasonable suspicion infection is not staphylococcal or if antibacterial therapy is ineffective
- Simple test

Disadvantage: Result is not immediate

Normal
No growth of bacterial colonies.

Abnormal
- Growth of bacterial colonies
- Antibiotic disks to which bacteria are sensitive will demonstrate a zone of no growth around them; thus, identifying bacterial sensitivity
- *Candida* may grow if present; though may be laboratory contaminate, may also be pathogenic
- Keep in mind the possibility of a false-positive or false-negative result

Cause of abnormal result
Bacterial infection.

Drugs, disorders and other factors that may alter results
- If patient has self-treated with topical antibiotic ointment, culture may be negative despite infection
- Laboratory technique may affect result

POTASSIUM HYDROXIDE (KOH) TEST
Description
- Swab of purulent discharge from perionychium collected and placed on glass slide
- Mixed with KOH
- Slide is covered and exposed to gentle heat
- Microscopic examination for fungi, fungal elements, or budding yeast

Advantages/Disadvantages
Advantages:
- Useful if there is reasonable suspicion infection is chronic and less likely to be bacterial, or if antibiotic therapy has failed
- Simple test
- Reasonably fast result

Normal
No pathogens seen.

Abnormal
- Yeast buds, fungi, or fungal elements seen
- Keep in mind the possibility of a false-positive or false-negative result

Cause of abnormal result
Infection with yeast or fungi.

Drugs, disorders and other factors that may alter results
- Topical or systemic antimycotic therapy may produce false-negative result
- Laboratory technique may affect result

FUNGAL CULTURE
Description
- Swab of purulent discharge from perionychium placed in sterile specimen cup
- Purulent drainage aspirated through needle and syringe, then submitted to laboratory in same syringe (cap replaces needle)

Advantages/Disadvantages
Advantages:
- Useful if there is reasonable suspicion infection is chronic and less likely to be bacterial, or if antibiotic therapy has failed
- Will identify specific type of fungus

Disadvantage: Results may take up to 4 weeks

Normal
No fungi present.

Abnormal
- Growth of fungi
- Keep in mind the possibility of a false-positive or false-negative result

Cause of abnormal result
Fungal infection.

Drugs, disorders and other factors that may alter results
- Topical or systemic antifungal therapy may produce false-negative result
- Laboratory technique may affect result

TREATMENT

CONSIDER CONSULT
- Despite traditional treatment, patients with chronic, recurrent paronychia may benefit from referral to a dermatologist to consult on prolonged treatment
- Refer if malignant tumor is suspected (usually to a surgeon or dermatologist)

IMMEDIATE ACTION
- Empiric antibiotic therapy may be necessary before causative organism is determined, especially if osteomyelitis is suspected
- Incision and drainage indicated if suppuration is present

PATIENT AND CAREGIVER ISSUES
Patient or caregiver request
- How did I contract this infection? Explain that trauma allows entry of pathogens; infection is not necessarily a reflection of patient's personal hygiene
- Is it contagious? Likelihood of passing on infection to another person is low

Health-seeking behavior
- Have you been to the emergency department? Often acute pain will cause the patient to visit the emergency department for treatment
- Have you attempted self-treatment with antibiotic creams or ointments? This can affect culture results
- Have you tried to clip or 'dig out' an ingrown toenail? Will cause tissue damage and often introduces pathogens
- Have you ignored symptoms in order to keep artificial nails?
- Have you delayed seeking treatment because of a lack of health insurance? Infection could spread into deeper tissues

MANAGEMENT ISSUES
Goals
- Reduce pain and swelling
- Facilitate drainage of purulent exudate
- Prevent complications, such as extension of infection into digit
- Prevent recurrence – change of lifestyle

Management in special circumstances
COEXISTING DISEASE
- Patients with diabetes are at risk for mixed bacterial infection and may need extended antibiotic treatment and more aggressive follow up, particularly if paronychia involves a toe or is associated with an ingrown toenail
- Patients with peripheral vascular insufficiency are more prone to severe disease course and possible side effects, therefore extended antibiotic treatment and more aggressive follow up may be needed
- In immunocompromised patients the clinical signs of inflammation may be less prominent (and more likely to be overlooked) despite serious disease. Extended antibiotic treatment is usually required

SUMMARY OF THERAPEUTIC OPTIONS
Choices
- Warm soaks promote drainage and provide symptom relief in acute paronychia. Mild topical steroids may help reduce inflammation. They should be used in combination with antifungal and antibacterial agents
- Acute paronychia is often treated with oral antibiotics, such as cephalexin and dicloxacillin

- Incision and drainage with or without partial nail removal relieves pain and removes pus
- Presence of paronychia will impact on treatment decisions for ingrown toenail, including surgical approach; incision and drainage of toe paronychia may include removing part of nail
- Chronic paronychia is more often caused by fungal infections and treated with topical antifungals, e.g. ketoconazole cream. Mild topical steroids, e.g. hydrocortisone (in combination with antifungal and antibacterial agents) may help reduce inflammation

Guidelines:
The American Academy of Family Physicians has produced the following: Acute and chronic paronychia. [1]

Clinical pearls
In immunocompetent individuals, prevention of recurrence should focus on reducing behaviors such as nail/hang nail manipulation, drying, and use of moisturizers after washing.

Never
- Never perform incision and drainage if there is any question that diagnosis might be herpetic whitlow
- Never miss a neoplastic lesion

FOLLOW UP
Patients with diabetes may need more extensive follow up, particularly if paronychia is related to an ingrown toenail.

Plan for review
Patient should be re-examined between 2 and 5 days after treatment.

Information for patient or caregiver
- If antibiotics are prescribed, the patient must know to take the entire course as prescribed
- Acute paronychia of the fingernail should dramatically improve within 24–48h of treatment. If not, the patient should call the physician promptly
- Notify the physician if there are red streaks up the arm, fever, chills, joint or muscle pain, or pain in the pad of the finger

DRUGS AND OTHER THERAPIES: DETAILS
Drugs
CEPHALEXIN
First-generation cephalosporin.

Dose
250mg orally four times daily until symptoms resolve.

Efficacy
Destroys *Staphylococcus aureus* by inhibiting bacterial cell wall synthesis.

Risks/benefits
Risks:
- Use caution in patients with penicillin hypersensitivity
- Use caution in renal impairment, history of gastrointestinal disease
- Use caution in breast-feeding

Side effects and adverse reactions
- Central nervous system: headache, sleep disturbance, confusion, dizziness
- Gastrointestinal: anorexia, nausea, diarrhea, abdominal pain

■ Hematologic: pancytopenia
■ Skin: rashes, erythema multiforme

Interactions (other drugs)
■ Warfarin ■ Aminoglycosides ■ Loop diuretics ■ Probenecid ■ Polymixin B
■ Vancomycin ■ Penicillins

Contraindications
■ Penicillin and cephalosporin hypersensitivity ■ Children less than one month of age
■ True penicillin allergy (anaphylaxis, respiratory compromise) ■ True cephalosporin allergy

Acceptability to patient
■ Four times daily dose administration may be difficult for patients to remember
■ Gastrointestinal upset may limit patient compliance
■ Incision and drainage may provide enough relief that patient doesn't see need to take antibiotics

Follow up plan
Examine affected digit within a week to ensure resolution of paronychia.

Patient and caregiver information
■ Patient must take entire course of antibiotics as directed, regardless of improvement in symptoms
■ If rash develops, patient should call physician
■ If side effects are not tolerable, patient should call physician so an alternative antibiotic can be prescribed

DICLOXACILLIN
Penicillin derivative effective against Gram-positive bacteria.

Dose
125mg orally four times daily until symptoms resolve.

Efficacy
Destroys *Staphyloccis aureus* and other Gram-positive organisms by inhibiting bacterial cell wall synthesis.

Risks/benefits
Risks:
■ Use caution in patients with a history of gastrointestinal disease
■ Use caution in patients with eczema or asthma
■ Use caution in breast-feeding

Side effects and adverse reactions
■ Central nervous system: seizures, anxiety, lethargy
■ Gastrointestinal: nausea, vomiting, diarrhea, pseudomembranous colitis, abdominal discomfort, gastrointestinal bleeding, elevated hepatic enzymes
■ Hematologic: thrombocytopenia, leukopenia, neutropenia
■ Skin: purpura, rashes, vasculitis, exfoliative dermatitis, maculopapular rash, Stevens-Johnson syndrome

Interactions (other drugs)
- Aminoglycosides ▪ Chloramphenicol ▪ Macrolide antibiotics ▪ Methotrexate
- Oral contraceptives ▪ Probenecid ▪ Tetracycline antibiotics ▪ Warfarin

Contraindications
- Hypersensitivity to penicillins

Acceptability to patient
- Four times daily dose administration may be difficult for patients to remember
- Gastrointestinal upset may limit patient compliance
- Incision and drainage may provide so much relief that patient doesn't see need to take antibiotics

Follow up plan
Examine affected digit within one week to assure resolution of paronychia.

Patient and caregiver information
- Patient must take entire course of antibiotics as directed, regardless of improvement in symptoms
- If rash develops, patient should call physician
- If side effects are not tolerable, patient should call physician so an alternative antibiotic can be prescribed

KETOCONAZOLE CREAM
Used for chronic paronychia caused by infection with *Candida*.

Dose
Apply thin film of 2% cream to affected area once daily (may use twice daily for more resistant cases). Treatment is continued until symptoms resolve.

Efficacy
Damages fungal cell membrane, altering permeability, and inhibits fungal enzymes.

Risks/benefits
Risk: sulfite sensitivity.

Side effects and adverse reactions
Minimal with topical preparation.

Interactions (other drugs)
- None listed

Contraindications
- None in this setting

Acceptability to patient
Creams have fewer systemic effects and tend to be well tolerated by patients.

Follow up plan
- Examine within 2 weeks. If clinical improvement is not seen, consider change of treatment

- If condition is not resolved within 4 weeks, explore other possible underlying diseases, such as malignancies

Patient and caregiver information
- Patient should continue applying cream as directed until physician tells them to stop
- Only a thin layer of cream should be applied to affected area
- Should be applied after a shower when affected area is clean and when cream will not be washed off

Surgical therapy
INCISION AND DRAINAGE
- In many cases of acute paronychia, blade may be used to elevate lateral nail fold, allowing drainage of purulent material without requiring an incision
- Partial removal of the affected nail may be needed if infection is more extensive

Efficacy
Once area is fluctuant, incision and drainage is usually curative.

Risks/benefits
Risk: incision and drainage is contraindicated for herpetic whitlow; herpes infection must be ruled out before this therapy is carried out.

Acceptability to patient
- Some patients may be reluctant to have a minor surgical procedure in any situation. Once they realize pain is relieved when pressure around the nail is removed, acceptance is high
- Adequate local anesthesia is critical to patient acceptance

Follow up plan
- If a wick is placed for drainage, it should be kept in place for 24–48h; physician will need to assess whether patient should return for wick removal or if the patient can accomplish this at home
- After wick removal, warm soaks (warm water for 10min) three or four times each day
- Recheck in 2–4 days

Patient and caregiver information
- Patient should leave wick in place and follow removal instructions from physician
- Warm soaks are very important in cure of acute paronychia

Other therapies
WARM SOAKS
Warm soaks (warm water for 10min) three or four times each day.

Efficacy
For acute paronychia; chronic paronychia should be kept dry.

Risks/benefits
Benefits:
- Symptom relief
- Promotes drainage

Acceptability to patient
- Simple and easy to perform

- As it is so simple (soaking the digit in warm water) patients may not believe it is important therapy

Follow up plan
Same follow up as for general treatment of acute paronychia; follow up in 2–5 days after treatment is started.

Patient and caregiver information
- Soak affected digit in warm water for 10min three or four times daily
- Make sure water is not so hot it could cause burns

EFFICACY OF THERAPIES

In the normal course, drainage of purulent material, antibiotics (as indicated by individual patient need), and warm soaks should lead to resolution within 5–10 days.

Evidence

PDxMD are unable to cite evidence that meets our criteria for evidence.

Review period

Typically, 2–5 days.

PROGNOSIS

- Complete cure is usual for acute paronychia
- Chronic paronychia is more difficult to cure and depends in large part on avoidance of predisposing factors where possible

Clinical pearls

Recurrence is common if precipitating behaviors are repeated.

Therapeutic failure

- Consider referral to dermatologist or hand surgeon if no clinical improvement
- Investigate whether patient followed instructions and took antibiotics (if prescribed) as directed
- Consider possible underlying condition (malignancy, psoriasis)

Recurrence

If paronychia recurs, review and modify risk factors with patient; try to determine if there are factors preventing lifestyle changes.

Deterioration

- Infection may spread deeper into tissues leading to osteomyelitis
- Urgent treatment with antibiotics and referral are necessary

COMPLICATIONS

- Felon
- Osteomyelitis
- Nail loss

CONSIDER CONSULT

- Refer to a hand surgeon if inflammation is accompanied by proximal spread or discharging sinus develops (osteomyelitis)
- Refer to a hand surgeon if underlying bone, joint, or tendons become affected (severe pain, fever, and malaise may be present)

RISK FACTORS

- **Trauma:** biting or picking at nails or cuticles increases the risk of introducing breaks in skin through which pathogens may enter
- **Artificial nails:** poor salon hygiene increases risk of introducing pathogens when fixing or removing nails
- **Continual immersion of hands in water:** occupational exposure to water increases risk for chronic infection
- **Coexisting disease, e.g. diabetes:** increases risk for chronic infection

MODIFY RISK FACTORS

- Do not bite or pick at nails and cuticles – carefully push back cuticles to prevent hangnail formation; carefully trim hangnails
- Evaluate cleanliness procedures at nail salons and change salons if necessary
- Try to avoid soaking hands in water without protection of waterproof gloves
- Control diabetes

ASSOCIATIONS

American Academy of Dermatology
930 East Woodfield Road
Schaumburg, IL 60173-4927
Mailing address:
PO Box 4014
Schaumburg, IL 60168-4014
Tel: (847) 330-0230
Fax: (847) 330-0050
http://www.aad.org

American College of Foot and Ankle Surgeons
515 Busse Highway
Park Ridge, IL 60068
Tel: (847) 292-2237
Fax: (800) 421-2237
E-mail: mail@acfas.org
http://www.acfas.org

KEY REFERENCES

- Ingrown toenails. Philadelphia (PA): Academy of Ambulatory Foot and Ankle Surgery; 2000. Available at the National Guidelines Clearinghouse
- Antosia RE, Lyn E. The hand: infections of the hand. In: Rosen P, ed. Emergency medicine: concepts and clinical practice, 4th edn. St. Louis: Mosby-Year Book: 1998, p662–3
- Drake LA. Guidelines of care for superficial mycotic infections of the skin: onychomycosis. J Am Acad Dermatology 1996;34:116–21
- Ellsworth AJ, Witt DM, Dugdale DC, Oliver LM. Mosby's 1999–2000 medical drug reference. St. Louis: Mosby-Year Book, 1999
- Fischbach F. A manual of laboratory & diagnostic tests, 5th edn. Philadelphia: Lippincott-Raven, 1996

EVIDENCE REFERENCES AND GUIDELINES

1   The American Academy of Family Physicians has produced the following: Rockwell PG. Acute and chronic paronychia. Am Fam Physician 2001;63:1113–6

CONTRIBUTORS

Fred F Ferri, MD, FACP
Seth R Stevens, MD
Rolland P Gyulai, MD, PhD

PEMPHIGOID

DESCRIPTION

- Chronic autoimmune bullous disease in which the lesion is at the basement membrane between the dermis and epidermis
- Prodomal pruritus for a few weeks
- Eczema and urticarial rashes may precede bullae
- Tense bullae subsequently appear on the trunk and to a lesser extent on the limbs
- Rapidly healing mucosal ulceration occurs rarely (10%)
- Affects the elderly predominately

ICD9 CODE
694.5 Pemphigoid

SYNONYMS
- Subepidermal autoimmune bullous dermatoses
- Pemphigoid

CARDINAL FEATURES
- Chronic autoimmune bullous disease in which the lesion is at the basement membrane between the dermis and epidermis
- Prodromal pruritus for a few weeks
- Eczema and urticarial rashes precede bullae
- Tense bullae subsequently appear one week to several months later
- The bullae can be provoked by trauma
- The surrounding skin shows erythematous patches
- Nikolsky's sign negative
- The large tense subepidermal bullae have less tendency to break than pemphigus
- Symmetrical bullae present on flexor surfaces of limb and trunk areas
- Head and neck areas spared
- Twice as common as pemphigus
- Acantholysis is not a histologic feature
- Rapidly healing oral lesions occasionally occur
- Affects elderly predominately
- Mortality varies between 6% and 36%

CAUSES
Common causes
- Autoimmune disease with IgG and C3 complement component reacting with antigens located in the basement membrane zone
- Two large epidermal polypeptides are the major antigenic target of the autoantibodies

Contributory or predisposing factors
The following diseases have been associated to pemphigoid: diabetes, multiple sclerosis, pernicious anemia, rheumatoid arthritis, lichen planus, psoriasis, and vitiligo.

EPIDEMIOLOGY
Incidence and prevalence
Most common of the autoimmune bullous dermatoses.

INCIDENCE
10/1,000,000.

Demographics
AGE
Commonly seen in elderly over 70 years old.

GENDER
Females more commonly affected.

RACE
No racial predilection.

GENETICS

- Two large epidermal polypeptides are the major antigenic target of the BP antibodies
- The BP230 gene is localized to the short arm of chromosome 6
- The BP180 gene is localized to the long arm of chromosome 10
- Both proteins are components of the hemidesmosome
- BP180 is a transmembrane glycoprotein with an external ectodomain consisting of collagen triple helical domains. It binds keratin to the hemidesmosome

DIFFERENTIAL DIAGNOSIS
Cicatrical pemphigoid
Benign mucosal pemphigoid with similar autoimmune etiology as bullous pemphigoid.

FEATURES
- Subepidermal bullae
- Present in mouth, conjunctiva, and perineal orifices
- Base of lesions is heavily infiltrated with lymphocytes and plasma cells leading to eventual fibrosis
- Skin lesions are usually localized with a tendency to recur at the same site
- Conjunctival involvement leads to corneal ulceration, entropion, symblepheron, ankyloblepheron, and blindness
- Direct and indirect immunofluorescent findings are similar to those of bullous pemphigoid, but fewer than 50% patients give positive results
- Rare and uncommon
- Low mortality

Gestational pemphigoid
FEATURES
- Presents in late second or third trimester
- Resolves on delivery
- Immunologically identical to bullous pemphigoid

Pemphigus
Pemphigus is a chronic autoimmune disease characterized by intraepidermal blister formation.

FEATURES
- Affects predominately 40- to 60-year-olds
- Oral lesions common
- Superficial bullae can occur anywhere on body
- Nikolsky's sign – the epidermis is easily detached from the underlying skin
- Bullae flaccid and superficial
- Bullae are fragile and often rupture
- Denuded and crusted lesions occur after rupture

Dermatitis herpetiformis
Dermatitis herpetiformis is an uncommon irritative skin condition associated with gluten-sensitive enteropathy – celiac disease.

FEATURES
- Irritative grouped vesicles
- Especially present on elbows, knees, and buttocks
- Numerous excoriations with blister crustation
- Histology reveals small subepidermal blisters
- Direct immunofluorescence reveal granular deposits of IgA in dermal papillae

Drug eruptions
Skin eruptions due to medication.

FEATURES
- Common causes of blisters
- Any medication can lead to skin lesions

- Blood-borne and have symmetrical patterns determined by vasculature
- Likely offenders include digoxin, tylenol, sulfonamides, and penicillins
- Identifying and removing cause will lead to resolution

Erythema multiforme

Erythema multiforme is an inflammatory disease secondary to immune complex formation and subsequent deposition in the skin and mucous membranes.

FEATURES
- Symmetrical skin lesions with a classic 'target' appearance
- Lesions most common on dorsum of hand and feet, and extensors of limbs
- Rarely involves trunk
- Bullae and erosions may be present in oral cavity
- Lesions heal within 2 weeks without scarring

SIGNS & SYMPTOMS
Signs
- Prodromal pruritus for a few weeks
- Eczema and urticarial rashes precede bullae
- Tense bullae subsequently appear one week to several months later
- The bullae can be provoked by trauma and can be hemorrhagic
- The surrounding skin shows erythematous patches and vesicles
- Nikolsky's sign negative – when firm sliding finger pressure is applied over the skin, the superficial layer should not move over deeper layers unlike pemphigus
- The large tense subepidermal bullae have less tendency to break than pemphigus
- Symmetrical bullae present on flexor surfaces of limb and trunk areas
- Head and neck areas spared
- Rapidly healing oral lesions occasionally occur (10%)
- Patient not systemically unwell even with secondary infections, which are common

Symptoms
- Prodromal intense itching
- Eczema and urticarial rash precede blister formation
- Large tense blisters occur on the trunk and limbs
- Rarely the patient complains of mouth ulcers (10%)

CONSIDER CONSULT
- All patients should be referred to a dermatologist with experience treating immunobullous disorders for full evaluation, confirmation of diagnosis, and appropriate management

INVESTIGATION OF THE PATIENT
Direct questions to patient
Q Is your skin irritating? An intense prodromal itch precedes blister formation.
Q Do you suffer from eczema or rashes? Eczema and urticarial rashes can precede the bullae formation especially at the peripheries.
Q Are there ulcers in your mouth? Only 10% of patients with pemphigoid suffer oral ulceration, which is rapidly healing.
Q Where are the blisters? The flexor surfaces of the limbs, groin, and axilla favor pemphigoid; the head and neck are spared.
Q Do blisters form where pressure or trauma has been applied to the skin? Bullae can be provoked by trauma.
Q Do you feel unwell? The patient normally feels well with pemphigoid, although secondary skin infection is common.

Examination

- **Does the patient have eczema?** Eczema and urticarial rashes on the extremities precede bullae
- **Are the bullae tense and intact?** Classical tense bullae are characteristic of pemphigoid that have less tendency to break than pemphigus
- **Can the bullae be provoked by trauma?** The bullae can occur at pressure points of the body and can be hemorrhagic
- **Is the surrounding skin to the vesicles normal?** The surrounding skin shows erythematous patches and vesicles
- **Is Nikolsky's sign negative?** When firm sliding finger pressure is applied over the skin, the superficial layer should not move over deeper layers, which occurs with pemphigus
- **What is the distribution of the bullae?** Symmetrical bullae present on flexor surfaces of limb and trunk areas with sparing of the head and neck areas
- **Has the oral cavity ulceration?** Rapidly healing oral lesions can occur (10%)
- **Is the patient systemically unwell?** The patient with pemphigoid is not usually ill even with secondary infection, which is common

Summary of investigative tests

- Serology for circulating IgG and C3 antibody to basement membrane zone is found in 75% of patients with pemphigoid
- Direct immunofluorescence: 70% show linear deposition of specific IgG for the basement membrane zone of the epidermis
- Skin biopsy of a fresh lesion demonstrates a split at the level of the basement membrane, commonly with a mixed inflammatory infiltrate rich in eosinophils at the base

DIAGNOSTIC DECISION

Diagnosis is based on the presence of appropriate binding of IgG and complement along the dermal-epidermal junction.

CLINICAL PEARLS

- There is clinical overlap between bullous pemphigoid and cicatricial pemphigoid. Appropriate history and physical examination of the skin, conjunctivae, and oral cavity should be performed on all patients with known or suspected bullous pemphigoid
- Urticaria confined to buttocks, groins, and/or periaxillary areas in older adults should raise question of bullous pemphigoid

THE TESTS
Body fluids
SEROLOGY
Description
Indirect immunoflurescence: a venous blood sample is taken to collect serum, which is placed on appropriate tissue substrate (e.g. guinea pig esophagus, human skin, rat tongue, or rat bladder). Antibodies recognizing cutaneous antigens (e.g. bullous pemphigoid antigens) are identified by fluorescenated antihuman IgG antibodies.

Advantages/Disadvantages
Advantages:
- Serum easily accessible
- Diagnostic for pemphigoid

Disadvantage: Requires a specialized laboratory to the immunofluorescent testing

Abnormal
IgG and C3 antibodies to basement membrane zone in the serum sample is diagnostic for pemphigoid group (bullous pemphigoid, cicatricial pemphigoid, gestational pemphigoid) or epidermolysis bullosa acquisita.

Biopsy
SKIN BIOPSY

Description
Skin biopsy of a lesion is taken for microscopy.

Advantages/Disadvantages
Advantages:
- Skin lesions easily accessible
- Inexpensive
- Diagnostic for pemphigoid

Abnormal
- Subepidermal blister on histology with no acantholysis
- Split at the level of the basement membrane with a mixed inflammatory infiltrate rich in eosinophils at the base

DIRECT IMMUNOFLUORESCENCE
Description
Direct immunofluorescent testing of a perilesional skin uses patient skin as substrate, exposed to fluorescein-conjugated antibodies directed against human immunoreactants (e.g. IgG or C3). In vivo deposition of immunoreactants is reflected as specific patterns of immunofluorescence when examined with a fluorescence microscope.

Advantages/Disadvantages
Advantages:
- Provides very specific information
- Performing skin biopsy is uncomplicated primary care office procedure

Disadvantage: Requires specialized skills, reagents, and equipment for processing of specimen

Abnormal
Direct immunofluorescent testing of a perilesional skin shows a linear band of immunofluorescence with IgG and C3 antibodies to the basement membrane zone.

Cause of abnormal result
Epidermolysis bullosa acquisita – a similar result can be obtained in epidermolysis bullosa acquisita and can be distinguished by splitting the skin with one molar NaCl either on direct or indirect immunofluorescence.

CONSIDER CONSULT

- Pemphigoid is a chronic treatment requiring careful management and close follow up. At the minimum, patients will need to be followed by those familiar with the use of steroid-sparing immunosuppressants

IMMEDIATE ACTION

Distinction from evolving Stevens-Johnson syndrome/toxic epidermal necrolysis should be made. If extensive blistering is present, hospital admission for wound care and fluid and electrolyte management is required.

PATIENT AND CAREGIVER ISSUES
Patient or caregiver request

- **Is this skin disease infectious?** Pemphigoid is not infectious
- **What is the cause of this disease?** Pemphigoid is due to an aberrant immune reaction that affects part of the skin
- **Is the disease serious?** Pemphigoid is serious, requiring careful management and follow up. Medications used to treat pemphigoid are associated with significant adverse effects and need to be monitored
- **Will I have to be hospitalized?** Most patients can be managed in the community
- **Will I gain weight with the steroid therapy?** Weight gain is common on steroids and good dietary advice is needed
- **Will the lesions scar?** Pemphigoid blisters do not scar, even with denudation, unless they get secondarily infected or are vigorously scratched
- **Will I get better?** Pemphigoid is usually a self-limiting disease and treatment can be stopped within 1–2 years

Health-seeking behavior

Have you tried over-the-counter remedies? Patients may have tried creams to reduce the urticarial itching and blister formation.

MANAGEMENT ISSUES
Goals

- Reduce the morbidity and mortality of pemphigoid
- Reduce the risk of sepsis
- Prevent new lesion formation
- Give support to the patient, especially as pemphigoid predominantly affects elderly patients over 70 years
- Prevent adverse effects of medications used to treat pemphigoid

SUMMARY OF THERAPEUTIC OPTIONS
Choices

- Morbidity and mortality are mainly secondary to treatment, so less aggressive regimens have been used
- Patients can use topical steroids for localized disease, e.g. triamcinolone acetonide
- Systemic steroids are the usual treatment for more advanced pemphigoid
- Pemphigoid can be treated using the combination of tetracycline and nicotinamide
- Steroid-sparing medication includes dapsone
- Pemphigoid is usually a self-limiting disease and treatment can be stopped within 1–2 years

Clinical pearls

Mild cases can be treated topically, though these are rare at presentation. At presentation, most patients will require systemic corticosteroids.

Never

Never ignore ocular symptoms in pemphigoid patients – scarring of ocular pemphigoid can lead to blindness.

FOLLOW UP

Careful follow up of pemphigoid patients is required, especially as the disease affects the elderly population. Monitoring for skin integrity, sequelae of loss of skin integrity, and adverse effects of immunosuppressants is required.

Plan for review

- Systemic steroids should be used in the lowest dose once new blisters cease to appear
- Occasional new lesions should not equate to an increase in steroids unless the benefits of the treatment outweigh the risks associated with steroids
- Topical steroids may be useful for occasional lesions

Information for patient or caregiver

- The importance of treatment compliance must be emphasized to patients and their caregivers as pemphigoid has high morbidity and mortality
- The side effects of steroids should be explained carefully and reduced to the minimum
- Weight gain is common with steroids and good dietary advice is needed
- Antiosteoporotic treatment is required if patient is to be started on systemic steroids

DRUGS AND OTHER THERAPIES: DETAILS
Drugs
PREDNISONE

- Systemic steroid required for more advanced pemphigoid
- It should be initiated in high doses and once new blister formation ceases, tapering off the dose to the minimum maintenance dose required

Dose
- Adult: initiate with 60–100mg orally, once daily, continue until new blister formation ceases
- Then taper to 20–40mg orally, once daily
- Gradually taper according to clinical response

Efficacy
- The mainstay of treatment in pemphigoid
- Prevents morbidity and mortality from pemphigoid

Risks/benefits
Risks:
- Use caution in congestive heart failure, renal disease, or diabetes mellitus
- Use caution in the elderly
- Use caution in glaucoma
- Use caution in ulcerative colitis or peptic ulcer
- Prednisone taken in doses higher than 7.5mg for a period of 3 weeks or longer may lead to clinically relevant suppression of the pituitary-adrenal axis

Benefit: Prevents morbidity and mortality from pemphigoid

Side effects and adverse reactions
- Side effects are minimized by short duration of therapy
- Cardiovascular system: hypertension, thromboembolism
- Central nervous system: insomnia, euphoria, depression, psychosis, seizures
- Endocrine: adrenal suppression, impaired glucose tolerance, growth suppression in children
- Eyes, ears, nose, and throat: cataract, glaucoma, blurred vision
- Gastrointestinal: dyspepsia, peptic ulceration, esophagitis, oral candidiasis
- Musculoskeletal: proximal myopathy, osteoporosis
- Skin: delayed healing, acne, striae, fragile skin

Interactions (other drugs)
- Aminoglutethimide (increased clearance of prednisone) ■ Antidiabetics (hypoglycemic effect inhibited) ■ Antihypertensives (effects inhibited) ■ Barbiturates (increased clearance of prednisone) ■ Cardiac glycosides (toxicity increased) ■ Cholestyramine, colestipol (may reduce absorption of corticosteroids) ■ Clarithromycin, erythromycin, troleandomycin (may enhance steroid effect) ■ Cyclosporine (may increase levels of both drugs; may cause seizures) ■ Diuretics (effects inhibited) ■ Isoniazid (reduced plasma levels of isoniazid) ■ Ketoconazole ■ NSAIDs (increased risks of bleeding) ■ Oral contraceptives (enhanced effects of corticosteroids) ■ Rifampin (may inhibit hepatic clearance of prednisone) ■ Salicylates (increased clearance of salicylates) ■ Warfarin (alters clotting time)

Contraindications
- Systemic infection ■ Avoid live virus vaccines in those receiving immunosuppressive doses ■ History of tuberculosis ■ Cushing's syndrome ■ Recent myocardial infarction

Acceptability to patient
- Some patients do not like taking steroids
- Compliance must be carefully monitored

Follow up plan
Careful monitoring of compliance and side effects is needed.

Patient and caregiver information
- The patient and caregiver must be informed of the potentially serious nature of this disease
- Compliance is important
- Weight gain is common with steroids, and good dietary advice is needed
- Discussion of the side effects and prevention of osteoporosis is needed

TRIAMCINOLONE ACETONIDE
Useful for localized disease with few lesions.

Dose
0.1% cream applied to affected areas twice daily.

Efficacy
Useful for localized disease.

Risks/benefits
Risks:
- The potential for systemic absorption must be considered
- Use with caution in children

Benefit: Useful for localized disease and spares the use of systemic steroids

Side effects and adverse reactions
- Eyes, ears, nose, and throat: conjunctivitis
- Skin: rash, dermatitis, pruritus, atrophy, hypopigmentation, striae, xerosis, burning, stinging upon application, alopecia

Interactions (other drugs)
- None listed

Contraindications
- Do not use on axilla, face, or groin

Acceptability to patient
Topical steroids are more acceptable to the patient as they have fewer side effects.

TETRACYCLINE
- Tetracycline is given in combination with nicotinamide to treat pemphigoid
- This combination may reduce the need for systemic steroids

Dose
Usual adult dose: 1–2g/day in two or four equally divided doses.

Efficacy
Tetracycline in combination with nicotinamide can be an effective treatment for pemphigoid.

Risks/benefits
Risks:
- Compliance can be a problem
- Use caution in patients with hepatic impairment
- Use caution with repeated or prolonged doses

Benefit: Tetracycline has far fewer side effects than steroids

Side effects and adverse reactions

- Cardiovascular system: pericarditis
- Central nervous system: headache, paresthesia, fever
- Gastrointestinal: abdominal pain, diarrhea, heartburn, hepatotoxicity, vomiting, nausea, dental staining, anorexia
- Genitourinary: polyuria, polydipsia, azotemia
- Hematologic: blood cell dyscrasias
- Skin: pruritus, rash, photosensitivity, changes in pigmentation, angioedema, stinging

Interactions (other drugs)
- Antacids ■ Atovaquone ■ Barbiturates ■ Bismuth subsalicyclate ■ Calcium, iron, magnesium, zinc ■ Cephalosporins ■ Cholestyramine, colestipol ■ Carbamazepine ■ Digoxin ■ Ethanol ■ Methoxyflurane ■ Oral contraceptives ■ Penicillins ■ Phenytoin ■ Quinapril ■ Sodium bicarbonate ■ Vitamin A ■ Warfarin

Contraindications
- Pregnancy and breast-feeding ■ Children less than 8 years ■ Severe renal disease

Acceptability to patient
Tetracycline and nicotinamide have far fewer side effects than systemic steroids.

Follow up plan
Careful follow up to check that combination treatment is effective in preventing new blister formation.

Patient and caregiver information
■ Patients should not take tetracyclines with milk or antacids
■ A full glass of water is needed when taking tetracyclines

NICOTINAMIDE
■ Nicotinamide is given in combination with tetracycline to treat pemphigoid
■ This combination may reduce the need for systemic steroids

Dose
500mg three times daily.

Efficacy
Tetracycline in combination with nicotinamide can be an effective treatment for pemphigoid.

Risks/benefits
Risks:
■ Use with caution in patients with a history of jaundice, hepatitis, or diabetes mellitus
■ Use caution in the elderly and children
■ Avoid large doses in pregnancy (US recommended daily amount is 20mg/day)

Benefit: Has demonstrated anti-inflammatory actions

Side effects and adverse reactions
Gastrointestinal: gastrointestinal distress including nausea and vomiting, transient elevations of liver function tests.

Interactions (other drugs)
■ Primidone ■ Carbamazepine

Contraindications
■ Hypersensitivity to nicotinamide ■ Breast-feeding

Acceptability to patient
Tetracycline and nicotinamide have far fewer side effects than systemic steroids.

Follow up plan
Careful follow up to check that combination treatment is effective in preventing new blister formation.

DAPSONE
■ Competitive antagonist of para-aminobenzoic acid
■ May be used instead of systemic steroids for pemphigoid

Dose
50–200mg daily.

453

Efficacy
- Can reduce blister formation
- Useful steroid-sparing agent
- Use in conjunction with topical steroids has benefit relative to topical steroids alone

Risks/benefits
Risks:
- Use caution in renal impairment and hepatic impairment
- Use caution in glucose-6-phosphate dehydrogenase deficiency
- Fatal agranulocytosis, aplastic anemia, and other blood dyscrasias reported
- Complete blood counts should be performed frequently

Benefit: Can reduce blister formation

Side effects and adverse reactions
- Central nervous system: headache, insomnia, paresthesia, peripheral neuropathy, psychosis, vertigo
- Eyes, ears, nose, and throat: blurred vision, optic neuritis, photophobia, tinnitus
- Gastrointestinal: abdominal pain, anorexia, nausea, vomiting
- Genitourinary: nephrotic syndrome, renal papillary necrosis, proteinuria
- Hematologic: agranulocytosis, aplastic anemia, hemolytic anemia
- Skin: lupus erythematosus, photosensitivity

Interactions (other drugs)
- Amprenavir (may increase dapsone levels) ■ Didanosine (may inhibit effect of dapsone) ■ Rifampin (decreased dapsone levels) ■ Folic acid antagonists (may increase risk of hematologic reactions) ■ Trimethoprim (increased levels of both drugs) ■ Probenecid (increased dapsone levels)

Contraindications
- Hypersensitivity to dapsone ■ Pregnancy and breast-feeding

Follow up plan
Careful follow up to check for prevention of new blister formation.

PROGNOSIS

- Pemphigoid will normally go into remission with immunosuppressant treatment
- Low-dose steroid therapy may be required for years
- Pemphigoid is normally a self-limiting disease and often goes spontaneously within a few years of onset

Clinical pearls

- Steroid-sparing agents should be begun early as they typically take a month or more to begin to be effective
- Distinction from other immunobullous diseases can at times be problematic and should be made by someone (usually a dermatologist) familiar with the differential diagnosis

Therapeutic failure

- If new blister formation occurs then increasing the immunosuppression is necessary
- Increasing systemic steroid dosage or adding a steroid-sparing agent
- Referral to a dermatologist is usually mandatory

Recurrence

Frequent attempts to reduce immunosuppressants should be attempted throughout the course of treatment. These will frequently be met with recurrence. These can be managed by reverting back to previously successful treatment. Rebound worsening is not the norm with pemphigoid.

Deterioration

- If new blister formation occurs then increasing the immunosuppression is necessary
- Increasing systemic steroid dosage or adding a steroid-sparer
- Referral to a dermatologist is mandatory

COMPLICATIONS

- Secondary skin infections are common: they require antimicrobial therapy and close follow up by a dermatologist
- Systemic complications of the disease are rare

CONSIDER CONSULT

- Localized pemphigoid can be treated with topical steroids. All other pemphigoid patients need a dermatology referral

PREVENTION

- There are no preventative measures known to pemphigoid
- There are no identifiable risk factors that can be modified
- The following diseases have been associated to pemphigoid: diabetes, multiple sclerosis, pernicious anemia, rheumatoid arthritis, lichen planus, psoriasis, and vitiligo

PREVENT RECURRENCE
Reassess coexisting disease
Oral or ocular disease suggests oral or ocular cicatricial pemphigoid and will need to be watched for.

KEY REFERENCES

■ Buxton PK. ABC of dermatology – blisters and pustules. BMJ (Clin Res Ed) 1987;295:1399–402
■ Korman NJ. Bullous pemphigoid. The latest in diagnosis, prognosis, and therapy. Arch Dermatol 1998;134:1137–41
■ Joly P. Autoimmune bullous skin diseases. Rev Med Interne 1999;20:26–38

FAQS
Question 1
How quickly is a patient presenting with bullae likely to become seriously ill? How rapidly should a consultation be scheduled?

ANSWER 1
Frequently, the patient presents with a fairly rapid (a few days) onset of numerous blisters and the need for consultation is immediately apparent. The primary care physician should expect the patient to be evaluated by the dermatologist within 36h, if not immediately. Occasionally, but not rarely, the patient may present with pruritus, an eruption (classically urticarial plaques), and few to no blisters, then develop blisters over the next 48h or so. The time between presentation and decrudescence to severe illness depends on the rapidity of blister formation and the general health of the patient. Within these parameters, patients generally become seriously ill between a day or two to a week after the onset of blisters.

Question 2
Should a primary care physician obtain a routine skin biopsy in the office at presentation or wait for the dermatologic consultant to see the patient first?

ANSWER 2
The techniques required for taking and transporting biopsies for direct immunofluorescence and routine histology are different from each other and are also different from some of the other elements of the differential diagnosis. Only someone knowledgeable about these differences should perform the skin biopsies. In general, primary care physicians lack the expert training to make these distinctions and the appropriate transport media to send a specimen for immunofluorescence.

CONTRIBUTORS
Dennis F Saver, MD
Seth R Stevens, MD
Richard Averitte, MD

PEMPHIGUS

SUMMARY INFORMATION

DESCRIPTION

- Autoimmune blistering disease
- Affects patients in middle age, predominantly 40-60 years
- Oral lesions common
- Superficial bullae can occur anywhere on body
- Bullae are superficial and flaccid

URGENT ACTION

- Hospitalization and high-dose steroids are indicated for patients with widespread disease
- May be fatal if treated inadequately

KEY! DON'T MISS!

- Pemphigus vulgaris should be suspected in any bullous or chronic mucosal ulceration
- Widespread skin involvement with erosions and bullae requires urgent hospitalization and systemic treatment as morbidity and mortality are high
- Severe oral ulceration spreading past the vermilion border should raise suspicion of paraneoplastic pemphigus

ICD9 CODE
694.4 Pemphigus

SYNONYMS
- Autoimmune bullous dermatoses
- Pemphigus vulgaris

CARDINAL FEATURES
- Autoimmune blistering disease
- Affects patients in middle age, predominantly 40-60 years
- Oral lesions common
- Superficial bullae can occur anywhere on body
- Nikolsky's sign - epidermis is easily detached from underlying skin
- Bullae are superficial and flaccid
- Bullae are fragile and often rupture
- Denuded and crusted lesions occur after rupture
- Acantholysis is diagnosed on histology of skin lesions

CAUSES
Common causes
- Pemphigus is an autoimmune disease
- Caused by autoantibodies against keratinocyte proteins desmoglein-1 and desmoglein-3

Rare causes
- Penicillamine: 9% of rheumatoid arthritis patients develop pemphigus
- Captopril, rifampin, and meprobromate have been associated with pemphigus

Contributory or predisposing factors
- Pemphigus can occur in systemic lupus erythematosus and myasthenia gravis
- Certain human leukocyte antigen (HLA) types predispose: HLA DR4 and HLA A10

EPIDEMIOLOGY
Incidence and prevalence
Pemphigus is uncommon.

INCIDENCE
1/100,000 population.

FREQUENCY
9% of rheumatoid arthritis patients taking penicillamine will develop pemphigus.

Demographics
AGE
- 40-60 years
- Rare in children

GENDER
Occurs in equal numbers in men and women.

RACE
More common in Ashkenazi Jews.

GENETICS
Associated with HLA DR4 and HLA A10.

GEOGRAPHY
- Higher incidence in South America, especially Brazil
- Most common reason for admission to a skin hospital in India

DIFFERENTIAL DIAGNOSIS
Pemphigus vegetens
Clinical variant of pemphigus where a reaction to the erosions causes the repairing epidermis to hypertrophy.

FEATURES
- Granulomata formation
- Occurs in axilla, groin, and angles of mouth and nose
- Small pustules may develop around the lesions
- Steroid suppression may increase granulomata formation

Pemphigus folliaceus
Benign variant of pemphigus in which lesions occur only on the skin.

FEATURES
- Lesions occur only on the skin
- Mucous membranes are never affected
- Lesions are very superficial
- Scaling and crusting often principal feature
- Mainly face and upper trunk affected
- Localized forms may look like seborrheic warts
- Antibodies are targeted against desmoglein-1 (intercellular surfaces of epithelial cells)
- Endemic form in Brazil and Columbia (*fogo selvagem*)
- Triggered by certain drugs, including penicillamine
- Associated with systemic lupus erythematosus and myasthenia gravis
- Requires less aggressive treatment than pemphigus vulgaris

Paraneoplastic pemphigus
Occurs with occult and known neoplasms, especially B-cell lymphoproliferative disorders such as non-Hodgkin's lymphoma, chronic lymphocytic leukemia, or thymomas.

FEATURES
- Painful bullae on mucous membranes
- Generalized pleomorphic blistering
- Lichenoid skin lesions
- Autoantibodies to desmoglein-3 and desmoglein-1 and against complex proteins (plakins)
- Usually progressive disease course
- Almost always fatal within 2 years
- Internal organs can be affected: progressive respiratory failure leads to death in about 30% of cases
- No effective treatment
- Chemotherapy to underlying tumor does not influence disease activity
- Thymoma excision will resolve the disease
- Some relief may occur with steroids and cyclosporine

Bullous pemphigoid
Bullous pemphigoid is the most common blistering skin disease, being twice as common as pemphigus.

FEATURES
- Most common in elderly patients
- Typical lesions are large tense blisters on urticarial base leading to intense irritation

- Symmetrical eruption
- Affects trunk and limbs, especially over flexures
- Face and scalp are usually spared
- Chronic condition with some cases of spontaneous remission

Drug eruptions

Any drug can cause skin lesions.

FEATURES

- Common cause of blisters and other skin lesions
- Lesions have symmetrical patterns determined by vasculature
- Likely offenders include digoxin, acetaminophen, sulfonamides, penicillins
- Identifying and removing the cause will lead to resolution

Erythema multiforme

Erythema multiforme is an inflammatory skin disease, probably due to immune complex formation.

FEATURES

- Predominant age group affected is 20-40 years
- Immune complexes deposit in the skin and mucous membranes leading to lesion formation
- Symmetrical skin lesions with a classic 'target' appearance
- Lesions most common on dorsum of hands and feet and extensor areas of limbs
- Rarely involves trunk
- Urticarial papules, vesicles and bullae are rare and indicate serious disease
- Lesions heal within 2 weeks without scarring
- Bullae and erosions may be present in oral cavity

Dermatitis herpetiformis

Dermatitis herpetiformis is associated with gluten intolerance.

FEATURES

- Irritative grouped vesicles
- Present especially on elbows, knees, and buttocks
- Numerous excoriations with blister crustation
- Histology reveals small subepidermal blisters
- Direct immunofluorescence reveals granular deposits of immunoglobulin A (IgA) in dermal papillae
- Responds dramatically to treatment with dapsone
- Patients should follow a gluten-free diet

Behçet's syndrome

Behçet's syndrome is an inflammatory disorder characterized by the presence of oral aphthous ulcers, genital ulcers, uveitis, and skin lesions.

FEATURES

- Affects adults typically between 30-40 years
- Initially presents with painful aphthous ulcers, 2-10mm diameter
- Genital ulcers are similar to oral ulcers
- Skin lesions include papules, vesicles and erythema nodosum
- Constitutional features include headaches, fevers, and neck stiffness
- Vasculitis can lead to signs of myocardial infarction, deep vein thrombosis, intermittent claudication, aneurysm formation, and hemoptysis
- Unknown etiology and no specific diagnostic tests

Herpes gestationis
Variant of pemphigoid, also known as gestational pemphigoid.

FEATURES
- Presents in second or third trimester
- Resolves on delivery
- Immunologically identical to bullous pemphigoid

SIGNS & SYMPTOMS
Signs
- Skin or mucosae can just shear off leaving widespread painful erosions
- Nikolsky's sign - epidermis is easily detached from underlying skin
- Flaccid bullae of various sizes
- Bullae arise from 'healthy' skin, rupture and leave crusting and denuded skin
- Any area of stratified epithelium can be affected
- Lesions appear first in the mouth prior to skin involvement
- Extent of skin and mucosal involvement varies
- Eyes, nasal mucosa, and genitalia may be affected
- Lesions may occur in oropharynx and upper esophagus
- Pyrexia and systemic features common
- Secondary infection is common

Symptoms
- Painful blisters in the mouth appear first, and may lead to weight loss
- Blisters occur on the skin and mucosal areas, especially where trauma and pressure applied
- Large areas of affected skin seep and crustation occurs
- Fever and malaise
- Pruritus normally absent

KEY! DON'T MISS!
- Pemphigus vulgaris should be suspected in any bullous or chronic mucosal ulceration
- Widespread skin involvement with erosions and bullae requires urgent hospitalization and systemic treatment as morbidity and mortality are high
- Severe oral ulceration spreading past the vermilion border should raise suspicion of paraneoplastic pemphigus

CONSIDER CONSULT
- All suspected cases of pemphigus should be referred to a dermatologist for confirmation of diagnosis

INVESTIGATION OF THE PATIENT
Direct questions to patient
Q **Have you noticed blisters in your mouth?** Usually oral lesions precede the skin lesions.

Q **Are the blisters painful?** Blisters are usually very painful.

Q **Do the blisters seep and leave the skin exposed?** Blisters are fragile, leaving the skin denuded.

Q **Do you feel generally unwell?** Constitutional symptoms and secondary infections are common.

Q **How long have you had these skin blisters?** Pemphigus is a chronic disease but patients usually present early due to pain.

Q **Where are the skin blisters?** Can be anywhere on the body including oropharynx, eyes, genitalia, and anus.

Contributory or predisposing factors

Q Have you been diagnosed with any of the following diseases? Systemic lupus erythematosus, thymoma, non-Hodgkin's lymphoma, carcinoma - all are associated with pemphigus.

Q Are you taking penicillamine for rheumatoid arthritis? 9% of these patients develop pemphigus.

Family history

Q Are there members of your family who have these skin lesions? Pemphigus vulgaris is associated with HLA DR4 and A10.

Examination

- Examine the oral cavity: lesions first arise in the mouth and may stay localized to the oral cavity for months to years before skin lesions appear
- Examine all mucosa membranes: including the pharynx, larynx, nasal mucosa, genitalia, anus; all are susceptible to pemphigus
- Check for Nikolsky's sign: the epidermis at the side of a blister is easily detached from the underlying skin by firm sliding pressure with a finger
- Look for constitutional signs such as pyrexia: common with pemphigus vulgaris
- Look for secondary skin infections: common with pemphigus vulgaris

Summary of investigative tests

- Skin biopsy of a lesion can be diagnostic for pemphigus as it will show acantholysis and intraepidermal separation of keratinocytes
- Direct immunofluorescence of the perilesional skin detects antibody deposition in the intercellular spaces of keratinocytes
- Serology (indirect immunofluorescence) can be diagnostic as it identifies pemphigus antibodies - desmoglein 1 and 3 - in serum
- The Tzanck test indicates the presence of acantholysis, although it has no diagnostic value as it is not specific for pemphigus; however, it can diagnose herpes simplex virus infection, another cause of oral ulceration
- Complete blood count has no diagnostic value, but may be useful to monitor drug side effects

DIAGNOSTIC DECISION

A patient with oral and cutaneous bullae and erosions, plus a skin biopsy that shows acantholysis and intraepidermal separation of keratinocytes, is likely to have pemphigus vulgaris. Diagnosis is confirmed by direct or indirect immunofluorescence.

CLINICAL PEARLS

Most PCPs will see few cases of pemphigus vulgaris and may never see a case of such important variants as paraneoplastic pemphigus. Therefore, most patients with suspected pemphigus vulgaris should be evaluated by a dermatologist or, if available, an Immunodermatologist.

THE TESTS
Body fluids
COMPLETE BLOOD COUNT
Description
Sample of venous blood.

Advantages/Disadvantages
Advantages:
- Quick and easy to perform
- Inexpensive
- Allows monitoring of drug side effects

Disadvantage: Not diagnostic for pemphigus

Normal
White blood cell (WBC) count 3200-9800/mm³.

Abnormal
- Raised WBC count >9800/mm³
- Reduced WBC count <3000/mm³

Cause of abnormal result
- Raised WBC count may indicate secondary skin infection leading to constitutional signs
- Reduced WBC count may indicate leukocytosis resulting from treatment with systemic steroids, azathioprine, or cyclophosphamide therapy

Drugs, disorders and other factors that may alter results
Laboratory technique may affect results.

SEROLOGY (INDIRECT IMMUNOFLUORESCENCE)
Description
- Sample of venous blood
- Monkey esophagus (as substrate) is incubated with patient's serum. If circulating antikeratinocyte antibodies are present, they bind to the epidermis of the monkey esophagus. These tissue-bound antibodies are detected by fluorescein-labeled antihuman antibodies

Advantages/Disadvantages
Advantages:
- Easy to access venous blood
- Diagnostic for pemphigus if antikeratinocyte (desmoglein 1 and 3) antibodies are detected
- Antibody titer may correlate with disease severity
- Positive in more than 90% patients with active disease
- Positive even with local lesions in the oral cavity

Disadvantages:
- Expensive
- Requires laboratory analysis

Normal
Undetectable pemphigus antibodies.

Abnormal
- Antikeratinocyte antibodies are detected on monkey esophagus or human skin (the intercellular space shows antibody binding)
- Similar findings can be present in patients with other pemphigus variants (paraneoplastic, or foliaceus); therefore, patient care is optimized by close collaboration of a knowledgeable clinician and the immunopathologist

Cause of abnormal result
Circulating antikeratinocyte (desmoglein 1 and 3) antibodies are present in patient's serum. Desmoplakin antibodies in paraneoplastic pemphigus serum can also yield similar fluorescence patterns.

Drugs, disorders and other factors that may alter results
Laboratory technique may affect results.

Biopsy
SKIN BIOPSY
Description
- Early skin lesion is removed
- Skin sample is stained with hematoxylin and eosin and examined by direct microscopy

Advantages/Disadvantages
Advantages:
- Skin readily accessible
- Easy to perform
- Does not require specialized laboratory

Disadvantage: Not diagnostic of pemphigus, but provides useful information towards diagnosis

Abnormal
- Intraepidermal separation of keratinocytes, forming a split between lower and upper portions of epidermis
- Acantholysis - separation of individual epidermal cells from surrounding cells
- Mild or absent inflammatory infiltrate

Cause of abnormal result
Pemphigus - autoimmune reaction separates epidermal cells from each other.

Drugs, disorders and other factors that may alter results
Biopsy and histologic technique can affect results.

DIRECT IMMUNOFLUORESCENCE
Description
Sample of perilesional skin is removed and incubated with fluorescein-labeled antihuman anti-Ig or anticomplement antibodies to detect tissue-bound antibodies or complement.

Advantages/Disadvantages
Advantages:
- Easy to access perilesional skin
- Highly diagnostic of pemphigus

Disadvantages:
- Specialized laboratory required
- Expensive

Normal
Antibodies are not detected in the skin.

Abnormal
- Direct detection of tissue-bound antikeratinocyte (desmoglein) antibodies on perilesional skin of the patient
- Antihuman IgG and C3 binding detected at epidermal cell surfaces; no deposition along basement membrane

Cause of abnormal result
Pemphigus vulgaris. Other pemphigus variants can yield a positive test (see indirect immunofluorescence, above).

Drugs, disorders and other factors that may alter results
Biopsy and laboratory technique can affect results.

TZANCK TEST
Description
Scraping from the base of a skin lesion is stained with Wright's or Giemsa stain.

Advantages/Disadvantages
Advantages:
- Noninvasive
- Easy to access skin sample
- Relatively inexpensive
- May yield specimen diagnostic for herpes virus infection, another cause of blistering

Disadvantage: Not diagnostic of pemphigus as other skin diseases with acantholysis can also give positive result

Abnormal
Acantholytic cells detected.

Cause of abnormal result
- Pemphigus vulgaris
- Other bullous skin diseases

Drugs, disorders and other factors that may alter results
Sampling and laboratory technique can affect results.

TREATMENT

CONSIDER CONSULT

- Patients with widespread disease should be referred to hospital for treatment
- Localized oral disease should be kept under close observation and referral made if the disease spreads

IMMEDIATE ACTION

- Patients with widespread disease should be referred for hospitalization and immediate treatment, as morbidity and mortality are high
- If secondary skin infection is suspected, immediate antimicrobial treatment should be commenced
- Fluid and electrolyte normalization should be achieved

PATIENT AND CAREGIVER ISSUES

Patient or caregiver request

- **Will steroids make me gain weight?** Steroids are likely to cause weight gain; dietary advice is needed
- **What are the side effects of steroids?** Careful counseling concerning steroid use and side effects will be needed to attain optimal compliance
- **Is this disease infectious?** Information concerning the cause of the disease is needed to prevent patients feeling ostracized
- **Will the skin lesions cause scarring?** Full information concerning treatment and compliance will minimize scarring
- **Will I get better?** Disease is chronic but resolution may occur and good treatment and follow up is imperative

Health-seeking behavior

- **Has the patient tried over-the-counter products?** Common for patients to attempt to treat themselves prior to seeking medical advice
- **Has the patient tried alternative treatments?** There is much misinformation concerning skin diseases and some 'remedies' can have deleterious effects, such as drastic dietary manipulation leading to malnutrition

MANAGEMENT ISSUES
Goals

- Prevent new lesions forming
- Prevent scarring
- Prevent secondary infections
- Minimize effects of disease on patient's lifestyle

Management in special circumstances
COEXISTING DISEASE

If there is coexisting disease, e.g. thymoma, carcinoma or non-Hodgkin's lymphoma, specialist opinions should be sought for their treatment. The presence of lymphoproliferative disorder should heighten suspicion of paraneoplastic pemphigus.

COEXISTING MEDICATION

Certain medications can cause pemphigus and should be stopped immediately; most likely is penicillamine for rheumatoid arthritis.

SUMMARY OF THERAPEUTIC OPTIONS
Choices

- Aim of treatment is to prevent eruption of new lesions
- Specific therapy depends on the extent and severity of the disease
- Corticosteroids: topical steroids such as triamcinolone can be used in mild disease but most patients require systemic steroids, which have adverse effects
- Nonalkylating agents (e.g. azathioprine, mycophenolic acid, cyclosporine) are steroid-sparing agents and are important in chronic disease
- Alkylating agents (e.g. cyclophosphamide, chlorambucil) are steroid-sparing agents and are important in chronic disease
- Antibiotics (e.g. tetracycline) have been used in pemphigus, usually in combination with other agents
- Local antiseptics and analgesics can give symptomatic relief
- Anti-inflammatory drugs, such as gold or dapsone, are disease-modifying drugs for severe cases of pemphigus vulgaris
- Other therapies include plasmapheresis, an inpatient procedure performed by a specialist. It is used only for refractory cases and results are variable
- Dietary modification may benefit patients with oral lesions
- Among immunodermatologists, the choice of steroid-sparing agent usually depends upon their training and personal experiences. There have been no head-to-head randomized trials to address preferred treatment protocols in the use of steroid-sparing agents

Clinical pearls

- One should anticipate long-term immunosuppression in pemphigus vulgaris patients, therefore, osteoporosis prophylaxis should be started early. Steroid-sparing agents should also be considered at the time of initial diagnosis. Appropriate laboratory evaluation to define risks of adverse drug reaction (e.g. glucose-6-phosphate dehydrogenase for dapsone and thiopurine methyl transferase for azathioprine) should be obtained early
- Whereas systemic steroids usually control disease in a few days, if used in adequate doses, steroid-sparing agents often take 4-6 weeks to become effective. Therefore, adequate overlap of therapy with both agents will be required before attempting to taper corticosteroids

Never

Never ignore hip or gastrointestinal pain, mood changes, tinnitus in a patient taking systemic steroids.

FOLLOW UP

- Pemphigus vulgaris is a serious disease with an inconsistent and unpredictable response to therapy, a prolonged course, and virtually inevitable complicating drug side effects
- Careful follow up is mandatory
- Pemphigus is fatal if inadequately treated

Plan for review

- Severe disease requires hospitalization with daily review
- Outpatients should be reviewed regularly to check on treatment response and adverse drug reactions
- Pemphigus is a chronic disease and requires careful follow up even when the treatment regimen is successful
- Steroid reduction to the minimal dose is needed to minimize side effects

Information for patient or caregiver

- Patients should be informed that a prolonged treatment course is required
- Compliance is important and motivation should be optimized
- Patients need time and much support to help them through this potentially serious disease
- Extensive discussion of potential adverse effects of therapies is required, balanced with the recognition that prior to the advent of corticosteroids, pemphigus vulgaris was usually fatal

DRUGS AND OTHER THERAPIES: DETAILS
Drugs
TRIAMCINOLONE

- Useful for minor disease with few lesions
- Rarely controls the disease, except in pemphigus foliaceus

Dose
Apply once or twice daily to the affected areas.

Efficacy
Topical corticosteroid treatment has very limited value in pemphigus vulgaris. It is effective only in pemphigus foliaceus.

Risks/benefits
Risks:

- Does not provide quick response; may take several hours for relief
- Risk of infection with intra-articular injection
- Use caution with glomerulonephritis, ulcerative colitis, renal disease
- Use caution with AIDS, tuberculosis, ocular herpes simplex, live vaccines, viral and bacterial infections
- Use caution in diabetes mellitus, glaucoma, osteoporosis, hypertension
- Use caution in children and the elderly
- Use caution in recent myocardial infarction
- Use caution in psychosis
- Do not withdraw abruptly

Benefits:

- Reduction in skin lesions
- Fewer side effects compared with systemic steroids

Side effects and adverse reactions

- Side effects are minimized by short duration of therapy
- Cardiovascular system: hypertension, thromboembolism
- Central nervous system: insomnia, euphoria, depression, psychosis, seizures
- Endocrine: adrenal suppression, impaired glucose tolerance, growth suppression in children
- Eyes, ears, nose, and throat: cataract, glaucoma, blurred vision
- Gastrointestinal: dyspepsia, peptic ulceration, esophagitis, oral candidiasis, nausea, vomiting
- Musculoskeletal: proximal myopathy, osteoporosis
- Skin: delayed healing, acne, striae, transient atrophy at injection site

Interactions (other drugs)

- Aminoglutethimide ▪ Antidiabetics ▪ Barbiturates ▪ Carbamazepine ▪ Cholestyramine
- Cholinesterase inhibitors ▪ Cyclosporine ▪ Diuretics ▪ Estrogens ▪ Isoniazid
- Isoproterenal ▪ Nonsteroidal anti-inflammatory drugs (NSAIDs) ▪ Phenytoin ▪ Rifampin
- Salicylates

Contraindications
- Local or systemic infection ▪ Peptic ulcer ▪ Pregnancy and breast-feeding

Acceptability to patient
- Patients may be reluctant to use steroid cream because of side effects
- Compliance needs to be monitored

Follow up plan
Careful follow up is needed to check that pemphigus is not deteriorating.

Patient and caregiver information
- Patients must be told to report new lesions
- Compliance is important to reduce lesions
- Side effects of steroid cream must be discussed with patients

SYSTEMIC STEROIDS
- Mainstay of treatment for pemphigus
- High doses are needed to suppress the disease
- Dose depends on activity of the disease
- Aim is to gain control of the disease and then reduce dose to the minimum to reduce side effects
- All details in this section relate to prednisone

Dose
- Prednisone: initial dose is 1mg/kg/day
- Dose should be tapered to 5-10mg on alternate days within 9-12 months

Efficacy
- Systemic steroids form the basis of treatment and are extremely effective
- Prior to steroids, 75% of patients with pemphigus vulgaris died

Risks/benefits
Risks:
- Use caution in congestive heart failure, renal disease
- Use caution in diabetes mellitus, glaucoma, ulcerative colitis, peptic ulcer
- Use caution in the elderly
- Prednisone taken in doses higher than 7.5mg for a period of 3 weeks or longer may lead to clinically relevant suppression of the pituitary-adrenal axis

Benefit: Prevention of morbidity and mortality of pemphigus

Side effects and adverse reactions
- Side effects are minimized by short duration of therapy
- Cardiovascular system: hypertension, thromboembolism
- Central nervous system: insomnia, euphoria, depression, psychosis, seizures
- Endocrine: adrenal suppression, impaired glucose tolerance, growth suppression in children
- Eyes, ears, nose, and throat: cataract, glaucoma, blurred vision
- Gastrointestinal: dyspepsia, peptic ulceration, esophagitis, oral candidiasis
- Musculoskeletal: proximal myopathy, osteoporosis
- Skin: delayed healing, acne, striae, fragile skin

Interactions (other drugs)

Prednisone:

■ Aminoglutethimide (increased clearance of prednisone) ■ Antidiabetics (hypoglycemic effect inhibited) ■ Antihypertensives (effects inhibited) ■ Barbiturates (increased clearance of prednisone) ■ Cardiac glycosides (toxicity increased) ■ Cholestyramine, colestipol (my reduce absorption of corticosteroids) ■ Clarithromycin, erythromycin, troleandomycin (may enhance steroid effect) ■ Cyclosporine (may increase levels of both drugs; may cause seizures) ■ Diuretics (effects inhibited) ■ Isoniazid (reduced plasma levels of isoniazid) ■ Ketoconazole ■ NSAIDs (increased risks of bleeeding) ■ Oral contraceptives (enhanced effects of corticosteroids) ■ Rifampin (may inhibit hepatic clearance of prednisone) ■ Salicylates (increased clearance of salicylates) ■ Warfarin (alters clotting time)

Contraindications

Prednisone:

■ Systemic infection ■ Avoid live virus vaccines in those receiving immunosuppressive doses ■ History of tuberculosis ■ Cushing's syndrome ■ Recent myocardial infarction

Acceptability to patient

■ Systemic steroids have numerous well publicized side effects
■ Compliance with high doses of steroids can be poor
■ Antiosteoporotic medication should be coadministered with steroids
■ Information on potential effects of the disease is important to keep patients motivated

Follow up plan

■ Careful follow up is required to monitor the patient while on steroids
■ Once the disease is under control, dose should be tapered to the minimum needed to keep the disease in remission
■ If a dose of 5-10mg on alternate days cannot be achieved within 9-12 months, combination therapy is indicated. Many experts begin combination therapy earlier in order to minimize steroid use

Patient and caregiver information

■ The patient must be given information concerning steroid side effects
■ A steroid card containing information about the effects of steroids is needed

AZATHIOPRINE

■ Immunosuppressive by inhibiting purine synthesis in cells
■ Used concomitantly with steroids for chronic disease
■ Used as a steroid-sparing medication
■ Careful monitoring of complete blood count (CBC) is needed due to bone marrow suppression

Dose

■ 3-5mg/kg/day, decrease according to response
■ Maintenance dose is 1-3mg/kg/day

Efficacy

Effective in conjunction with systemic steroids.

Risks/benefits

Risks:

■ Use caution with bone marrow suppression and infection
■ Use caution in renal or hepatic impairment
■ Severe blood cell disorders may occur
■ May increase risk of neoplasia

Benefit: Allows reduction of systemic steroid dose

Side effects and adverse reactions
- Gastrointestinal: nausea, vomiting, diarrhea, abdominal pain, hepatic failure, jaundice
- Genitourinary: depression of spermatogenesis
- Hematologic: anemia, leukopenia, pancytopenia, thrombocytopenia
- Musculoskeletal: arthralgia, myalgia, malaise
- Skin: rash, alopecia
- Miscellaneous: fungal, bacterial, protozoal and viral infections, may increase risk of neoplasm (skin cancer, reticulocyte or lymphomatous tumors)

Interactions (other drugs)
- Angiotensin-converting enzyme (ACE) inhibitors ▪ Allopurinol ▪ Anticoagulants
- Carbamazepine ▪ Clozapine ▪ Co-trimoxazole (TMP-SMX) ▪ Cyclosporine
- Methotrexate ▪ Nondepolarising muscle blockers ▪ Vaccines ▪ Warfarin

Contraindications
- Intramuscular injections ▪ Pregnancy or breast-feeding ▪ Vaccines

Acceptability to patient
Side effects are serious, but most patients will accept treatment to control pemphigus.

Follow up plan
- Careful follow up required, with monthly CBC
- Discontinue if leukocytes <3000/mm^3 (<3.0x10^9/L)

Patient and caregiver information
Compliance with blood tests and medication is important to control disease with minimal side effects.

CYCLOPHOSPHAMIDE
- Active metabolites alkylate DNA and RNA, causing immunosuppression
- Activity is not linked to cell cycle
- Steroid-sparing medication

Dose
1-5mg/kg orally, proportional to disease activity.

Efficacy
- One of the most effective drugs used to control pemphigus
- Used only in severe and refractory cases

Risks/benefits
Risks:
- Use caution with radiation therapy
- The risks of bone marrow suppression and hepatotoxicity must be weighed against the limited evidence for real therapeutic benefit in established renal involvement in Henoch-Schönlein purpura

Benefit: One of the most effective drugs used to control pemphigus vulgaris and to reduce systemic steroid use and complications

Side effects and adverse reactions
- Cardiovascular system: cardiotoxicity (at high doses)
- Central nervous system: dizziness, headache
- Gastrointestinal: nausea, vomiting, diarrhea
- Genitourinary: amenorrhea, azoospermia, ovarian fibrosis, sterility, hematuria, hemorrhagic cystitis, neoplasms
- Hematologic: leukopenia, myelosuppression, panycytopenia, thrombocytopenia
- Metabolic: bone marrow supression
- Respiratory: fibrosis
- Skin: alopecia, dermatitis

Interactions (other drugs)
- Allopurinol (increased cyclophosphamide toxicity) ■ Clozapine (may cause agranulocytosis) ■ Digoxin (decreased digoxin absorption from tablet form) ■ Pentostatin (increased toxicity with high-dose cyclophosphamide) ■ Phenytoin (reduced absorption of phenytoin) ■ Succinylcholine (prolonged neuromuscular blockade) ■ Suxemethonium (enhanced effect of suxemethonium) ■ Warfarin (inhibits hypoprothrombinemic response to warfarin)

Contraindications
- Serious infections, including chicken pox and herpes zoster ■ Myelosuppression

Acceptability to patient
Patients may find side effects difficult to tolerate, but most will accept treatment as necessary to control severe disease.

Follow up plan
- CBC weekly
- Discontinue if white blood cell count <4000/mm^3 (<4.0x10^9/L) or platelet count <75x10^3/mm^3 (<75x10^9/L)

Patient and caregiver information
Compliance with blood tests, medication, and proper hydration are important.

TETRACYCLINE
Antibiotic that may help to control pemphigus disease activity.

Dose
Adult dose: 250-500mg four times daily.

Efficacy
- Effective medication for pemphigus
- Can be given in combination with nicotinamide

Risks/benefits
Risk:
- Compliance can be a problem
- Use caution in patients with hepatic impairment
- Use caution with repeated or prolonged doses

Benefits:
- Few side effects and good drug profile
- Can be given long-term

Side effects and adverse reactions
- Cardiovascular system: pericarditis
- Central nervous system: headache, paresthesia, fever
- Gastrointestinal: abdominal pain, diarrhea, heartburn, hepatotoxicity, vomiting, nausea, dental staining, anorexia
- Genitourinary: polyuria, polydipsia, azotemia
- Hematologic: blood cell dyscrasias
- Skin: pruritus, rash, photosensitivity, changes in pigmentation, angioedema, stinging

Interactions (other drugs)
- Antacids ■ Atovaquone ■ Barbiturates ■ Bismuth subsalicyclate ■ Calcium, iron, magnesium, zinc ■ Cephalosporins ■ Cholesytramine, colestipol ■ Carbamazepine ■ Digoxin ■ Ethanol ■ Methoxyflurane ■ Oral contraceptives ■ Penicillins ■ Phenytoin ■ Quinapril ■ Sodium bicarbonate ■ Vitamin A ■ Warfarin

Contraindications
- Pregnancy ■ Nursing mothers ■ Children <8 years ■ Severe renal disease

Acceptability to patient
Generally acceptable.

Follow up plan
- Review to check drug effectiveness
- Steroids may need to be added to regimen

DAPSONE
- Competitive antagonist of para-aminobenzoic acid (PABA)
- Steroid-sparing agent

Dose
Adult oral dose: 25-100mg/day.

Efficacy
Effective steroid-sparing medication.

Risks/benefits
Risks:
- Use caution in renal and hepatic impairment
- Use caution with glucose-6-phosphate dehydrogenase deficiency
- Fatal agranulocytosis, aplastic anemia, and other blood dyscrasias reported
- CBCs should be performed frequently

Benefit: Steroid-sparing

Side effects and adverse reactions
- Central nervous system: headache, insomnia, paresthesia, peripheral neuropathy, psychosis, vertigo
- Eyes, ears, nose, and throat: blurred vision, optic neuritis, photophobia, tinnitus
- Gastrointestinal: abdominal pain, anorexia, nausea, vomiting
- Genitourinary: nephrotic syndrome, renal papillary necrosis, proteinuria
- Hematologic: agranulocytosis, aplastic anemia, hemolytic anemia
- Skin: lupus erythematosis, photosensitivity

Interactions (other drugs)
- Amprenavir (may increase dapsone levels) ■ Didanosine (may inhibit effect of dapsone)
- Rifampin (decreased dapsone levels) ■ Folic acid antagonists (may increase risk of hematologic reactions) ■ Trimethoprim (increased levels of both drugs) ■ Probenecid (increased dapsone levels)

Contraindications
- Hypersensitivity to dapsone ■ Pregnancy and breast-feeding

Acceptability to patient
Used only for severe cases of pemphigus vulgaris; patients are generally willing to accept all treatments offered.

Follow up plan
- Careful follow up of patient with weekly CBC for one month, then once monthly for 6 months, then twice yearly
- Periodic liver function tests are required

Patient and caregiver information
Compliance with blood tests and medication is important.

LIFESTYLE
- Soft diet for patients with oral lesions may be beneficial
- Low osmosis fluids may help reduce exudation from skin lesions

EFFICACY OF THERAPIES

In the era before corticosteroid therapy, the vast majority of patients died from the disease. Mortality has reduced to <10% due to significant improvement in therapy over the past decades. Many of the deaths associated with pemphigus are now iatrogenic in nature.

Review period

Monthly review of disease response, laboratory evaluations, and medication modifications are required. Active management is required to minimize risk/benefit ratios.

PROGNOSIS

- If untreated, death occurs approx. 2 years after the first lesions appear
- Combined use of steroids and steroid-sparing medications has reduced mortality to <10%
- Pemphigus vulgaris patients usually die from sepsis or complications from therapy

Clinical pearls

Watch patients with pemphigus carefully or refer to a specialist.

Therapeutic failure

- Pemphigus refractory to treatment regimens requires expert opinion
- Plasmapheresis may be indicated

Recurrence

- Systemic steroids are required to gain control and reduce further lesions
- Dose should be increased until control is gained and then gradually tapered

Deterioration

- Referral for expert opinion is needed
- Plasmapheresis may be indicated

COMPLICATIONS

- Secondary skin infection is common
- Complications from steroid and steroid-sparing medications are common

CONSIDER CONSULT

- All patients with pemphigus vulgaris must be referred for treatment due to the high morbidity and mortality associated with this disease. Treatment regimens are complicated and require close observation of the patient's disease and blood counts

PREVENTION

Remove known causes of pemphigus, including penicillamine. Otherwise, there is little that affects the pathogenesis of this disease.

PREVENT RECURRENCE

- Correct compliance with treatment regimen
- Careful follow up of patient's disease status

ASSOCIATIONS
American Academy of Dermatology
930 N Meacham Road
PO Box 4014
Schaumburg, IL 60168-4014
Tel: (847) 330-0230
Fax: (847) 330-0050
www.aad.org

KEY REFERENCES
- Bean SF. Diagnosis and management of chronic oral mucosal bullous diseases. Derm Clin 1987;5:751-60
- Burns T. Recognizing blisters: causes and treatment. Practitioner 2000;244:850-62
- Collier, et al. Blistering diseases. Medicine 1997;25:51-5
- Hope, et al. Oxford handbook of clinical specialties. 4th edn. New York: Oxford University Press, 1995
- Joly P. Autoimmune bullous skin disorders. Rev Med Intern 1999;20:26-8
- Merck manual of diagnosis and therapy centennial edition 2000. Available from the Merck homepage
- Younger IR, Harris DW, Colver GB, et al. Azathioprine in dermatology. J Am Acad Dermatol 1991;25:281-6

FAQS
Question 1
How do I find a qualified expert to assist in the treatment of my patient with pemphigus?

ANSWER 1
Most academic centers will have an immunodermatologist who can assist with the care of these patients. The American Board of Dermatology certifies immunodermatologists and may be able to provide assistance.

CONTRIBUTORS
Fred F Ferri, MD, FACP
Seth R Stevens, MD
Rolland P Gyulai, MD, PhD

PHOTODERMATITIS

DESCRIPTION

- Painful or pruritic erythema, edema, or vesiculation on the surface of the skin that is induced by normal exposure to ultraviolet (UV) light
- Polymorphous light eruptions are the second most common light-induced skin disorder (after sunburn) seen by the primary care physician
- Phototoxic reactions are nonimmunologic cutaneous responses resulting from the effects of UV light in association with a photosensitizing substance
- Photoallergic reactions are immunologic cutaneous responses resulting from the combined effects of UV light and a photosensitizing substance
- Phytophotodermatitis refers to skin eruptions induced by the combination of exposure to sunlight and to plants that contain light-sensitizing compounds

URGENT ACTION

No specific measures necessary. Sun avoidance may be instituted until a diagnosis can be confirmed. The possibility of lupus erythematosus should be considered if systemic signs and symptoms are present in the context of photosensitivity, and appropriate action should be taken.

BACKGROUND

ICD9 CODE
- 692.79 Due to solar radiation
- 692.89 Due to other specified agents (some photodermatoses are exacerbated by light sources with high UV output, such as photocopiers and arc-welding machines)

SYNONYMS
Sun poisoning.

CARDINAL FEATURES
Polymorphous light eruption:
- After sunburn, this is the most common type of photosensitivity disease seen by the primary physician
- Usually occurs in spring or summer (after first exposure to significant light, but usually NOT with significant exposures afterward during the same season)
- Often transient (2 or 3 days), manifests with initial sun exposure in the spring, then subsides spontaneously with continued exposure (hardening)
- The most common initial symptoms are burning, itching, and erythema, which typically occur within 2h of sun exposure
- Sun-exposed surfaces, e.g. the face, the nape of the neck, the tips of the ears, the 'V' of the chest, the back of the hands, and the forearms, are the areas most frequently involved
- Involvement can spread to nonexposed areas
- Women are affected more often than men

Phototoxic reactions:
- Nonimmunologic cutaneous responses resulting from effects of UV light in association with a photosensitizing substance, e.g. certain drugs, topical agents, or plants
- Systemic route of exposure is most common
- Occurs after a first exposure
- Reactions usually occur between 1h and 24h (can be up to 72h until maximal severity) after exposure
- Typical clinical manifestations include erythema resembling sunburn, limited to areas exposed to sunlight
- Usually reactions quickly desquamate within several days
- Drug-related phototoxic reactions are dose-related
- Postinflammatory dyspigmentation may persist for one year or more

Photoallergic reactions:
- Immunologic (delayed type IV hypersensitivity) cutaneous responses resulting from effects of UV light in association with a photosensitizing substance, e.g. certain drugs or topical agents
- Less common than phototoxic reactions
- Topical route of exposure is most common
- No response with first sensitizing exposure
- Reactions typically occur with a delay of 24–48h after exposure
- Reactions can spread to areas that have not been exposed to sun
- Eruptions are usually pruritic and eczematous, consisting of papules with erythema and occasionally vesicles
- Drug-related photoallergic reactions are not dose-related
- On rare occasions, the reaction can persist for years when exposed to sunlight, even in the absence of additional drug exposure (persistent light reaction)

Phytophotodermatitis:

- Induced by a combination of exposure to plants that contain light-sensitizing compounds, e.g. furanocoumarins (psoralens), and UV light
- Distribution of reaction is sharply limited to areas of sun exposure
- May take on unique clinical forms, e.g. criss-cross linear streaks of erythema, vesicles, and bullae associated with meadow grass

CAUSES
Common causes

- Sunlight
- Drugs, including chlorothiazides, retinoids, quinolones, psoralens, tetracyclines, amiodarone, sulfonamides, sulfonylureas, furosemide, tricyclic antidepressants, vinblastine, some nonsteroidal anti-inflammatory drugs (NSAIDs)(piroxicam, naproxen), oral contraceptives
- Dyes, including anthraquinone, eosin, methylene blue, rose bengal
- Topical agents, including coal tar derivatives, antifungals, fragrances, sunscreens (PABA, cinnamates, benzophenones)
- Plants containing psoralen compounds (e.g. celery, gas plant, meadow grass, parsnip, lime, cow parsley, carrot, and fig) can produce phytophotodermatitis. This can occur systemically if ingested in sufficient quantity or locally at sites exposed to both the photosensitizing plant product and to sunlight

Rare causes

- Erythropoietic protoporphyria: a rare childhood disorder
- Pellagra: not commonly seen in the US

Serious causes

- Lupus erythematosus
- Porphyria cutanea tarda
- Variegate porphyria

Contributory or predisposing factors

Those who frequently use multiple topical or systemic prescriptions or over-the-counter drugs, herbal remedies, or many different cosmetic products may increase their risk of encountering a photosensitizing compound. One commonly encountered occupational phytophotodermatitis occurs in outdoor bartenders exposed to lime juice and sun.

EPIDEMIOLOGY
Incidence and prevalence
INCIDENCE

Unknown: incidence is dependent upon a number of factors, including the season, latitude, thickness of the ozone layer, and topographic features of the area.

PREVALENCE

The reported prevalence of polymorphous light eruption ranges between 10 and 20% depending on geographic location, with higher rates in temperate climates. Populations with increased risk are various Native American groups from both North and South America.

Demographics

AGE

- Photosensitization can occur at all ages
- Polymorphous light eruption often has its onset in the first three decades, except in Native Americans in whom it frequently presents in childhood
- Elderly people are more likely to experience adverse reactions to causative drugs

GENDER

Polymorphous light eruptions are more common in women than men.

RACE

Hereditary polymorphous light eruption occurs in the Inuit of North America and in Native Americans of North, Central, and South America.

GENETICS

Inbred populations, e.g. Pima Indians, are predisposed to photosensitive reactions.

GEOGRAPHY

Latitude, the thickness of the ozone layer, and the topographic features of the area affect risk.

DIAGNOSIS

DIFFERENTIAL DIAGNOSIS
Systemic lupus erythematosus (SLE)
Systemic lupus erythematosus is an inflammatory autoimmune disorder that may affect multiple organ systems.

FEATURES
- SLE plaque-like lesions and histology may be identical to polymorphous light eruption
- Occurs predominantly in women
- The malar (butterfly) rash is a fixed erythematous rash, flat or raised, over the cheeks and bridge of the nose
- Rash is photosensitive
- A more diffuse maculopapular rash is also common in sun-exposed areas and usually indicates disease flare
- Joint symptoms in 90% of patients
- A positive antinuclear antibody test supports the diagnosis; antibodies to double-stranded DNA and to Sm are relatively specific for SLE; antibodies to Ro/SS-a are common in photosensitive LE patients and may be the only positive serologic test in patients with subacute cutaneous LE (formerly termed ANA-negative LE)
- May have other associated features of LE, such as discoid lesions, oral ulcerations, hematologic, renal, or neurologic abnormalities

Porphyria cutanea tarda
Porphyria cutanea tarda is the most common type of porphyria.

FEATURES
- Defect in uroporphyrinogen decarboxylase
- Manifests clinically (in order of frequency) as blistering in sun-exposed areas, crusting, erosions, increased skin fragility, facial hypertrichosis, hyperpigmentation, scleroderma-like induration, and dystrophic calcification with ulceration
- May be associated with hepatitis C virus infection
- May be brought to clinical attention after ingestion of drugs such as NSAIDs or ethanol
- Biochemical confirmation of the diagnosis can be obtained by measurement of urinary uroporphyrins and coproporphyrins. Uroporphyrins are elevated 2- to 5-fold above coproporphyrins

Variegate porphyria
Variegate porphyria is a hepatic porphyria resulting from deficient activity of protoporphyrinogen oxidase.

FEATURES
- Can present with neurologic symptoms, photosensitivity similar to porphyria cutanea tarda, or both
- When variegate porphyria is symptomatic, fecal protoporphyrin and coproporphyrin and urinary coproporphyrin are increased
- Precipitating factors include infections, starvation, stress, alcohol
- Can be distinguished rapidly from all other porphyrias by examining the fluorescence emission spectrum of porphyrins in plasma at neutral pH
- Urinary uroporphyrins are equal to or less than coproporphyrins

Atopic dermatitis
The papular form of polymorphous light eruption resembles atopic dermatitis.

FEATURES
- Pruritic, exudative, or lichenified eruption on face, neck, upper trunk, wrists, and hands, and in the antecubital and popliteal folds
- Can be exacerbated by light or heat, which can mimic photosensitivity because they are often present simultaneously
- Personal or family history of allergic manifestations, including asthma or allergic rhinitis
- Tendency to recur, with remission from adolescence to age 20
- Polymorphous light eruption is less pruritic than atopic dermatitis and occurs in a sun-exposed distribution, not in crease areas (as is common in atopic dermatitis)

Solar urticaria
Solar urticaria is precipitated by radiation in the UV and/or visible spectrum.

FEATURES
- Manifests 1–30min following exposure and lasts 15min to 3h
- Locally, pruritic wheals or morbilliform erythema over exposed areas
- Anaphylactic symptoms may occur when large body areas are involved
- Elevated blood histamine levels have been reported

DNA repair defects
Xeroderma pigmentosum and Cockayne syndrome are both rare autosomal recessive disorders involving defective ability to repair DNA damage, such as that produced by UV radiation.

FEATURES
Dermatologic manifestations include hypersensitivity of skin to sunlight and skin lesions.

SIGNS & SYMPTOMS
Signs
Polymorphous light eruptions:
- Small papules, either disseminated or densely aggregated on patchy erythematous skin
- Affects sun-exposed areas but can spread to nonexposed areas
- Papulovesicular lesions are less common and usually begin with urticarial plaques from which groups of vesicles form
- Plaques are less common and may be either superficial, urticarial, or eczematous

Phototoxic reactions:
- The eruption is confined to light-exposed areas and often resembles an exaggerated sunburn
- More severe cases may be urticarial or bullous
- There may be postinflammatory hyperpigmentation that can persist for a year or more
- Onycholysis may be present
- Chronic reactions may be associated with epidermal thickening, elastosis, telangiectasia, and pigmentary changes

Phytophotodermatitis:
- Can take on unique clinical forms depending on exposure (e.g. pigmentation on the hands of bartenders exposed to Persian limes)

Photoallergic reactions:

- Eruptions mimic other cutaneous hypersensitivity eruptions; usually consist of papules with erythema and occasionally vesicles
- Eczematous changes
- Reactions can spread to areas that have not been exposed to sun
- Pruritus

Symptoms

- Patients with polymorphous light eruption may experience malaise, chills, headache, and nausea starting approximately 4h after exposure but lasting for only 1–2h
- Most common initial symptoms are burning, itching, and erythema, which typically occur within 2h of exposure
- Photosensitivity reactions are often associated with pain

ASSOCIATED DISORDERS

- Solar urticaria: a rare photosensitive disorder. Pruritic wheals form within minutes of sun exposure and last up to 3h only
- Several genetic disorders associated with photosensitivity include xeroderma pigmentosum, Bloom syndrome, Cockayne syndrome, Rothmund-Thomson syndrome

CONSIDER CONSULT

- Refer to dermatologist if diagnosis, treatment, prognosis, or preventive measures are uncertain
- Referral to dermatologist is appropriate for identification of an inciting agent; further diagnostic testing; counseling to prevent recurrences

INVESTIGATION OF THE PATIENT
Direct questions to patient

Q Is there seasonal variation in the eruption? Some may be perennial, or exacerbated during spring and summer.

Q How old were you when the symptoms began? Childhood onset is common for hereditary variants and the porphyrias.

Q How long after exposure to UV light does the eruption occur? This may help distinguish between phototoxic (immediate) and photoallergic (delayed) reactions.

Q Have you had any history of sun exposure or spent time outdoors recently? UV light is a precipitant.

Q What is your occupation and what leisure activities or hobbies do you pursue? These relate to UV light exposure.

Q Are you currently taking any prescribed, alternative, or over-the-counter medications? Many substances can be involved in photodermatitis reactions.

Q Have you used any creams or lotions recently? Many topical agents can precipitate photodermatitis reactions.

Q Have you been in contact with any unusual plant material? Many plants (e.g. celery, Queen Anne's lace, limes) contain psoralen compounds that can produce phytophotodermatitis.

Q Do you have any other medical conditions? Other conditions, such as systemic lupus erythematosus and atopic dermatitis, can produce signs and symptoms similar to those of photodermatitis.

Contributory or predisposing factors

Skin type does not seem to play a role in susceptibility, and fair or darker skin types are similarly affected. Native Americans are at increased risk.

Family history

A family history is usually negative except in the hereditary variant of polymorphous light eruption.

Examination

- Examine skin to determine the form of photodermatitis. Are there papules, plaques, or vesicles? Is there erythema?
- Examine pattern and distribution of reactions. Is the affected area restricted to (or markedly worse in) regions of sun exposure such as nape of the neck or 'V' on the chest? Typically, shaded areas of the face (e.g. under the nose, eyelids, under the chin) are spared or much less involved
- Examine nails for signs of onycholysis. This can occur with drug-induced photosensitivity

Summary of investigative tests

- Antinuclear antibody test helps determine whether photosensitivity reaction is associated with systemic lupus erythematosus
- A punch-type skin biopsy can provide diagnostic information and help exclude other diagnoses with typical histologic findings. Interpretation of the skin biopsy may require special stains or the opinion of a dermatopathologist
- Urinary uroporphyrin and coproporphyrin are used to determine whether the photosensitivity reaction is associated with porphyria cutanea tarda or variegate porphyria. This is a very uncommon etiology, and ordering should await the recommendation of a specialist
- Photopatch testing is used to provide diagnostic confirmation of phototoxicity, and photoallergy can often be identified; usually performed by a dermatologist
- Phototesting/photoprovocation testing is used to demonstrate abnormal sensitivity to UV light and identify the causal wavelengths; usually performed by a dermatologist

DIAGNOSTIC DECISION

- Physical examination and medical history with empiric removal of suspected agent is often all that is needed
- Histologic features are characteristic but not pathognomonic for polymorphous light eruptions; histology may help in excluding other diagnoses such as lupus or porphyria
- Suspect photodermatitis if patients have used any photosensitizing agents, e.g. medications or topical agents, or have been in contact with plants that are known to produce phytophotosensitivity reactions
- Diagnostic confirmation of phototoxicity and photoallergy can often be obtained using phototest procedures

CLINICAL PEARLS

- Do not be fooled by a history of eruption only once per year, despite frequent exposure to sunlight. This is a typical history for polymorphous light eruption
- Sunscreens themselves can be photoallergens, and thus attempts to treat or prevent photodermatitis may in fact worsen the disease
- Although considered a genetic disease, porphyria can be acquired, particularly as a drug-induced phenomenon or secondary to liver dysfunction
- Photoallergic eruptions can be found at sites of mild trauma (e.g. scratching) in sun-protected areas as part of the so-called isomorphic response or Koebner phenomenon

THE TESTS
Body fluids
ANTINUCLEAR ANTIBODY (ANA)
Description
Serum sample.

Advantages/Disadvantages
Advantages:
- A positive ANA test supports the diagnosis of SLE
- A negative ANA test makes the diagnosis unlikely

Disadvantage: Nonspecific

Normal
Absence of ANA, or low titer positive.

Abnormal
- Presence of ANA, while not specific for SLE, increases post-test probability of SLE
- Keep in mind the possibility of a false-positive result, especially in the elderly

Cause of abnormal result
Probable SLE or other autoimmune disorder.

Drugs, disorders and other factors that may alter results
- Many other immunologically mediated medical conditions can yield a positive ANA result (e.g. rheumatoid arthritis)
- Results must be interpreted in conjunction with the patient's medical history because infections, hematologic or oncologic conditions, and endocrine or gastrointestinal diseases may result in a positive ANA
- In healthy people, pregnancy, older age, and drugs such as hydralazine or procainamide may give a positive ANA

Biopsy
SKIN BIOPSY: PUNCH TYPE
Description
A punch-type skin biopsy, usually 4mm in size.

Advantages/Disadvantages
Advantages:
- Relatively easy and quick to perform
- May provide diagnostic information and help exclude other diagnoses with typical histologic findings

Disadvantages:
- Some pain, usually minimal, during initial injection of anesthesia at biopsy site
- If closed by suture, will need to be removed after healing
- Knowledge is necessary to choose site for biopsy

Normal
No histologic pathology.

Abnormal
Specific histologic pattern of a disease entity:
- Polymorphous drug eruption: upper and mid-dermal perivascular infiltrate, predominantly of T cells with some polymorphonuclear cells. Upper and mid-dermal edema and endothelial swelling
- Phototoxic: epidermal necrosis/apoptosis with or without spongiosus, dermal edema, and polymorphous infiltrate
- Photoallergy: spongiosus and dermal infiltrate of mononuclear cells

Histologic information will come from the pathologist on the biopsy report; thus it is not generally necessary to identify the presence or absence of these features.

Cause of abnormal result

- Specific skin diseases such as polymorphous light eruption, phototoxicity and photoallergic eruptions, SLE, and porphyria often have specific abnormalities on biopsy
- Keep in mind the possibility of a falsely abnormal result

Drugs, disorders and other factors that may alter results

- Ulceration and coexistent unrelated skin disease may alter histologic interpretation
- Biopsy of an old lesion may have undergone secondary changes due to such factors as rubbing or scratching
- Biopsy of eruption near some other lesion, such as a nevus or seborrheic keratosis, may distract the pathologist from the inflammatory component
- The most important issue is to ensure that biopsy tissue is interpreted by a qualified dermatopathologist

TREATMENT

CONSIDER CONSULT

- Refer to dermatologist if patient has severe pain or extensive blisters or erythema
- Refer if patient has systemic symptoms such as fever, chills, high-output cardiac failure, severe edema, or third spacing of fluids secondary to generalized vasodilation or fluid loss

PATIENT AND CAREGIVER ISSUES
Patient or caregiver request

- **How long will this condition last?** Polymorphous light eruption usually lasts for many years but may decrease in intensity over time
- **Where should I go for treatment?** If desensitization with phototherapy is required, then a dermatologist who has phototherapy equipment is needed
- **How can I avoid further flares of the disease?** Avoidance of the sensitizing compounds in phototoxic and photoallergic diseases and the sun are necessary. Desensitizing regimens should be prescribed by a dermatologist who is knowledgeable regarding photomedicine

Health-seeking behavior

- Use of emollients may help with pruritus
- Education about substances to avoid, with handouts listing photosensitive compounds
- Use of special glass that screens UVA light. Normal window glass screens UVB light

MANAGEMENT ISSUES
Goals

- To resolve the skin reactions
- To prevent further attacks

Management in special circumstances
COEXISTING DISEASE

- It is important to distinguish from other photoexacerbated diseases such as SLE and dermatomyositis
- Medical conditions, such as hepatic disease and alcohol and estrogen use that are associated with porphyria cutanea tarda, should be identified
- Neurologic manifestations may be associated with variegate porphyria

COEXISTING MEDICATION
A careful review of all medications taken by the patient may reveal a causal agent.

PATIENT SATISFACTION/LIFESTYLE PRIORITIES
Patients must address lifestyle factors to reduce the chance of further attacks. These include minimizing sunlight exposure, using sunscreen with maximum sun protection factor (SPF) in conjunction with protective clothing, and discontinuing use of photosensitizing agents.

SUMMARY OF THERAPEUTIC OPTIONS
Choices
Polymorphous light eruption:

- First treatment option is symptomatic relief with topical corticosteroids and lifestyle changes to avoid excessive sunlight. Sunscreens can be useful but should be broad spectrum because UVA contributes significantly to this disease. Symptoms subside with repeated exposure to sunlight (hardening) in many patients, but excessive exposure can prompt a flare, which may require systemic corticosteroids

- Patients who do not respond to first treatment options and those who experience significant eruptions each summer may receive phototherapy, such as UVB, or preferably psoralen plus UVA (PUVA) phototherapy. This is usually done under the supervision of a dermatologist
- Antimalarials (e.g. hydroxychloroquine) may be effective for patients who are not protected by sunscreens and who do not respond to UVB or PUVA phototherapy. This is an off-label indication, and such treatment is usually given by a specialist. Other similar off-label therapies include thalidomide, beta-carotene, and nicotinamide
- Severe, nonresponsive cases may require systemic immunosuppressants such as azathioprine or cyclosporine. This is an off-label indication, and such treatment is usually given by a specialist

Phototoxic, photoallergic, and phytophotoallergic reactions:
- Eliminate exposure to chemical agents responsible for photosensitivity reaction and institute lifestyle changes to minimize sun exposure
- Acute symptoms of photosensitivity may be treated with cool moist compresses
- Short, intermittent, 3- to 14-day courses of topical corticosteroids (e.g. betamethasone valerate) are effective for photoallergic and phytophotoallergic eruptions
- For more severe reactions, prednisone for 3–10 days is effective
- Antihistamines (e.g. hydroxyzine) are effective for pruritus
- NSAIDs (e.g. indomethacin) for pain relief
- Cyclo-oxygenase-2 inhibitors (e.g. rofecoxib and celecoxib) are relatively new drugs and, because photodermatoses are relatively uncommon, there are no data evaluating these drugs in these conditions, although they may prove to be efficacious

Clinical pearls
Many photosensitive patients react to wavelengths in the UVA range. Sunscreens with high SPF (UVB protection) without UVA protection may worsen certain conditions (e.g. polymorphous light eruption) by allowing prolonged sun exposure and thus increased UVA exposure without concomitant sunburn to warn the patient of unsafe exposure.

FOLLOW UP
Plan for review
If potent topical corticosteroids are used, close monitoring every few weeks is necessary to avoid cutaneous side effects, particularly if the face is involved.

Information for patient or caregiver
Alert patients to the following information:
- Sunscreens with maximum SPFs and broad-spectrum coverage should be used
- Be aware that some sunscreens (those containing PABA and/or benzophenones) can sometimes cause photosensitivity or allergic contact dermatitis
- Avoiding exposure to sunlight between 11 a.m. and 2 p.m. (when 50% of the daily UV light is emitted) may minimize photoreactions
- Sitting in the shade does not protect against UV exposure (50% of the ambient UV light is received)
- 90% of UV light penetrates clouds, so wear protection even on cloudy days
- Most sensitivities are triggered, at least in part, by long wavelength ultraviolet light (UVA), which is most intense in suntan parlor lamps and can also pass through the glass of cars and building windows

DRUGS AND OTHER THERAPIES: DETAILS
Drugs
BETAMETHASONE VALERATE
Topical corticosteroid.

Dose
0.1% cream applied to the affected areas twice daily for a short course of treatment. Usually one week is sufficient; more than 2 weeks is rarely required.

Efficacy
- Limited benefit in phototoxic reactions; helpful in treatment of photoallergic reactions and polymorphous light eruptions
- Reduces pruritus and hastens resolution

Risks/benefits
Risk: long-term use of potent topical corticosteroids can result in permanent thinning of sensitive skin, telangiectasis, or redness.

Side effects and adverse reactions
- Systemic absorption of betamethasone is minimal but theoretical
- Endocrine: Cushing's syndrome; inhibition of the hypothalamic-pituitary-adrenal axis can occur if applied over large surface areas
- Metabolic: hyperglycemia, glucosuria, if used chronically (unlikely in these photodermatoses); growth retardation can occur in children
- Skin: rash, dermatitis, pruritus, atrophy, hypopigmentation, striae, xerosis, burning, stinging upon application, alopecia, conjunctivitis, cutaneous atrophy can occur after a few weeks

Interactions (other drugs)
- No known interactions with topical betamethasone

Contraindications
- Rosacea ▪ Pruritus ▪ Acne vulgaris

Acceptability to patient
- Acceptability to patient is a balance between severity of symptoms and potential side effects of steroids. Side effects are variable depending on dosing, duration, and place of application
- It is important to discuss pros and cons of steroid therapy in order to allow patient to make an informed decision about treatment

Follow up plan
- Close monitoring every 3 weeks required
- Review for symptom resolution and to avoid side effects, particularly when the face is involved

Patient and caregiver information
- Patients are often cautious about corticosteroid use, and benefits need to be explained
- The role of long-wave (UVA) radiation, its relationship to sunscreen SPF (UVB protection), and the fact that it is not filtered by window glass need to be explained

PREDNISONE
This is an off-label indication

Dose
0.5–1mg/kg per day for 3–9 days (doses should be individualized).

Efficacy
- Useful for patients with severe photosensitivity reactions
- Short courses useful for very itchy, widespread eruptions or for patients who flare during a course of phototherapy
- With properly educated, otherwise healthy patients, a short course can be used during predictable sun exposure (e.g. during a tropical vacation)

Risks/benefits
Risks:
- Overwhelming septicemia if patient has an infection
- Loss of control of blood glucose in those with diabetes
- Prolonged use causes adrenal suppression
- Use caution in elderly due to risk of diabetes and osteoporosis
- Use caution in patients with psychosis, seizure disorders, or myasthenia gravis
- Use caution in patients with congestive heart failure, hypertension, ulcerative colitis, peptic ulcer, or esophagitis

Side effects and adverse reactions
- Side effects are minimized by short duration of therapy
- Cardiovascular system: hypertension, thromboembolism
- Central nervous system. insomnia, euphoria, depression, psychosis
- Endocrine: adrenal suppression, impaired glucose tolerance
- Eyes, ears, nose, and throat: cataract, glaucoma, blurred vision
- Gastrointestinal: dyspepsia, peptic ulceration, esophagitis, oral candidiasis
- Musculoskeletal: proximal myopathy, osteoporosis
- Skin: delayed healing, acne, striae

Interactions (other drugs)
- Aminoglutethamide (increased clearance of prednisone) - Antidiabetics (hypoglycemic effect inhibited) - Antihypertensives (effects inhibited) - Barbiturates (increased clearance of prednisone) - Cardiac glycosides (toxicity increased) - Cholestyramine, colestipol (my reduce absorption of corticosteroids) - Clarithromycin, erythromycin, troleandomycin (may enhance steroid effect) - Cyclosporine (may increase levels of both drugs; may cause seizures) - Diuretics (effects inhibited) - Isoniazid (reduced plasma levels of isoniazid) - Ketoconazole - Nonsteroidal antiinflammatory drugs (increased risks of bleeeding) - Oral contraceptives (enhanced effects of corticosteroids) - Rifampin (may inhibit hepatic clearance of prednisone) - Salicylates (increased clearance of salicylates) - Warfarin (alters clotting time)

Contraindications
- Systemic infection - Avoid live virus vaccines in those receiving immunosuppressive doses

Acceptability to patient
Patients are often cautious about corticosteroid use, and benefits need to be explained.

Follow up plan
Review after a few days to check for symptom resolution and side effects.

Patient and caregiver information
- Notify clinician if signs and symptoms appear following dose reduction or withdrawal of therapy
- May cause sensitivity to bright light; sunglasses should be worn

HYDROXYZINE
Antihistamine.

Dose
25–50mg by mouth, four times a day.

Efficacy
- Effective in treating pruritus
- Relief from symptoms within 30min

Risks/benefits
Risks:
- Can cause sedation, which may be dangerous depending on the patient's occupation
- Use caution in pregnancy and the elderly
- Use caution in hepatic and renal disease

Benefit: Can greatly reduce the symptom of itch

Side effects and adverse reactions
- Central nervous system: confusion, depression, dizziness, drowsiness, headache, seizures, tremor
- Gastrointestinal: dry mouth
- Genitourinary: urinary retention

Interactions (other drugs)
- Alcohol

Contraindications
- Hypersensitivity to hydroxyzine

Acceptability to patient
Good.

Follow up plan
Therapy can be ceased when symptoms resolve.

INDOMETHACIN
NSAID.

Dose
25mg three times a day.

Efficacy
Pain and inflammation should begin to ease within 2h.

Risks/benefits
Risks:
- Use caution in hepatic and cardiac failure, epilepsy, psychiatric disorders, and parkinsonism
- Use caution in pregnancy and breast-feeding patients
- Use caution in bleeding disorders

Benefits:
- Usually very well tolerated
- Good analgesic effect
- Easy to take and widely available
- Good dose flexibility

Side effects and adverse reactions
- Cardiovascular system: cardiac abnormalities, congestive heart failure
- Central nervous system: headache, dizziness, tinnitus, somnolence
- Gastrointestinal: anorexia, nausea, vomiting, abdominal pain, diarrhea, constipation, dyspepsia, peptic ulceration, gastritis, gastrointestinal bleeding
- Genitourinary: renal dysfunction, hyperuricemia
- Hematologic: blood cell disorders
- Hypersensitivity: rashes, bronchospasm, angioedema

Interactions (other drugs)
- Aminoglycosides ▪ Anticoagulants ▪ Antidiabetics ▪ Antihypertensives ▪ Baclofen ▪ Corticosteroids ▪ Cidofovir ▪ Cyclosporine, tacrolimus ▪ Digoxin ▪ Diuretics ▪ Ethanol ▪ Gentamicin ▪ Haloperidol ▪ Lithium ▪ Methotrexate ▪ Phenylpropanolamine ▪ Probenecid ▪ Triamterene ▪ Vancomycin ▪ Warfarin

Contraindications
- Severe renal, hepatic, or cardiac disease ▪ Hypertension ▪ Peptic ulceration, gastrointestinal bleeding, ulcerative colitis ▪ Hypersensitivity to NSAIDs ▪ Coagulation defects ▪ Untreated infection ▪ Thrombocytopenia ▪ Cidofovir

Acceptability to patient
Good.

Follow up plan
Cease medication when symptoms resolve.

Patient and caregiver information
Take with food.

Other therapies
COOL MOIST COMPRESSES
Efficacy
Can provide good relief from the acute symptoms of photosensitivity, although requires frequent application and results are modest at best.

Risks/benefits
Benefits:
- Treatment is simple, cheap, and easy for patients to self-administer as required
- Few risks, if any

Acceptability to patient
Good.

Follow up plan
Review after several days in order to ascertain whether symptoms have persisted and need additional therapy.

LIFESTYLE

- Avoid or limit sunlight exposure
- Sunscreens with maximum SPFs and high UVA protection should be used in conjunction with protective clothing
- Avoiding exposure to sunlight between 11 a.m. and 2 p.m. (when 50% of the daily UV light is emitted) may minimize photoreactions

RISKS/BENEFITS
Benefit: should help reduce the incidence of photodermatitis.

ACCEPTABILITY TO PATIENT
Good.

EFFICACY OF THERAPIES

- The treatment of polymorphous light eruption by phototherapy generally provides symptom relief
- Mild cases of polymorphous light eruption may benefit simply from behavioral changes such as UV avoidance and sunscreen use
- Phototoxic and photoallergic reactions respond well to the avoidance of the implicated agent

Evidence
PDxMD are unable to cite evidence that meets our criteria for evidence.

PROGNOSIS

- Polymorphous light eruption and photoallergy can persist for many years
- The most common phototoxic reactions are usually benign and self-limiting, except in instances where they are associated with a more serious disorder or when the burn is severe

Clinical pearls
Rule out LE, including chronic cutaneous and subacute cutaneous lupus, before embarking on phototherapy.

Therapeutic failure
- Systemic medications may be tried if patients do not improve with phototherapy and their disease state is severe
- Some medications that have been tried include hydroxychloroquine, thalidomide, corticosteroids, and azathioprine. These are all off-label indications

Recurrence
- All of the photodermatoses may recur after a quiescent period, although the factors leading to a recurrence are unknown
- Management should be the same as for the initial presentation

COMPLICATIONS
Some patients continue to experience photosensitivity reactions even when they are no longer exposed to photosensitizing agents.

CONSIDER CONSULT

- Referral to dermatologist is indicated in cases where the course is refractory to first-line treatment options or if patient is unable to tolerate or is not a suitable candidate for treatment options
- Dermatologists are more likely to have phototherapy units and the knowledge to provide the appropriate regimen
- A rheumatologist or dermatologist may be required if a connective tissue disease, such as LE, needs to be excluded

RISK FACTORS

- Sunlight, tanning parlors: avoid when possible
- Photosensitive agents: avoid exposure to these agents

MODIFY RISK FACTORS

- Avoid or limit sun exposure
- Wear protective clothing and a sunscreen with a high SPF when exposed to sunlight
- Be aware that some sunscreens (those containing PABA and/or benzophenones) can sometimes cause photosensitivity or allergic contact dermatitis
- Avoid medications or other agents known to cause photosensitivity reactions

PREVENT RECURRENCE

- If exposed to sunlight, wear protective clothing and sunscreen with a high SPF
- Be aware that some sunscreens (those containing PABA and/or benzophenones) can sometimes cause photosensitivity or allergic contact dermatitis
- Avoid using photosensitizing agents

RESOURCES

ASSOCIATIONS
American Academy of Dermatology
930 N. Meacham Road
PO Box 4014
Schaumburg, IL 60168-4014
Tel: 847-330-0230
Fax: 847-330-0050
http://www.aad.org

KEY REFERENCES
- Habif TP. Clinical dermatology, 3rd ed. Philadelphia: Mosby, 1995
- Tierney LM, McPhee S, Papadakis M. Current medical diagnosis and treatment. New York: McGraw-Hill, 2001
- Behrman RE, Kliegman RM, Arvin AM. Nelson textbook of pediatrics, 16th ed. Philadelphia: WB Saunders, 1999

Diagnostic Guidelines
- Kim JJ, Lim HW. Evaluation of the photosensitive patient. Semin Cutan Med Surg 1999;18(4):253–6. Medline
- Roelandts R. The diagnosis of photosensitivity. Arch Dermatol 2000;136:1152–1157. Medline

FAQS
Question 1
Does window glass protect against photodermatoses?

ANSWER 1
No. UVA is not filtered by glass and can contribute greatly to a patient's disease.

Question 2
If a patient can tolerate a compound (e.g. toxins in limes), does that mean it cannot be the cause of the patient's eruption?

ANSWER 2
No. Photosensitivity disorders are caused by simultaneous exposure to the chemical (either topically or systemically) and light of the appropriate wavelength.

CONTRIBUTORS
Dennis F Saver, MD
Seth R Stevens, MD
Albert Peng, MD

Photodermatitis – RESOURCES

PILONIDAL CYST

DESCRIPTION

- Common, acquired condition
- Midline tract lined by granulation tissue
- Majority occur in skin of natal cleft
- Solitary or as a row in the midline
- Tufts of hair may be found lying in the midline
- Hairs penetrate subcutaneous tissue, leading to formation of a cyst or a sinus
- Suppuration, tenderness, and swelling may indicate abscess formation

URGENT ACTION

Acute abscess of the pilonidal sinus with systemic features requires urgent incision and drainage with antibiotic treatment.

KEY! DON'T MISS!

- Abscess formation, which will require incision and drainage
- Systemic features indicate more severe infection and will require both surgical and antibiotic treatment

ICD9 CODE
685.1 Pilonidal cyst

SYNONYMS
- Pilonidal sinus
- Jeep driver's/rider's disease: term originates from the Second World War, during which it was common in US Army personnel, causing more than 80,000 soldiers to be hospitalized
- Coccygeal sinus
- Piliferous cyst
- Described in 1830 by Herbert Mayo as a 'hair-containing sinus'

CARDINAL FEATURES
- Midline tract lined by granulation tissue
- Majority occur in skin of natal cleft
- Can occur between fingers and at the umbilicus
- Solitary or as a row in the midline
- Tufts of hair may be found lying in the midline
- Suppuration, tenderness, and swelling indicates abscess formation
- Systemic reaction can occur infrequently

CAUSES
Common causes
- The exact etiology is unknown
- Congenital sinuses occur, but most are acquired
- Hair appears to be a causal factor, but the exact mechanism for the sinus formation is unknown
- Hair may be driven into the skin by sitting or the shearing action of buttocks
- Hair implantation into the skin sets up a foreign body reaction and produces a short tract (the sinus)
- Infection by skin organisms (fecal contamination) occurs, causing rupture of the sinus into the surrounding adipose tissue
- A chronic pilonidal abscess occurs where the tract's wall contains fibrous tissue

Contributory or predisposing factors
The following risk factors have been noted:
- Male sex
- Dark hair
- Obesity
- Sedentary lifestyle
- Local hirsutism
- Occupations requiring prolonged sitting
- Poor hygiene and increased sweating
- Barbers and hairdressers (clefts between fingers)

EPIDEMIOLOGY
Incidence and prevalence
INCIDENCE
26 cases/100,000 people in the US.

Demographics

AGE

- Rarely presents before adolescence
- Average age of presentation is 21 years
- Most present between ages of 20 and 40 years

GENDER

Male:female ratio is 2.2:1.0.

RACE

Caucasians are more at risk for developing a pilonidal cyst.

GENETICS

There is a familial predisposition, although the genetic theory of congenital origin is disfavored. Most cases of pilonidal cysts are acquired.

DIFFERENTIAL DIAGNOSIS
Anal fistula
An anal fistula is a track of granulation tissue between the perianal skin and the anal or rectal lumen, which is constantly infected.

FEATURES
- Originate as abscesses that drain
- Persistence of purulent discharge
- Perianal irritation and discomfort
- Pain develops when orifice becomes occluded

Furuncle
A furuncle is an infection of hair follicle that results in boil formation.

FEATURES
- Infection of hair follicle
- Boil formation results
- Can occur anywhere on skin with hair follicles
- Staphylococcal bacteria are the causal agent
- Coalescence of boils results in caruncle formation

Caruncle
A caruncle is a coalescence of boils that results from infected hair follicles.

FEATURES
- Multiple boils in hair follicles
- Caused by infections with staphylococci
- A caruncle is formed from coalescence of these boils

SIGNS & SYMPTOMS
Signs
- Small midline tract that is usually easy to see
- Majority occur in the skin of the natal cleft
- Can occur in clefts between fingers, at the umbilicus, and the perineum
- Solitary or as a row of sinuses in the midline
- Gentle pressure may produce serous discharge
- Tufts of hair may be found lying in the midline, with hair often visible at the orifice
- The skin around the sinus is normal until infection causes it to become red and tender; there may be pain in the area
- Suppuration, tenderness, and swelling indicates abscess formation
- Systemic reaction can occur infrequently, leading to the patient being febrile with or without chills

Symptoms
- Asymptomatic until infection occurs, leading to pain and discharge: pain may vary from a dull ache to an acute throbbing pain; discharge will vary from small amount of serous fluid to a sudden gush of pus
- Acute exacerbations (infections) occur at irregular intervals

KEY! DON'T MISS!

- Abscess formation, which will require incision and drainage
- Systemic features indicate more severe infection and will require both surgical and antibiotic treatment

CONSIDER CONSULT

- Pilonidal sinus will require surgical referral for excision to prevent later complications of abscess and cyst formation
- Complications of the pilonidal sinus (abscess and cyst formation) will require urgent surgical referral for incision and drainage

INVESTIGATION OF THE PATIENT
Direct questions to patient

Q How long have you noticed pain and discharge? Often, recurrent infections occur in the pilonidal sinus.

Q Have you had a previous operation for similar symptoms? Recurrence of the pilonidal sinus is common, and may occur even after surgical intervention.

Q Do you have fever and chills? Systemic reaction can occur with fever, leukocytosis, and malaise.

Contributory or predisposing factors

Q Do you have a sedentary lifestyle? This is associated with pilonidal sinus formation.

Q Does your occupation require prolonged sitting? Prolonged sitting is associated with pilonidal sinus formation.

Q Are you a barber or hairdresser? Pilonidal sinus formation can occur in the clefts between the fingers.

Q What kind of clothes do you wear? Tight clothing may predispose to pilonidal cyst.

Family history

Q Has anyone in your family had a similar disease? Pilonidal sinus formation has a familial predisposition.

Examination

- Is the sinus in the natal cleft at the midline? This is the classic site for pilonidal sinus formation
- Are hair follicles visible at the orifice? This is indicative of pilonidal sinus formation
- Is the skin around the sinus tender, hot, red, and swollen? These features indicate that infection and/or abscess formation has occurred
- Does the sinus discharge serous fluid or pus? Infection and/or abscess formation has occurred
- Are there scars around the natal cleft? Previous abscesses may have discharged or been incised

Summary of investigative tests

- The diagnosis is usually clear from the patient's history and physical examination, and diagnostic tests are not usually required
- If the patient feels ill or is febrile, then a complete blood count (CBC) for leukocytosis may be ordered, to identify whether any systemic infection is present or an abscess has formed

DIAGNOSTIC DECISION

- Diagnosis is based on history and physical examination
- Midline pits present behind the anus overlying the sacrum and coccyx
- Insert probe in pilonidal sinus to examine cavity fully

CLINICAL PEARLS

Diagnosis is apparent from the emergence of hairs. Most patients benefit from a surgical evaluation.

THE TESTS
Body fluids
COMPLETE BLOOD COUNT
Description
- A venous sample of blood should be taken
- Pathology laboratory analysis is needed

Advantages/Disadvantages
Advantages:
- Quick and simple
- Inexpensive

Normal
White blood cells (WBCs): 3200–9800/mm^3 (3.2–9.8x10^9/L)

Abnormal
WBCs: >9800/mm^3 (>9.8x10^9/L).

Cause of abnormal result
- Infection of the pilonidal sinus
- Abscess formation

Drugs, disorders and other factors that may alter results
Corticosteroids or infection elsewhere in the body may have an impact on findings.

CONSIDER CONSULT

- Definitive treatment can be difficult, and most patients should be referred to a surgical specialist
- Pilonidal sinus will require surgical referral for excision to prevent later complications of abscess and cyst formation
- Complications of the pilonidal sinus (abscess and cyst formation) will require urgent surgical referral for incision and drainage

IMMEDIATE ACTION

Complications of the pilonidal sinus (abscess and cyst formation) will require urgent surgical referral for incision and drainage.

PATIENT AND CAREGIVER ISSUES
Patient or caregiver request

- **Do I need to have surgery for this condition?** Unless the sinus is fully excised, there is a significant risk for recurrence
- **What is the likelihood of recurrence?** Recurrence rate following excision is up to 6%
- **Is the condition contagious?** There is no risk of infectivity
- **Is the condition due to an underlying disease?** The condition is benign

Health-seeking behavior

- **Have you experienced this problem before?** The pilonidal sinus may have been infected repeatedly before presentation. In between acute exacerbations, symptoms would be minimal
- **Have you taken any medications?** The patient may have self-treated with analgesia, delaying presentation to the physician

MANAGEMENT ISSUES
Goals

- To reduce pain and swelling
- To prevent further acute exacerbations
- To prevent complications of infection and abscess formation
- To inform the patient of the importance of undergoing surgical excision

Management in special circumstances

Surgical excision of the tract will be needed.

COEXISTING DISEASE
Surgery requires anesthesia, which could compromise patients with comorbidities, including:
- Ischemic heart disease
- Respiratory disease
- Malignancy
- Immune compromise

COEXISTING MEDICATION
Certain medications could cause complications. For example, warfarin and aspirin can lead to prolonged bleeding.

SPECIAL PATIENT GROUPS
Surgery in children and the elderly requires specialist input to plan the anesthesia and after care. Antibiotics will be needed for comorbid conditions, including:
- Rheumatic heart disease
- Immunosuppression

PATIENT SATISFACTION/LIFESTYLE PRIORITIES
- Consent for surgery will be needed
- Surgery and wound management will require the patient to be absent from work for at least 2 weeks
- Patients should be told that scarring will occur from the pilonidal sinus and surgery
- General anesthesia may compromise the patient's car insurance, and the patient should be advised to refrain from driving for this time period
- Strong analgesia will be required initially, which could cause drowsiness

SUMMARY OF THERAPEUTIC OPTIONS
Choices
Surgical treatment:
- Incision and curettage with drainage is required for acute exacerbations and is an urgent procedure. An asymmetric excision with primary closure with suction drain, with the aim of eliminating the causative factors, has been described
- Excision of the pilonidal sinus is an elective procedure for chronic pilonidal disease; laser surgery for the excision of pilonidal cysts has also been used
- Postoperative care includes: keeping the open granulation tissue meticulously clean; allowing the tissue to heal by complete granulation of the wound; and skin grafting, which may be needed if complete healing does not occur

Acute general treatment will require:
- Analgesia: codeine or nonsteroidal anti-inflammatory drugs (NSAIDs) (e.g. ibuprofen, naproxen)
- Antibiotics are not required for incision and drainage unless comorbidity is present

Chronic treatment of the pilonidal sinus requires wide excision down to the presacral fascia:
- Analgesia: codeine or ibuprofen
- Antibiotics for 24h: ampicillin/sulbactam (for *Staphylococcus* spp.) and metronidazole (for *Bacteroides* spp.)

Lifestyle:
- In addition to the treatments above, there are certain lifestyle measures that will reduce the occurrence of exacerbations

FOLLOW UP
Regular wound management will be needed for both acute treatment (incision and drainage) and elective treatment (wide excision).

Plan for review
Daily wound dressings will be needed:
- Keep the wound meticulously clean
- Check for good healing
- Check for infection
- Check for good pain control
- Check that the patient is coping and give advice

Information for patient or caregiver
- Pilonidal sinus will require surgical referral for excision to prevent later complications of abscess and cyst formation
- Good wound management will be required to allow for granulation to completely obliterate the tract
- Recurrence will be kept to the minimum if full granulation takes place

DRUGS AND OTHER THERAPIES: DETAILS
Drugs
CODEINE
Narcotic analgesic.

Dose
Adult oral dose: 15–60mg every 4h.

Risks/benefits
Risks:
- Use caution in the elderly
- Use caution in renal and hepatic disease
- Use caution in Addison's disease and hypothyroidism
- Use caution in recent head injury
- Use caution in patients with a history of drug abuse
- Use caution in gastrointestinal and cardiac disease
- Use caution in pregnancy and breast-feeding
- Small risk of dependency

Side effects and adverse reactions
- Cardiovascular system: bradycardia, tachycardia, palpitations, hypotension
- Central nervous system: headache, drowsiness, dizziness, dysphoria, addiction
- Gastrointestinal: nausea and vomiting, constipation, diarrhea, paralytic ileus, abdominal cramps
- Respiratory: respiratory depression
- Skin: rashes, urticaria

Interactions (other drugs)
- Alcohol Antidepressants (tricyclics and monoamine oxidase inhibitors) Antipsychotics Anxiolytics and hypnotics Cimetidine Ciprofloxacin Domperidone Metoclopramide Moclobemide Ritonavir

Contraindications
- Hypersensitivity to codeine or other opioids Colitis Liver failure Diarrhea secondary to poisoning or infectious diarrhea Severe pulmonary disease or respiratory failure Children under one year of age

NONSTEROIDAL ANTI-INFLAMMATORY DRUGS
NSAIDs with analgesic and antipyretic properties, such as ibuprofen and naproxen.

Dose
- Ibuprofen: adult oral dose: 200–600mg up to three times daily
- Naproxen: 375–500mg orally, twice daily

Risks/benefits
Risks:
- All currently available NSAIDs have unwanted effects, especially in the elderly
- Substantial individual variation in clinical response to NSAIDs
- Use caution in renal, cardiac, and hepatic impairment

Benefit: Have a range of actions: anti-inflammatory, analgesic, antipyretic

Side effects and adverse reactions
- Gastrointestinal: diarrhea, dyspepsia, nausea, vomiting, gastric bleeding and perforation
- Skin: rashes, urticaria, photosensitivity
- Genitourinary: reversible renal insufficiency, renal disease (high doses over long periods)
- Respiratory: worsening of asthma
- Ears, eyes, nose, and throat: tinnitus, decreased hearing
- Central nervous system: headache, dizziness

Interactions (other drugs)
- Antihypertensives (angiotensin-converting enzyme (ACE) inhibitors, adrenergic neurone blockers, alpha-blockers, angiotensin-II receptor antagonists, beta-blockers, clonidine, diazoxide, diuretics, hydralazine, methyldopa, minoxidil, nitroprusside)
- Antidysrhythmics (calcium channel blockers, cardiac glycosides) ▪ Antiplatelet agents (clopidogrel, ticlopidine) ▪ Aspirin ▪ Baclofen ▪ Cyclosporine ▪ Corticosteroids ▪ Heparins ▪ Ketorolac ▪ Lithium ▪ Methotrexate ▪ Moclobemide ▪ NSAIDs ▪ Nitrates ▪ Pentoxifylline (oxpentifylline) ▪ Phenindione ▪ Phenytoin ▪ Quinolones ▪ Ritonavir ▪ Sulfonylureas ▪ Tacrolimus ▪ Zidovudine

Contraindications
- Pregnancy and breast-feeding ▪ Coagulation defects ▪ Active peptic ulceration

AMPICILLIN/SULLBACTAM
Aminopenicillin/penicillinate antibiotic.

Dose
- Augmentin (amoxicillin/clavulanate) 875mg orally twice daily
- Unasyn (ampicillin/sulbactam) – adult dose: 1.5–3.0g intravenously every 6h

Risks/benefits
Risk: use caution with mononucleosis.

Side effects and adverse reactions
- Central nervous system: seizures, fatigue, headache, malaise
- Eyes, ears, nose, and throat: pseudomembranous colitis, vomiting, diarrhea, epitaxis
- Genitiurinary: dysuria, increased blood urea nitrogen/creatinine, urinary retention
- Hematologic: bone marrow depression
- Skin: exfoliative dermatitis, pain at injection site, thrombophlebitis, urticaria

Interactions (other drugs)
- Chloramphenicol (inhibits effect of ampicillin/sulbactam) ▪ Macrolides, tetracyclines (inhibits effect of ampicillin/sulbactam) ▪ Methotrexate (increases serum levels of methorexate) ▪ Oral contraceptives (may impair effectiveness of contraception)

Contraindications
- Hypersensitivity to penicillins or sulbactam ▪ The efficacy and safety of ampicillin sodium/sulbactam sodium have not been established in infants and children under the age of 12

METRONIDAZOLE
Antibiotic against anaerobic bacteria, including *Bacteroides* spp.

Dose
Adult dose: 7.5mg/kg (approx. 500mg) not to exceed 4.0g/day intravenous, or oral dose three times daily.

Risks/benefits
Risks:

- Nausea and vomiting likely if alcohol is taken
- Use caution in hepatic and renal impairment
- Use caution in central nervous system disease or history of seizures

Side effects and adverse reactions

- Central nervous system: dizziness, headache, seizures, ataxia, peripheral neuropathy
- Gastrointestinal: nausea, vomiting, taste disturbance, diarrhea, abdominal pain, dry mouth, anorexia, constipation
- Genitourinary: urination difficulties, cystitis, vaginal dryness
- Hematologic: blood cell disorders
- Skin: rashes, itching, flushing

Interactions (other drugs)

- Alcohol ▪ Antiepileptics ▪ Anticoagulants ▪ Barbiturates ▪ Carbamazepine
- Cholestyramine ▪ Cimetidine ▪ Colestipol ▪ Disulfiram ▪ Fluorouracil ▪ Lithium

Contraindications

- Pregnancy and breast-feeding ▪ Blood dyscrasias

Surgical therapy
INCISION AND DRAINAGE

- Needed for acute exacerbations
- Allows for drainage of the pus through an incision into the tract

Efficacy

- Useful during the suppuration phase to allow for pus to be drained
- The recurrence rate of the pilonidal sinus is high because the tract is not excised completely

Risks/benefits
Risks:

- Carries a risk of infection and scarring
- Good wound management is needed to reduce these risks to a minimum

Acceptability to patient

- Relatively quick operation that allows for drainage of pus
- Postoperative pain needs good analgesia
- Wound management requires good compliance
- Scarring will occur due to both the disease and the operation

Follow up plan
Daily wound dressing is needed to check for:

- Good healing
- Infection
- Pain control
- Patient compliance with advice

Patient and caregiver information

- Good advice on postoperative care is needed to reduce risks of infection and enable good healing

- The patient will have to take leave from work while healing occurs
- Recurrence may occur because the tract is not completely excised
- Cure rate of 76% after 18 months

EXCISION

- Wide excision is the treatment of choice as an elective procedure
- Recurrence is minimal

Efficacy

- Recurrence rate is minimal if complete granulation occurs
- If complete granulation does not occur then skin grafting may be required to close the defect

Risks/benefits

Risks:

- Infection
- Scarring
- Poor healing, leading to skin grafting of defect

Acceptability to patient

- The procedure can be painful
- Postoperative pain needs good analgesia
- Wound management requires good compliance
- The procedure will leave scarring

Follow up plan

Daily wound dressing is needed to check for:

- Good healing
- Infection
- Pain control
- Patient compliance with advice

Patient and caregiver information

- Procedure of choice because the tract is completely excised
- Good advice on postoperative care is needed to reduce risks of infection and to enable good healing
- The patient will have to take leave from work while healing occurs
- Recurrence rate is between 1–6%

LIFESTYLE

Nonpharmacologic measures that prevent acute exacerbations include:

- Good local hygiene
- Avoidance of prolonged sitting position
- Weight reduction in obese patients

RISKS/BENEFITS

Benefit: all of these measures will benefit the patient's health and aid in preventing further infections and abscess formation of the pilonidal sinus.

ACCEPTABILITY TO PATIENT

- The patient will need good motivation to lose weight
- If the patient has employment that leads to prolonged sitting (driver, office worker), then compliance with this advice is difficult

FOLLOW UP PLAN

The patient can be monitored for weight loss if this helps with motivation and compliance.

PATIENT AND CAREGIVER INFORMATION

- The patient needs to be informed of the health benefits of losing weight
- Motivation to lose weight needs to be ongoing
- The patient needs to be informed of the benefits of avoiding prolonged sitting
- Good local hygiene prevents sweat and bacterial accumulation on the skin, thus preventing infection of the pilonidal sinus

EFFICACY OF THERAPIES
Efficacy regarding these treatments and the treatment of pilonidal cysts is highly variable.

Review period
Disease may recur following primary treatment:
- Patients should have a follow up examination within a week after the procedure. The week allows for resolution of inflammation and assessment of the likely success of the treatment
- Local hygiene has been shown to reduce recurrence rates. The PCP can check the patient's hygiene techniques on a weekly basis

PROGNOSIS
- Recurrence is relatively common
- Incision and drainage does not excise the tract
- Wide excision of the pilonidal sinus tract gives the highest cure rate
- Recurrence rates are in the region of 24% after 18 months with incision and drainage, and 1–6% after excision
- Pilonidal disease can rarely undergo malignant transformation, in those with chronic disease or in those with condylomata who are immunocompromised with HIV

Clinical pearls
Definitive treatment by a qualified surgeon improves prognosis.

Therapeutic failure
Surgical referral for excision of the pilonidal sinus is needed.

Recurrence
Surgical referral for excision of the pilonidal sinus is needed.

Deterioration
Surgical referral for excision of the pilonidal sinus is needed.

COMPLICATIONS
- Lumber osteomyelitis and epidural abscess can rarely complicate recurrent pilonidal cyst in a patient with diabetes mellitus
- Recurrent exacerbations may occur during the process that leads to sinus infection and abscess formation, requiring incision and drainage and elective excision

CONSIDER CONSULT

- Patients with recurrent exacerbations with pilonidal disease will require surgical referral

PREVENTION

Patients can prevent acute exacerbations by:

- Good local hygiene
- Avoiding prolonged sitting
- Weight reduction in obese patients

MODIFY RISK FACTORS
Lifestyle and wellness

There are lifestyle measures that can prevent acute exacerbations.

DIET

Good weight monitoring should prevent obesity, which can lead to acute exacerbations.

PHYSICAL ACTIVITY

Avoiding a sedentary lifestyle may prevent acute exacerbations.

ENVIRONMENT

- Avoiding prolonged sitting will help prevent acute exacerbations
- Good local hygiene can prevent acute exacerbations

PREVENT RECURRENCE

Patients can prevent acute exacerbations by:

- Good local hygiene
- Avoiding prolonged sitting
- Weight reduction in obese patients

ASSOCIATIONS

American Society of Colon and Rectal Surgeons
85 W. Algonquin Road, Suite 550
Arlington Heights, IL 60005
Tel: (847) 290-9184
Fax: (847) 290-9203
www.fascrs.org

KEY REFERENCES

■ Verdu A, Garcia-Granero E, Garcia-Fuster MJ, et al. Lumbar osteomyelitis and epidural abscess complicating recurrent pilonidal cyst: report of a case. Dis Col Rectum 2000;43:1015–7
■ da Silva JH. Pilonidal cyst: cause and treatment. Dis Colon Rectum 2000;43:1146–56
■ Akinci OF, Unzunkoy A. Simple and effective surgical treatment of Pilonidal sinus: asymmetric excision and primary closure using suction drain and subcuticular skin closure. Dis Colon Rectum 2000;43:701–6
■ Palesty JA, Zahir KS, Dudrick SJ, et al. Nd:YAG laser surgery for the excision pilonidal cysts: a comparison with traditional techniques. Lasers Surg Med 2000;26:380–5
■ Velitchklow N, Vezardova M, Losanoff J, et al. A fatal case of carcinoma arising from a pilonidal sinus tract. Ulster Med J 2001;70:61–3
■ Borges VF, Keating JT, Nasser IA, et al. Clinicopathologic characterization of squamous cell carcinoma arising from pilonidal disease in association with condylomata accuminatum in HIV-infected patients: report to two cases. Dis Colon Rectum 2001;44:1873–7
■ De Vos. Fistula-in-ano, abscess, pilonidal cyst aínd hidradenitis suppurativa. Available from the American Society of Colon and Rectal Surgeons website (http://www.fascrs.org/coresubjects/2000/devos.html)

FAQS
Question 1
How can a pilonidal cyst be prevented?

ANSWER 1
Keeping the skin clean with a daily bath or shower using soap. Avoid wearing tight-fitting clothing.

CONTRIBUTORS

Thompson H Boyd, III, MD
Seth R Stevens, MD
Richard Averitte, MD

PITYRIASIS ROSEA

DESCRIPTION

- Initial lesion is the 'herald' patch
- Eruption 1–2 weeks later of pink to salmon-colored oval lesions on trunk
- Up to 100 lesions with a 4–5mm diameter
- Lesions have a ring of scale around the border (collarette)
- Symmetrical lesions
- Occasional pruritus
- Resolves spontaneously

KEY! DON'T MISS!

History of 'herald' patch is diagnostic for pityriasis rosea.

BACKGROUND

ICD9 CODE
696.3 Pityriasis rosea

CARDINAL FEATURES
- Initial lesion is the 'herald' patch
- Eruption 1–2 weeks later of scaly pink to salmon-colored oval lesions on trunk
- Up to 100 lesions with a diameter of 4–5mm
- Lesions have a ring of scale around the border (collarette)
- Symmetrical lesions with longitudinal axes tending to follow cleavage lines of trunk, forming so-called Christmas-tree pattern
- Occasional pruritus
- Not highly infectious
- Most cases occur in spring or fall
- Resolves spontaneously

CAUSES
Common causes
- Exact cause is unknown
- Picornavirus has been implicated
- Various drugs have been implicated, including: bismuth, barbiturates, captopril, gold, organic mercurials, methoxypromazine, metronidazole, D-penicillamine, isotretinoin, tripelennamine hydrochloride, ketotifen, and salvarsan

EPIDEMIOLOGY
Incidence and prevalence
- Incidence is highest in spring and fall
- In the US incidence has been calculated as 1.3/1000 men and 1.4/1000 women

Demographics
AGE
- Most cases occur between 10 and 35 years
- Mean age of contraction is 23 years

GENDER
Female:male ratio is 1.5:1.

RACE
There is no racial variation.

GEOGRAPHY
There is no geographic variation.

DIFFERENTIAL DIAGNOSIS
Tinea corporis
Tinea corporis is a dermatophyte fungal infection of the skin.

FEATURES
- Annular lesions with scaly border
- Margin is red, and usually raised, occasionally pustular
- Hypopigmented central area
- Primarily trunk and legs involved
- Diagnosed using potassium hydroxide examination of scale scraping

Eczema
Eczema is an inflammatory disorder of the skin.

FEATURES
- Pruritis leading to scratching, which modifies skin surface
- Skin surface is dry, scaly, red, and lichenified
- Involves symmetrical flexure surfaces of extremities
- Face, neck, and upper trunk affected
- Oozing, crusting, and blistering may occur

Psoriasis
Psoriasis is a chronic skin disorder with excessive proliferation of keratinocytes. The guttate form, which usually follows a streptococcal infection, may appear similar to pityriasis rosea.

FEATURES
- Erythematous papules topped by loosely adherent scales, mostly over the trunk
- May be accompanied by chronic plaques that are symmetrical over elbows, scalp, nails, and knees
- Plaques can develop over areas of physical trauma – Koebner's phenomenon
- Pruritus may be a feature
- Joint involvement can occur

Secondary syphilis
Syphilis is a sexually transmitted disease that causes acute and chronic lesions of the skin and mucous membranes. The secondary stage may present with widespread lesions resembling pityriasis rosea.

FEATURES
- Diffuse or localized mucocutaneous lesions
- Generalized lymphadenopathy
- Systemic symptoms of fever and malaise
- Maculopapular lesions on soles and palms
- Lesions can occur on mucous membranes

SIGNS & SYMPTOMS
Signs
- Herald patch precedes eruption by 1–2 weeks
- Herald patch is round to oval and 3–6cm in diameter
- Eruptive phase follows within 2 weeks and peaks by 14 days
- Lesions on trunk have symmetrical appearance following cleavage lines

- Most lesions are 4–5mm in diameter with a ring of scale around the border (collarette)
- Lesion numbers vary from a few to hundreds

Symptoms
25% of patients may experience the following symptoms:
- Fever
- Malaise
- Headaches
- Sore throat
- Occasionally the skin will be irritative

KEY! DON'T MISS!
History of 'herald' patch is diagnostic for pityriasis rosea.

CONSIDER CONSULT
- Refer to a dermatologist if diagnosis is in doubt

INVESTIGATION OF THE PATIENT
Direct questions to patient
Q Did you notice an initial oval patch? The 'herald' patch is diagnostic.
Q Is the rash irritative? Pruritus can be a feature of pityriasis rosea.
Q Have you felt unwell recently? 25% of cases have systemic features of fever, malaise, headaches, and sore throat.
Q Have you had this rash before? Recurrence is rare (<2%).
Q Have you been taking any medication recently? A number of drugs are implicated in pityriasis rosea, including bismuth, barbiturates, captopril, gold, organic mercurials, methoxypromazine, metronidazole, D-penicillamine, isotretinoin, tripelennamine hydrochloride, ketotifen, and salvarsan.

Contributory or predisposing factors
Q Have you had a similar rash previously? Recurrence can take place over a few years but is rare (<2%).

Family history
Q Has anyone else in your family had a similar rash? Concurrence in household contacts has been reported.

Examination
- Is there evidence of a 'herald' patch? This is characteristic of pityriasis rosea
- Are the lesions pink and oval with a scaly border? Rash features characteristic of pityriasis rosea
- Is the rash symmetrical over the trunk following cleavage lines? 'Christmas-tree' pattern of pityriasis rosea
- Are the lesions multiple? Lesion number varies from a few to hundreds in pityriasis rosea

Summary of investigative tests
- Diagnostic test for pityriasis rosea generally not indicated unless for atypical cases
- Tinea infection can be excluded by using potassium hydroxide (KOH) to dissolve the keratin and look for hyphae under the microscope
- Syphilis serology should be done if clinically indicated
- Skin biopsy is reserved for atypical cases

DIAGNOSTIC DECISION
Presence of 'herald' patch and characteristic rash are diagnostic.

CLINICAL PEARL(S)

Once other elements of differential diagnosis have been excluded, the main issues with pityriasis rosea are patient comfort and reassurance that it is a self-limiting condition.

THE TESTS
Body fluids
SEROLOGY FOR SYPHILIS
Description
If syphilis is suspected as cause of rash, *Treponema pallidum* hemagglutination test will identify treponeme-specific antibodies in patient's blood.

Advantages/Disadvantages
Advantage: quick and easy to obtain
Disadvantage: requires pathologic analysis of blood

Normal
Negative for treponeme-specific antibodies.

Abnormal
- Positive for treponeme-specific antibodies
- Keep in mind the possibility of a false-positive result

Cause of abnormal result
Infection with *Treponema pallidum* or nonvenereal treponemes (yaws and pinta).

Biopsy
SKIN BIOPSY
Description
Skin lesion removed under local anesthetic undergoes histologic analysis to ascertain cause.

Advantages/Disadvantages
Advantage: can be diagnostic in atypical cases of pityriasis rosea
Disadvantage: can lead to scarring

Normal
Normal skin architecture.

Abnormal
Lesions show inflammation of dermis and epidermis.

Cause of abnormal result
Pityriasis rosea.

Drugs, disorders and other factors that may alter results
Multiple other pathologies may be found (e.g. psoriasis, tinea).

POTASSIUM HYDROXIDE TEST
Description
Test performed to exclude fungal infection. Skin scrapings of lesion placed on microscope slide and gently heated with KOH to clear keratin. If hyphae are present (indicating fungal infection), parallel lines will be seen on microscopic examination.

Advantages/Disadvantages
Advantage: simple and cheap
Disadvantage: not diagnostic for pityriasis rosea

Normal
No fungal elements seen.

Abnormal
Hyphae seen on microscopic examination.

Cause of abnormal result
Fungal infection.

TREATMENT

CONSIDER CONSULT
- Refer to a dermatologist for further assessment and treatment if lesions do not resolve within 8 weeks

PATIENT AND CAREGIVER ISSUES
Patient or caregiver request
- **Is the rash infectious?** The rash is not contagious
- **What causes the rash?** Unknown cause, but may be due to picornavirus
- **Will the rash scar?** Rash resolves without scarring
- **Will the rash recur?** Recurrence of rash can occur over a period of years
- **Is the rash due to underlying disease?** The rash is benign and not caused by a comorbid condition

Health-seeking behavior
- **Have you used topical creams?** The patient may have tried antifungal and anti-inflammatory creams on the lesions
- **Have you taken antihistamines?** Pruritus can be a symptom
- **When did you first experience symptoms?** Identify whether the patient has delayed seeking medical advice. Patients may not present until the eruptive phase

MANAGEMENT ISSUES
Goals
- A self-limiting disease; rash does not generally require medication
- Symptomatic treatment may be required if lesions are pruritic

Management in special circumstances
PATIENT SATISFACTION/LIFESTYLE PRIORITIES
Antihistamines can be sedating, so warn patients who drive or operate machinery.

SUMMARY OF THERAPEUTIC OPTIONS
Choices
- Ultraviolet light from direct sun exposure can reduce disease severity
- Various drugs have been implicated in causing pityriasis rosea, including: bismuth, barbiturates, captopril, gold, organic mercurials, methoxypromazine, metronidazole, D-penicillamine, isotretinoin, tripelennamine hydrochloride, ketotifen, and salvarsan. Check medication history – revision of patient's regimen may result in rapid resolution
- Symptomatic treatments include oral antihistamines (chlorpheniramine, loratadine) and topical steroids (hydrocortisone)

Clinical pearl(s)
Focus of therapy should be patient comfort. This is a self-limiting condition without long-term consequence. As all therapeutic approaches have potential adverse effects, possible benefit must be balanced against these risks.

FOLLOW UP
Follow-up required to check that lesions are resolving.

Plan for review
If treatment instituted, patient should be reviewed on a 2-week basis until disease has resolved.

Information for patient or caregiver
- Disease is self-limiting
- Rash does not generally require medication
- Symptomatic treatment may be required if lesions are pruritic

DRUGS AND OTHER THERAPIES: DETAILS
Drugs
CHLORPHENIRAMINE
Antihistamine.

Dose
Adult oral dose: 2–4mg four times daily

Efficacy
Unknown.

Risks/benefits
Risks:
- Use caution with raised intraocular pressure, asthma, cardiac, hepatic and renal disease, hypertension, seizures, hyperthyroidism, peptic ulcer stenosis, and bladder neck obstruction
- Use caution with pregnancy and the elderly

Side effects and adverse reactions
- Central nervous system: anxiety, drowsiness, dizziness, headache, paresthesia
- Gastrointestinal: diarrhea, nausea
- Hematologic: hemolytic anemia, thrombocytopenia, agranulocytosis
- Eyes, ears, nose, and throat: dilated pupils, dry nose and mouth, tinnitus

Interactions (other drugs)
- Alcohol ■ Antidepressants (tricyclics and MAOIs) ■ Antimuscarinics
- Anxiolytics and hypnotics

Contraindications
- Asthma ■ Respiratory tract disease ■ Pregnancy and nursing

Acceptability to patient
Drug has sedative properties, which can affect patient's ability to operate machinery and drive.

Patient and caregiver information
Advise patients of possible side-effects.

LORATADINE
Antihistamine.

Dose
- Adult and child over 12 years of age: 10mg/day orally
- Child 6–11 years of age: 10mg (2 teaspoonsful) once daily

Efficacy
Unknown.

Risks/benefits
Risks:
- Use caution in renal impairment, prostatic hypertrophy, urinary retention, glaucoma and hepatic disease
- May affect driving
- Avoid excess alcohol
- Use caution in children and the elderly

Side effects and adverse reactions
- Central nervous system: headache, dizziness, sedation, agitation
- Gastrointestinal: dry mouth, dyspepsia, diarrhea, nausea

Interactions (other drugs)
- Cimetidine ▪ Erythromycin ▪ Fluconazole ▪ Fluoxetine ▪ Itraconazole
- Ketoconazole ▪ Miconazole ▪ Quinidine

Contraindications
- Pregnancy and nursing ▪ Porphyria

Acceptability to patient
Generally acceptable.

Patient and caregiver information
Inform patients of possible side-effects.

HYDROCORTISONE
Topical corticosteroid.

Dose
Apply to affected area up to four times daily.

Efficacy
Unknown in pityriasis rosea.

Risks/benefits
Risks:
- Systemic absorption of topical corticosteroids has produced reversible hypothalamic-pituitary-adrenal (HPA) axis suppression, manifestations of Cushing's syndrome, hyperglycemia, and glucosuria in some patients
- Therefore, patients receiving a large dose of a potent topical steroid applied to a large surface area or under an occlusive dressing should be evaluated periodically for evidence of HPA axis suppression
- Pediatric patients may absorb proportionally larger amounts of topical corticosteroids and thus be more susceptible to systemic toxicity
- If irritation develops, topical corticosteroids should be discontinued

Benefit: Simple dosing regimen allows for better patient compliance, also allows for application directly to area affected

Side effects and adverse reactions
Skin: burning, itching, irritation, dryness, folliculitis, hypertrichosis, acneiform eruptions, hypopigmentation, perioral dermatitis, allergic contact dermatitis, maceration of the skin, secondary infection, skin atrophy, striae, miliaria

Interactions (other drugs)
■ No known interactions with topical hydrocortisone

Contraindications
■ Should be used during pregnancy only if the potential benefit justifies the potential risk to the fetus ■ Use on face, axilla or groin

Acceptability to patient
Generally acceptable.

Patient and caregiver information
Inform patients of possible side-effects.

EFFICACY OF THERAPIES

Complete resolution of rash occurs within 2–6 weeks.

Review period

- Patient should be reviewed weekly, especially if therapy is instituted
- Diagnosis should be reviewed if lesions do not improve

PROGNOSIS

- Spontaneous resolution of rash occurs within 4–8 weeks
- Recurrence is rare

Clinical pearl(s)

Reassurance is key to management of these patients, as the clinical appearance can at times be dramatic.

Therapeutic failure

Refer to a dermatologist to ensure that correct diagnosis has been made.

Recurrence

Refer to a dermatologist to ensure that correct diagnosis has been made

Deterioration

Refer to a dermatologist to ensure that correct diagnosis has been made.

CONSIDER CONSULT

- If lesions recur, refer to a dermatologist for further assessment and appropriate treatment

RISK FACTORS

- Low infectivity means that household contacts rarely contract the disorder
- There are no clear risk factors

ASSOCIATIONS
American Academy of Dermatology
930 N. Meacham Road
PO Box 4014
Schaumburg, IL 60168-4014
Phone: (847) 330-0230
Fax: (847) 330-0050
www.aad.org

KEY REFERENCES
- Burton J. Essentials of dermatology, 3rd edn. New York: Churchill Livingstone, 1990, p139, 161
- Hope R, et al. Oxford handbook of clinical medicine. New York: Oxford University Press, 1990
- Tierney L, Lawrence M., McPhee SJ, et al. Current medical diagnosis and treatment. New York: Appleton and Lange, 1993
- Weatherall D, Ledingham JGG, Warrell DG. Oxford textbook of medicine. New York: Oxford University Press, 1988

FAQS
Question 1
Are there behavioral recommendations to help with itch?

ANSWER 1
Water, wool, soap, and sweating can cause irritation and should be avoided during the acute stages of the disease.

Question 2
I gave my patient topical hydrocortisone and the itching got worse. Does this preclude a diagnosis of pityriasis rosea?

ANSWER 2
No. Exacerbations have been reported with corticosteroid use. If there are other features that raise questions about the diagnosis these should be pursued. In this example, the possibility of tinea corporis should be reconsidered.

CONTRIBUTORS
Dennis F Saver, MD
Seth R Stevens, MD
Elma D Baron, MD

PSORIASIS

DESCRIPTION

Common chronic skin disorder characterized by excessive proliferation of keratinocytes resulting in the formation of thickened, scaly plaques; itching; and inflammatory changes of epidermis and dermis.

Various forms:

- Chronic plaque psoriasis - most common
- Guttate psoriasis - distinctive acute form that characteristically occurs in children and young adults; closely associated with preceding sore throat or tonsillitis
- Pustular psoriasis - characterized by crops of sterile pustules that erupt repeatedly over months or years on the palms and soles. Affected areas tend to become red and scaly, and painful cracks often form. May rarely become generalized
- Arthritic variants
- Erythrodermic psoriasis - severe psoriasis; may involve most of the skin surface with systemic upset

URGENT ACTION

Refer acute erythrodermic psoriasis for urgent admission.

KEY! DON'T MISS!

- Erythrodermic psoriasis: emergent condition; immediate referral required to emergency medicine or dermatology section for admission
- Generalized pustular psoriasis: immediate referral to dermatology section necessary
- Mycosis fungoides: if suspected, referral for skin biopsy may be necessary for diagnosis; if available, referral to center with expertise in this disease is desirable

BACKGROUND

ICD9 CODE
- 696.0 Psoriasis, arthritis, arthropathic
- 696.1 Psoriasis, any type except arthropathic

SYNONYMS
- Chronic plaque psoriasis
- Guttate psoriasis
- Pustular psoriasis
- Psoriatic arthropathy
- Erythrodermic psoriasis

CARDINAL FEATURES
- Primary psoriatic lesion is an erythematous papule topped by loosely adherent scale that reveals several pinpoint bleeding points if scraped
- Generally a sharply demarcated, symmetric, erythematous, silver-scaled patch
- Occurs mainly on extensor surfaces, elbows, knees, and scalp; may also occur in flexures, intergluteal folds (scale is not prominent in these areas), and fingernails and toenails
- Nail involvement is common – pitting of the nail plate results in hyperkeratosis, onychodystrophy, and onycholysis
- Pruritus is variable
- Can develop at the site of any trauma – Koebner phenomenon
- Joint involvement can result in sacroiliitis and spondylitis
- Guttate psoriasis is generally preceded by 1–2 weeks by a streptococcal infection and manifests as multiple drop-like lesions on the extremities and trunk; may be mistaken for a drug eruption before the scale has a chance to develop

CAUSES
Common causes
- Etiology is unknown
- Previously thought to be a disease primarily of keratinocytes, but there is evidence to suggest that it is immunologically mediated

Contributory or predisposing factors
- Streptococcal infection
- Drugs – beta-blockers, lithium, antimalarials, withdrawal of oral steroids
- Alcohol
- Trauma
- HIV
- Endocrine – improves during pregnancy and relapses in the postpartum period
- Smoking – strong association with palmoplantar pustular psoriasis but no evidence that this improves if smoking is stopped

EPIDEMIOLOGY
Incidence and prevalence
INCIDENCE
Approximately 9.7–23/1000. Relatively rare in West African and North African-Americans.

PREVALENCE
Affects 1–3% of the world population.

Demographics
AGE
Peak age of onset in adolescence and at 60 years but may occur at any age.

GENDER
Men and women are equally affected.

GENETICS
- Strong association with HLA B13, B17, B27 (particularly pustular)
- Genetic linkage studies show susceptibility locus on chromosome 6q
- Familial clustering occurs – one-third of people have a positive family history
- An affected first-degree relative confers increased risk – 60% increase in risk if both parents are affected

DIFFERENTIAL DIAGNOSIS
Contact dermatitis
The key features of contact dermatitis are as follows:

FEATURES
- Redness and weeping followed by dryness and fissuring
- Common irritants include detergents, soaps, oils, solvents, alkalis, and nickel
- Occurs in the area of contact

Atopic dermatitis
The key features of atopic dermatitis are as follows:

FEATURES
- Skin dryness
- Red and weepy
- Itchy
- May become lichenified
- Nummular or discoid patches may resemble psoriatic plaques but are not usually so scaly and are usually poorly demarcated

Nummular dermatitis
The key features of nummular dermatitis are as follows:

FEATURES
- Skin dryness
- Red and weepy
- Itchy
- May become lichenified
- Nummular or discoid patches may resemble psoriatic plaques but are not usually so scaly

Seborrheic dermatitis
The key features of seborrheic dermatitis are as follows:

FEATURES
- May coexist with psoriasis
- Common red scaly rash
- Affects scalp, eyebrows, nasolabial folds, cheeks, flexures

Tinea fungal infections
The key features of tinea infections are as follows:

FEATURES
- Solitary or few lesions that are expanding and asymmetric
- Well-defined red lesions with peripheral scale and central clearing

Candidiasis
The key features of candidiasis are as follows:

FEATURES
- Typically found in mouth and vagina and around the nails, web spaces, and submammary areas, but also in flexures
- Skin is red, often moist, and there may be satellite lesions

Mycosis fungoides

The key features of mycosis fungoides are as follows:

FEATURES
- Cutaneous T-cell lymphoma
- Well-defined red scaly patches on trunk and limbs, which may initially be confused with psoriasis and biopsy at this point, may not be diagnostic
- Later, more typical patches develop with central clearing or arciform or polycyclic arrangement

Cutaneous lupus erythematosus

The key features of cutaneous lupus erythematous (LE) are as follows:

FEATURES
- Light exposure may trigger erythematous eruptions
- Malar rash typical – fixed erythematosus over cheeks and bridge of nose
- More diffuse maculopapular rash is also common
- Discoid lesions are circular with an erythematous rim; are raised and scaly with follicular plugging and telangiectasia; and occur over the scalp, ears, face, and sun-exposed areas of arms, back, and chest

Secondary/tertiary syphilis

The key features of secondary/tertiary syphilis are as follows:

FEATURES
- Secondary syphilis rash is macular, papular, papulosquamous, and occasionally pustular on palms, soles, and scalp
- Could be confused with palmopustular psoriasis in the early stages
- The gummas of tertiary syphilis in the skin are painless, nodular, papulosquamous lesions that may be red and ulcerated. They form characteristic arcs or circles with peripheral hyperpigmentation

Drug reaction

The key features of drug reactions are as follows:

FEATURES
- Macular erythema and red papules particularly affecting the trunk are the most common
- Guttate psoriasis may be mistaken for a drug reaction before the scale has had a chance to develop, especially if the patient has been given penicillin for a sore throat or tonsillitis
- Drugs such as beta-blockers, thiazides, gold, and antimalarials may produce lichenoid drug eruptions

SIGNS & SYMPTOMS
Signs
- Symmetric, well-defined plaques with silvery scale
- Characteristic scale is coarse and described as micaceous (like the mineral mica)
- Pinpoint bleeding on scraping
- Distribution: extensor surfaces, scalp, sacrum, and flexures
- Lesions in flexures are not scaly
- Nail changes – pepper pot nail pitting, onycholysis (separation from the nail bed), thickening, subungual hyperkeratosis, oil spotting may occur
- Guttate psoriasis – very small plaques often in young patients after streptococcal throat infection
- Pustular psoriasis – sterile pustules affecting palms and soles, often with fissuring

- Erythrodermic psoriasis and generalized pustular psoriasis may cause severe systemic upset with fever, dehydration, and raised white blood cell count. May be triggered by rapid withdrawal of systemic steroids
- Koebner phenomenon

Symptoms
Patients may present to the family physician with the following symptoms:
- Asymptomatic: typical rash identified coincidentally at consultation for another condition
- Rash
- Itching
- Joint pains
- Nail problems
- Systemic upset – generally unwell with fever in erythrodermic psoriasis

ASSOCIATED DISORDERS
- Arthropathy: distal interphalangeal joint disease, large single joint oligoarthritis, arthritis mutilans (telescoping fingers), sacroiliitis, and psoriatic spondylitis are all described. About 8% of patients with psoriasis develop arthropathy; of these, arthritis may precede skin involvement in about one in six. Males and females are equally affected
- Malabsorption: Crohn's disease and ulcerative colitis are both associated with psoriasis

KEY! DON'T MISS!
- Erythrodermic psoriasis: emergent condition; immediate referral required to emergency medicine or dermatology section for admission
- Generalized pustular psoriasis: immediate referral to dermatology section necessary
- Mycosis fungoides: if suspected, referral for skin biopsy may be necessary for diagnosis; if available, referral to center with expertise in this disease is desirable

CONSIDER CONSULT
- Skin biopsy is rarely necessary for diagnosis, but referral may be indicated in cases of doubt or if mycosis fungoides is suspected

INVESTIGATION OF THE PATIENT
Direct questions to patient
Q For how long have you had the rash? May have waxed and waned over long periods before the patient seeks treatment. Acute guttate psoriasis may appear a couple of weeks after a sore throat.

Q What is it like? Psoriasis is typically a well-demarcated silvery patch except in flexures. Fungal infections tend to be red and weepy, whereas eczema and dermatitis are erythematous and dry.

Q Where is it on your body? Typically the extensor surfaces are affected, although it may occur on the scalp and flexures too. Pustular psoriasis affects palms and soles; inverse psoriasis describes thinner, moist lesions of psoriasis in intertriginous areas. Fungal infections are often in moist, unexposed areas; contact dermatitis occurs in areas in contact with an allergen, often the hands, face, and umbilicus from the nickel button in a pair of jeans; discoid lupus occurs in sun-exposed areas; maculopapular drug eruptions often occur on the trunk.

Q Does it itch? Psoriasis is variably itchy. Contact and atopic dermatitis are often extremely itchy.

Q Does it bleed? Scraping a psoriatic lesion reveals little pinprick bleeding points.

Q Have you been unwell recently? Have you had a sore throat? Streptococcal infection may precede guttate psoriasis.

Q How do you feel now? A patient who is becoming erythrodermic may feel systemically unwell with fever and shivering.

Q Have you been in contact with any allergens? Contact dermatitis occurs in areas in contact with an allergen.

Q **Have you noticed any problems with your nails?** Pitting and separation from the nail bed may occur.

Q **Have you had any joint pains or backache?** 8% of patients develop psoriatic arthropathy.

Contributory or predisposing factors

Q **Are you taking any medication?** Beta-blockers, antimalarials, and lithium may all exacerbate psoriasis. In addition, these drugs, as well as gold, may provoke a lichenoid drug eruption. Antibiotics commonly cause maculopapular skin eruptions.

Q **How much alcohol do you drink?** There is a strong association with alcohol and a significant increase in risk for the development of psoriasis with excess alcohol; more pronounced for men.

Q **Do you smoke?** Smoking is associated particularly with pustular psoriasis.

Q **Are you pregnant or have you recently had a baby?** May improve during pregnancy and flare postpartum.

Q **Do you know your HIV status?** May become very severe in association with HIV infection.

Family history

Q **Have any members of your family had a similar rash?** Strong family history in psoriasis. There are two peaks in age distribution. Onset before the age of 40 is associated with familial psoriasis.

Examination

- **Complete physical examination:** should include the whole of the skin surface
- **General examination:** should include fever and hydration status because erythrodermic patients may be seriously unwell
- **Examine throat:** for tonsillitis or sign of possible streptococcal infection
- **Examine the rash:** also look for further lesions on the whole skin surface – description and distribution will aid diagnosis
- **Description of lesions:** the well-demarcated silvery-scaled lesion of psoriasis is fairly typical. Look for erythema, scaling, demarcation, whether macular or papular, central clearing
- **Distribution of lesions:** psoriasis occurs mainly on extensor surfaces, fungal infections are common in moist unexposed areas, and lupus erythematosus is more common in sun-exposed areas
- **Observe the Koebner phenomenon:** lesion may occur in site of trauma, e.g. further patches of psoriasis along scratch lines
- **Scrape some scale from a lesion:** Auspitz sign is pinpoint bleeding under the scale
- **Inspect nails:** may show pitting, separation from the bed (onycholysis), thickening and subungual hyperkeratosis, oil spots
- **Examine joints and back:** may be signs of arthropathy, e.g. deformities of fingers, and stiffness of lower spine and sacroiliac joints

Summary of investigative tests

- Laboratory tests are not required for positive diagnosis
- Some investigations may be useful to exclude differential diagnoses, e.g. swabs/skin scrapings may be useful to exclude fungal infection and skin biopsy may be required if there is doubt or it is reasonable to exclude mycosis fungoides (but may not always be diagnostic in the early stages of mycosis fungoides)

DIAGNOSTIC DECISION

Diagnosis is clinically based on history and examination of the lesions, with investigations to exclude differential diagnoses in doubtful cases.

CLINICAL PEARLS

The morphology of the primary lesions is usually key to the diagnosis. The silvery micaceous scale will show the laminations typical of this mineral.

THE TESTS
Biopsy
SKIN BIOPSY
Description
Surgical sampling of the skin.

Advantages/Disadvantages
Advantage: can distinguish other elements of the differential diagnosis
Disadvantages: those of minor surgery

Normal
Normal skin.

Abnormal
Inflammation, vascular ectasia, acanthosis.

Cause of abnormal result
Inflammatory component and epidermal hyperproliferative response.

Drugs, disorders and other factors that may alter results
Effective therapy.

TREATMENT

CONSIDER CONSULT

- All patients with generalized disease should be referred
- Admission may be necessary for severe diffuse or poorly responsive disease
- Patients not responding to intermittent topical treatment should be referred for consideration of systemic treatment
- Refer to dermatologist if adequate control is not obtained without significant adverse effects of therapy

IMMEDIATE ACTION

Erythrodermic patients and those with generalized psoriasis require immediate admission.

PATIENT AND CAREGIVER ISSUES
Impact on career, dependants, family, friends

May be stigmatizing for the patient and much more emotionally than physically disabling for most patients. Palmoplantar pustular psoriasis may cause minimal symptoms but is very often debilitating, interfering with work and everyday activities involving hands and mobility.

Patient or caregiver request

A common misconception is that psoriasis is contagious. Many patients may believe some infectious etiology to be responsible.

Health-seeking behavior

Self-management? Patients may have tried over-the-counter emollients, tar shampoos, exposure to sunlight, or other complementary therapies before seeking advice.

MANAGEMENT ISSUES
Goals

- To minimize the extent and severity of the condition
- To prevent substantial disruption of the patient's quality of life

Management in special circumstances

Erythrodermic patients may become extremely systemically unwell and should be admitted for treatment without delay.

COEXISTING DISEASE

- Patients with hypertension would be better treated with drugs other than beta-blockers
- Antimalarial agents may not be avoidable – patients with malaria should be informed of the risks. Antimalarials, specifically hydroxychloroquine, often cause psoriasis to flare. Ultimately, treatment of malaria in the setting of concomitant psoriasis should be managed by a specialist. Adverse side effects for hydroxychloroquine can include retinopathy, corneal opacities, blurred vision, hematologic, pigmentary, constitutional, myopathy, and toxic psychosis (rare)
- Coexisting psoriatic arthropathy may direct choice of treatment to oral medication such as methotrexate

COEXISTING MEDICATION

- Combinations such as keratolytics and oral retinoids should be avoided
- Other cutaneous eruptions, notably drug eruptions or contact dermatitis, may manifest as or evolve to typical lesions of psoriasis. Attention should be paid to identify such instances (e.g. unusual distribution of patient's usual psoriasis) and the offending agent avoided

SPECIAL PATIENT GROUPS
Women of childbearing years should be aware of the potential teratogenicity of retinoids, and these should not be used if pregnancy is desired within the next couple of years.

PATIENT SATISFACTION/LIFESTYLE PRIORITIES
- Creams and ointments may be messy and time-consuming to use
- Treatment should be tailored to fit in with the patient's lifestyle

SUMMARY OF THERAPEUTIC OPTIONS
Choices
May be a difficult condition to treat, and there are few evidence-based guidelines available to help make sensible choices for therapy. In particular, there is currently no firm evidence on which to base the treatment of acute guttate psoriasis, and studies comparing standard available therapies are required.

Palmoplantar pustular psoriasis tends to be unresponsive to topical therapy in most patients. Dermatologists have found topical psoralen, photochemotherapy, and systemic retinoids to be of most value.

Patient education is essential and aids compliance with prescribed therapy. Management options available include the following:

Removal of possible triggers:
- Streptococcal infection – antibiotics are widely advocated
- Drugs such as beta-blockers, lithium, antimalarials
- Stress
- Smoking
- Alcohol

Nondrug treatments:
- Heliotherapy
- Acupuncture
- Dietary manipulation

Topical drugs:
- Emollients and keratolytics: suitable for very mild psoriasis or as adjunct to other therapies
- Tar preparations: suitable for all types of psoriasis and may be used in conjunction with other treatments
- Anthralin: UVB radiation for more severe, extensive forms of psoriasis
- Calcipotriene: vitamin D derivative, indicated for mild to moderate chronic plaque psoriasis covering up to 40% of the body
- Topical steroids: may be useful for small areas for short periods in treatment of chronic plaque psoriasis. Probably best avoided due to adverse effects and potential severe flare on withdrawal
- Topical retinoids: indicated for mild to moderate psoriasis affecting up to 10% of the skin area

Phototherapy:
Indicated for moderate to severe psoriasis and extensive large plaque psoriasis, and requires referral to a specialist center. There are several different types and regimens, including broad- or narrow-band UVB and psoralens and ultraviolet A (PUVA)

Oral drugs:

These are second-line treatments and should be used under specialist supervision.

- Oral retinoids: acitretin is indicated for severe, resistant, extensive psoriasis. May be better for pustular and erythrodermic psoriasis than chronic plaque psoriasis. Not first-line treatment; should be used under the supervision of dermatologist only
- Methotrexate: indicated for use in severe resistant psoriasis under specialist direction. May also be used in psoriatic arthritis
- Cyclosporine and other immunosuppressants: also indicated for severe resistant psoriasis under specialist advice

Clinical pearls

Rotation of therapies may help avoid cumulative toxicities (e.g. skin cancers in PUVA-treated patients or renal complications in cyclosporine-treated patients).

Never

- Never withdraw oral steroids abruptly; always give reducing course over last weeks of treatment
- Anthralin is contraindicated in pustular psoriasis

FOLLOW UP
Plan for review

The frequency of consultation will be determined by the therapy used. Some require no specific follow up and consultation may be patient-initiated, whereas others will require intensive monitoring and weekly blood tests or hospital admission. It may be useful to see the patient 6 months after clearing has occurred to the patient's satisfaction to determine whether the condition has relapsed and other therapy may be indicated.

Information for patient or caregiver

Patients should be informed that psoriasis is a relapsing and remitting condition for which there is no permanent cure. A physician's advice should be sought if it flares or becomes unresponsive to the usual treatment.

DRUGS AND OTHER THERAPIES: DETAILS
Drugs
EMOLLIENTS AND KERATOLYTICS

- Many emollient preparations are available. Aqueous cream, emulsifying ointment, and petrolatum may also be bought over the counter. May be useful for mild psoriasis and soothing to itch
- Capsaicin is an alkaloid derivative of the *Solanaceae* plant family
- Keratolytics such as salicylates and urea can be used to enhance rate of loss of surface scale

Dose

- Emollients can be used topically as frequently as necessary
- Capsaicin applied three to five times daily for 3–5 months or as long as necessary
- Preparations containing salicylic acid 2% are used initially, gradually increased to 3–6% concentration. Urea creams come in strengths as high as 40%. Apply twice daily in a thin layer
- Preparations containing urea should be applied two or three times per day
- Preparations containing petrolatum should be applied following manufacturer's instructions

Efficacy

Emollients are not very efficacious alone but are a useful adjunct to other treatments.

Risks/benefits
Risks:
- Use caution in children
- Avoid contact with mucous membranes, eyes, and surrounding normal skin
- Use preparations containing urea with caution when hepatic disease, renal disease, electrolyte imbalance, cardiac disease, congestive heart failure, or hypovolemia is present
- Salicylate toxicity may occur when large areas are treated
- Do not take a bath or shower either before or after applying capsaicin

Benefit: Emollients are safe and easy to use

Side effects and adverse reactions
- Burning, itching of skin where applied
- Urea may cause extravasation and phlebitis
- Salicylics may cause skin irritation, sensitivity, and dryness
- Systemic effects after long-term use (salicylism: dizziness, confusion headache, tinnitus, hearing disturbances)

Interactions (other drugs)
- No recorded drug interactions

Contraindications
- Hypersensitivity to any component

Salicylic acid:
- Diabetes or other disorders with impaired blood circulation ▪ Warts on mucous membranes, facial areas, or genital areas ▪ Warts with hairs growing from them ▪ Moles, birthmarks ▪ Infected or irritated skin

Capsaicin:
- Broken or damaged skin

Evidence
Emollients may be effective in the management of psoriasis.
- A systematic review compared capsaicin with other treatments in the management of chronic plaque psoriasis. Erythema, scaling, and itching were improved in patients treated with capsaicin. There was significant heterogeneity in the trial results [1] *Level M*
- Another systematic review examined the efficacy of aloe vera in a number of conditions, including psoriasis. Although a clinically important effect was not excluded, the effectiveness of aloe vera in the treatment of psoriasis was not proven [2] *Level M*
- A blinded randomized controlled trial (RCT) compared a lubricating base (oil-in-water type) plus UVB exposure vs UVB alone in patients with stable plaque psoriasis. The combination treatment led to a significantly greater improvement in scaling, infiltration, and erythema [3] *Level P*

Acceptability to patient
- Emollients can often be greasy to use and uncomfortable to have on the skin, which may reduce compliance
- Capsaicin may burn, but topical lidocaine before treatment may relieve this

Patient and caregiver information
- Use emollients regularly for best effect

- Salicylic acid for external use only – avoid on face, eyes, genitalia, mucous membranes, and normal skin. Soaking skin for 5min prior to application may improve effect

TAR PREPARATIONS

- Tars are well established in the treatment of psoriasis and have antiscaling and anti-inflammatory properties
- Coal tar paste is suitable for most cases
- Also available with zinc, in bandage form, as tar shampoo, and as bath additives
- Preparations combined with zinc or salicylic acid have no advantage over simpler preparations
- May be used as part of the Ingram regimen, which involves a daily coal tar bath, UVB irradiation, and anthralin; also used in the Goeckerman treatment, which involves a daily coal tar bath followed by UVB irradiation

Dose

- Formulation and strength depend on patient acceptance and severity of the condition – the thicker the patch, the stronger the strength of tar required
- Apply one to three times daily

Efficacy
More effective than salicylic acid.

Risks/benefits
Risks:

- Messy to use
- Should not get into eyes or onto mucosal or genital areas
- Should not get onto broken or inflamed skin
- May need to use gloves to administer
- Stains hair, skin, and clothing

Side effects and adverse reactions
Skin: irritation, acne-like eruptions, photosensitivity.

Interactions (other drugs)

- No known interactions

Contraindications

- Skin infection ■ Pustular or acute psoriasis

Evidence
A small RCT compared tar with emollient in psoriasis patients. Tar was found to be more effective in improving disease activity scores [4] Level P

Acceptability to patient
Tar preparations are smelly, stain clothes and burn, and are generally disliked by patients.

Patient and caregiver information

- Do not use on face and avoid eye contact
- Wash hands immediately after use

ANTHRALIN

- Preparation is applied carefully to lesion
- Usual concentrations are 0.1–3%
- Lower concentrations may be applied overnight, but higher concentrations (1–3%) should be applied for shorter contact periods of 30–60min

- May be used in hospital as part of the Ingram regimen: coal tar bath, UVB irradiation, followed by anthralin paste applied to lesions. Normal skin is protected by talc

Dose
- Test skin sensitivity at 0.1% concentration before using higher strengths
- Further increases should be gradual – start with 0.1% and increase every 7 days until therapeutic effect without irritation is obtained

Efficacy
Good efficacy in the short-term.

Risks/benefits
Risks:
- Use caution in renal and hepatic impairment
- Use caution on inflamed skin and when applying to face or genitals

Side effects and adverse reactions
Skin: irritation, hypersensitivity, staining of nails and hair.

Interactions (other drugs)
- None recorded

Contraindications
- Acute or actively inflamed psoriasis ■ Safety and effectiveness in children not established
- Pregnancy category C

Evidence
Two small RCTs have found that anthralin improves chronic plaque psoriasis when compared with placebo [5] *Level P*

Acceptability to patient
Smell, staining, and burning may be a problem. May cause quite severe skin irritation to perilesional skin.

Follow up plan
Patient will need to be seen regularly to assess response and increase strength of preparation.

Patient and caregiver information
- Do not apply to flexures
- Wash hands after use
- Continued use in patients sensitive to anthralin can result in psoriasis becoming unstable; more likely in fair than in dark skin

CALCIPOTRIENE
- Vitamin D derivative used topically
- Widely used for mild to moderate psoriasis affecting up to 40% of skin area

Dose
Cream or ointment applied once or twice daily up to a maximum of 100g/week.

Efficacy
- Benefit in mild to moderate psoriasis
- Once-daily preparation slightly less effective
- Same as or slightly more effective than topical steroids, anthralin, and coal tar
- Combination of calcipotriene with topical steroids provides better clearance and maintenance

Risks/benefits
Risk: May cause transient skin irritation

Benefits:
- No unpleasant smell
- Does not stain clothing

Side effects and adverse reactions
Skin: irritation, rash, pruritus, dermatitis, possible worsening of psoriasis.

Interactions (other drugs)
- None recorded

Contraindications
- Should not be used by patients with hypercalcemia or vitamin D toxicity

Evidence
There is evidence for the use of calcipotriene in the management of chronic plaque psoriasis.
- A systematic review assessed the use of calcipotriene in patients with mild to moderate chronic plaque psoriasis. Calcipotriene was found to have similar or better efficacy compared with other medications used for psoriasis (including tar, topical steroids, and dithranol); however, it did cause more skin irritation than potent topical corticosteroids [6] *Level M*
- Calcipotriene has been found in RCTs to be as effective as or more effective than topical steroids, dithranol short contact treatment, and coal tar. Combination therapy with topical steroids leads to better clearance and maintenance [5] *Level P*

Acceptability to patient
Causes more irritation than potent topical steroids. Perilesional irritation in 25% of patients.

Follow up plan
Periodic review to assess response and continued need for treatment.

Patient and caregiver information
Do not use more than 100g/week. Adverse effects of hypercalcemia and hypercalciuria are dose-related.

TOPICAL STEROIDS
- Limited use
- Short periods of up to 4 weeks for flexural or facial psoriasis; no stronger than hydrocortisone on the face
- Mid- to high potency may be used in the treatment of chronic plaque psoriasis
- May be used in conjunction with calcipotriene
- Long-term use must be avoided – may cause atrophy, striae, telangiectasia, skin fragility, and dyspigmentation; mask local infections; and produce systemic side effects
- Severe flares may occur on withdrawal, and pustular psoriasis may be precipitated
- Tachyphylaxis (diminishing clinical response with repeated use) is described but no estimate of its frequency

Dose
- Studies have mainly examined courses of no longer than 8 weeks
- Betamethasone once weekly gave better control than placebo at 6 months when used for maintenance (but only assessed a target area)
- Actual dose will depend on the chosen preparation and is applied once or twice daily

Efficacy
- As effective as calcipotriene
- Improves psoriasis in the short term, reduction in erythema and scale

Risks/benefits
Benefit: will potentially improve psoriasis by thinning plaques.

Side effects and adverse reactions
Skin: rash, dermatitis, pruritus, atrophy, hypopigmentation, striae, xerosis, burning, stinging upon application, alopecia, conjunctivitis.

Interactions (other drugs)
- No known interactions with topical betamethasone

Contraindications
- Do not use on face, axilla, or groin

Evidence
Topical corticosteroids may be effective for the temporary treatment of psoriasis.
- RCTs have shown temporary improvement in psoriatic lesions with the use of mid- to high-potency topical corticosteroids [5] *Level P*
- Psoriasis patients with controlled disease after a 3- to 4-week course of topical corticosteroids (augmented betamethasone dipropionate) were entered into a blinded RCT. Patients were randomized to corticosteroid treatment once weekly for 6 months and placebo groups. Control of disease was better in the treatment group [7] *Level P*

Follow up plan
Careful follow up required to avoid prolonged use or abrupt withdrawal.

Patient and caregiver information
Stopping abruptly may cause severe disease flare.

TOPICAL RETINOIDS
- Tazarotene
- Indicated for mild to moderate psoriasis affecting up to 10% of skin area
- Retained in the skin for long periods

Dose
Apply once daily in evening.

Efficacy
Improves chronic plaque psoriasis in comparison with placebo.

Risks/benefits
Risks:
- Skin irritation
- Do not use on eczematous skin
- Avoid contact with eyes, eyelids, and mouth

Side effects and adverse reactions
Skin: irritation - desquamation, pruritus, burning, stinging, dryness, discoloration

Interactions (other drugs)
- Tetracyclines and sulfonamides (concomitant administration may increase risk of photosensitization)

Contraindications
- Pregnancy category X
- Safety and efficacy not established in children under 12 years

Evidence
RCTs have demonstrated that tazarotene is effective in the management of chronic plaque psoriasis. When used in combination with topical corticosteroids, further benefit may be achieved [5] *Level P*

Acceptability to patient
Patients may experience irritation – variable from patient to patient.

Follow up plan
Follow up required to assess response and continued need for treatment. Usual course up to 12 weeks.

Patient and caregiver information
- Wash hands after use
- Avoid contact with eyes
- Avoid excessive exposure to UV light
- Women should use effective contraception

ORAL RETINOIDS
- Acitretin
- Metabolite of etretinate, a vitamin A derivative
- Indicated for severe extensive resistant or complicated psoriasis, palmoplantar pustular psoriasis
- Prescribed only by or under supervision of a consultant dermatologist

Dose
- In accordance with expert's advice
- Initially 25–30mg/day for 2–4 weeks, then adjusted according to response
- Usual range 25–50mg/day

Efficacy
Marked effects on keratinizing epithelia.

Risks/benefits
Risks:
- Side effects can be significant
- Women of childbearing age should use contraception during and for 3 years after therapy
- Use caution in renal insufficiency, liver disease, hyperlipidemia, and pancreatitis
- Teratogenic – can be converted to etretinate in patients who consume alcohol. This metabolite persists in fat for many years and can be high enough to be teratogenic

Benefit: High efficacy

Side effects and adverse reactions
- Central nervous system: dizziness, fatigue, headache

- Eyes, ears, nose, and throat: cheilitis, dry eyes and nose, conjunctivitis, xerostomia
- Metabolism: abnormal liver function tests, hypertriglyceridemia, hyperglycemia
- Musculoskeletal: arthralgia, myalgia
- Skin: alopecia, dry skin

Interactions (other drugs)
- Methotrexate ▪ Alcohol ▪ Tetracyclines ▪ Progesterone

Contraindications
- Pregnancy ▪ Alcohol ▪ Use of vitamin A

Evidence

Oral retinoids may be effective for the clearance of psoriasis, but there is a high incidence of adverse effects.
- RCTs comparing etretinate with placebo or conventional therapy have found clearance rates between 15 and 90% [5] *Level P*
- An RCT compared acitretin and etretinate in the management of severe psoriasis. Similar efficacy was noted with both medications, but mucocutaneous adverse effects and the withdrawal rate were higher with acitretin [8] *Level P*
- Evidence from RCTs suggests that pustular and erythrodermic psoriasis are more responsive to oral retinoid than plaque psoriasis [5] *Level P*

Acceptability to patient
- Most patients suffer dry, cracked lips and mild transient increase in hair fall (reversible)
- May be unacceptable to women of childbearing years because it is teratogenic

Follow up plan
- Treatment period should be limited to 6–9 months with a 3- to 4-month rest period before commencing treatment again
- Contraception must be used one month before treatment begins and for 2 years after a course of the drug
- Monitor hepatic function and lipids at start, one month after initiating treatment, and then every 3 months

Patient and caregiver information
- Takes time to show effects – therapeutic effect after 2–4 weeks and maximum benefit after 4–6 weeks
- Avoid pregnancy for one month before and 2 years after treatment
- Avoid tetracycline
- Avoid use of keratolytics
- Do not donate blood for at least one year after treatment (teratogenic effect)
- Avoid excessive sunlight and unsupervised use of sunlamps

METHOTREXATE
- Indicated for severe resistant psoriasis
- Also for use in psoriatic arthropathy
- Given under specialist supervision

Dose
- Dose adjusted to severity of condition and in accordance with hematologic and biochemical measures
- Usual dose: 10–25mg once weekly, orally or intramuscularly

Efficacy
Improves skin lesions while therapy continues, but about one-half of patients relapse within 6 months of stopping treatment.

Risks/benefits
Risks:
- Use caution with infection and bone marrow depression
- Use caution in peptic ulceration and ulcerative colitis, and renal and hepatic impairment
- Use caution with the elderly and in pregnancy

Side effects and adverse reactions
- Central nervous system: headache, seizures, dizziness, drowsiness
- Eyes, ears, nose, and throat: visual disturbances, tinnitus
- Gastrointestinal: abdominal pain, diarrhea, hepatotoxicity, nausea, vomiting, stomatitis
- Genitourinary: renal failure, urinary retention, depression of and defective spermatogenesis, hematuria
- Hematologic: blood cell disorders
- Musculoskeletal: osteoporosis, muscle pain and wasting
- Respiratory: pulmonary fibrosis
- Skin: rashes, acne, dermatitis, alopecia, hyperpigmentation, vasculitis

Interactions (other drugs)
- Aminoglycosides ■ Antimalarials ■ Binding resins ■ Co-trimoxazole ■ Cyclosporine
- Ethanol ■ Etretinate ■ Live vaccines ■ NSAIDs ■ Omeprazole ■ Penicillins
- Probenecid ■ Salicylates ■ Sulfinpyrazone

Contraindications
- Severe renal and hepatic impairment ■ Profound bone marrow depression
- Nursing mothers, pregnancy, and avoid conception for 6 months after stopping

Evidence
Methotrexate may improve chronic plaque psoriasis.
- A small RCT compared methotrexate with placebo. The extent of skin lesions was reduced compared with placebo after 12 weeks [9] *Level P*
- An uncontrolled trial found that maintenance with weekly low dose methotrexate (not to exceed 15mg) provided skin control in 81% of patients over a mean of 8 years; 45% experienced a full relapse within 6 months of cessation of treatment [10] *This study does not meet the criteria for level P*

Acceptability to patient
- Potential serious adverse effects may prove unacceptable
- Strict follow up with regular venesection may be unattractive

Follow up plan
Monitor liver function, complete blood count, and renal function before starting treatment and weekly until therapy is stabilized, thereafter every 2–3 months.

Patient and caregiver information
- Limit alcohol consumption because it may potentiate liver toxicity
- Report all signs and symptoms suggestive of infection, especially sore throat
- Report cough or breathlessness (interstitial pneumonitis)
- Men and women should both avoid conception for at least 6 months after stopping treatment

CYCLOSPORINE

- Indicated for severe resistant psoriasis
- Specialist supervision required

Dose

- Initially 2.5mg/kg/day in two divided doses, increased gradually to maximum 5mg/kg/day if no improvement within one month
- Discontinue if response still insufficient after 6 weeks
- Reduce by 25–50% if serum creatinine increases 30% above baseline
- Discontinue if reduction not successful after one month

Efficacy

Clears psoriasis especially at higher doses, but toxicity is high.

Risks/benefits

Risks:

- Increased susceptibility to infection and possible development of neoplasia
- Bacterial, fungal, viral, and protozoal infections often occur and can be fatal
- Avoid excessive sunlight
- Use caution in children and the elderly
- Use caution in hypertension and hepatic or biliary tract disease
- Recent vaccinations will be rendered ineffective

Benefit: Has no depressant effects on bone marrow

Side effects and adverse reactions

- Cardiovascular system: hypertension
- Central nervous system: tremors, seizures, encephalopathy, confusion, depression, headache, dizziness, insomnia, paresthesias, fever
- Eyes, ears, nose, and throat: gingival hyperplasia
- Gastrointestinal: nausea, vomiting, diarrhea, elevated hepatic enzymes, hepatotoxicity, abdominal pain, gingivitis, stomatitis, anorexia, dyspepsia, flatulence
- Genitourinary: nephrotoxicity, hyperuricemia, menstrual irregularity, inhibition of spermatogenesis, gynecomastia
- Hematologic: thrombotic thrombocytopenic purpura, leukopenia
- Metabolic: hyperkalemia, hypercholesterolemia, hypomagnesemia, hyperglycemia
- Musculoskeletal: arthralgia, fatigue, weakness, dysarthria, myalgia
- Skin: hirsutism, acne, alopecia, rash, skin ulcers, flushing

Interactions (other drugs)

- Drugs utilizing cytochrome P-450 to be metabolized ■ Allopurinol, colchicine ■ Antidysrhythmics (amiodarone, calcium channel blockers, digoxin) ■ Antihypertensives (ACE inhibitors, acetazolamide, carvedilol, clonidine, potassium-sparing diuretics) ■ Antivirals (acyclovir, ganciclovir, antiretroviral protease inhibitors, foscarnet, nevirapine, delavirdine) ■ Antibiotics (aminoglycosides, ceftriaxone, ciprofloxacin, clarithromycin, clindamycin, erythromycin, dalfopristin, quinupristin, imipenem; cilastatin, nafcillin, norfloxacin, polymyxin B, sulfamethoxazole (SMX); trimethoprim (TMP), SMX-TMP, troleandomycin, vancomycin, sulfonamides) ■ Antifungals (amphotericin B, bacitracin, fluconazole, itraconazole, ketoconazole, griseofulvin) ■ Anticonvulsants (carbamazepine, fosphenytoin, phenobarbital, phenytoin, primidone) ■ Antineoplastics (daunorubicin, doxorubicin, epirubicin, docetaxel, etoposide, VP-16, melphalan, mitoxantrone, paclitaxel)

■ Antilipemics (fenofibrate, statins, probucol) ■ Antidiabetics (glipizide, glyburide, pioglitazone, troglitazone) ■ Antidepressants (fluoxetine, fluvoxamine, nefazodone, St. John's Wort) ■ Androgens ■ Bromocriptine ■ Cisplatin ■ Corticosteroids ■ Creatine ■ Danazol ■ Estrogens ■ Immunosuppressives ■ Methotrexate ■ Metoclopramide ■ Misoprostol ■ Modafinil ■ Mycophenolate ■ Neuromuscular blockers ■ NSAIDs ■ Omeprazole, rabeprazole ■ Orlistat ■ Rifampin ■ Sirolimus ■ Tacrolimus ■ Vinca alkaloids ■ Warfarin

Other:
■ Food (decreases cyclosporine levels) ■ Grapefruit juice (increases cyclosporine levels)

Contraindications
■ PUVA (psoriasis patients are at increased risk of developing skin cancer with this treatment) ■ Rheumatoid arthritis ■ Renal impairment ■ Known polyoxyethylated castor oil hypersensitivity ■ Pregnancy and breast-feeding

Evidence
There is evidence for the use of cyclosporine for clearance and maintenance in psoriasis.
■ Cyclosporine has been shown to effectively clear psoriasis in RCTs, especially at higher doses. There is a high incidence of adverse effects [5] *Level P*
■ A small RCT reported that low-dose cyclosporine is effective for maintenance in palmoplantar pustular psoriasis [11] *Level P*

Acceptability to patient
104 of 122 consecutive patients treated with cyclosporine for 3–76 months at dose not exceeding 5mg/kg discontinued treatment because of adverse effects, including renal dysfunction and hypertension (average is 2 years).

Follow up plan
■ Dermatologic and physical examination required at least twice before starting – must include blood pressure and renal function blood test
■ If hypertension develops that cannot be controlled by dose reduction or antihypertensive drug, cyclosporine must be discontinued
■ Monitor serum creatinine every 2 weeks throughout first 3 months, then every 3 months

Complementary therapy
HELIOTHERAPY
Efficacy
Significantly improves psoriasis and reduces use of routine treatment in the year after a 4-week course of therapy.

Risks/benefits
Risk: if UV rays are not administered in a controlled setting, may be difficult to assess long-term nonmelanoma skin cancer risk.

Evidence
An RCT compared heliotherapy vs no treatment. Psoriasis was significantly improved, and the use of routine treatment was reduced in the year after a 4-week course of heliotherapy [12] *Level P*

ACUPUNCTURE
Efficacy
Low.

Evidence
Acupuncture did not show any benefit over placebo in the management of chronic plaque psoriasis in one RCT [13] *Level P*

Other therapies
PHOTOTHERAPY
- Requires referral to specialist center
- Improves psoriasis in the short term and when used as maintenance treatment
- Indicated for moderate to severe psoriasis
- Narrow band UVB may be given three times a week for 6 weeks and is suitable for guttate and small plaque psoriasis
- PUVA with oral or topical psoralen (usually 8-methoxsalen) is suitable for extensive large plaque psoriasis; can also be combined with oral retinoids (RePUVA) to allow decrease in light dose
- Goeckerman regimen involves a daily application of coal tar followed by UVB radiation
- Ingram regimen consists of a daily coal tar bath followed by UVB irradiation and then the application of anthralin

Efficacy
May be effective for treatment and maintenance.

Risks/benefits
Risk: provides good clearance but risk of skin malignancies with prolonged use.

Evidence
UVB phototherapy may be effective as maintenance therapy. PUVA is effective for clearance and maintenance treatment.
- An RCT compared UVB radiation with PUVA in the treatment of patients with moderate to severe psoriasis. Clearance rates were similar between the two groups; however, UVB was less effective for patients with >50% body involvement [14] *Level P*
- Another RCT found PUVA to be superior to UVB for the clearance of psoriasis [15] *Level P*
- UVB phototherapy was found to be effective as maintenance compared with control when administered weekly to patients with cleared lesions in an RCT [16] *Level P*
- There is evidence from RCTs that PUVA is an effective treatment for chronic plaque psoriasis. There is a significant risk of developing cutaneous squamous cell carcinoma with long-term use of this treatment [5] *Level P*

Acceptability to patient
- UVB may increase photoaging and risk of skin cancer
- UVA has dose-dependent increased risk of squamous cell carcinoma, basal cell carcinoma, and possibly malignant melanoma, which may be unacceptable to patient
- Risk of cataract formation can be avoided if UVA opaque glasses worn 24h after psoralen ingestion

Follow up plan
Long-term follow up required to detect development of skin malignancies.

Patient and caregiver information
Regular hospital attendance required.

ANTISTREPTOCOCCAL INTERVENTIONS
Antibiotics and tonsillectomy have both been advocated for treatment of guttate psoriasis and chronic plaque psoriasis because it is well known that guttate psoriasis may be precipitated by streptococcal infection.

Efficacy
No evidence that either is helpful.

Risks/benefits
Benefit: most efficacious in patients with guttate psoriasis. Must correlate history of previous clinical symptoms, e.g. sore throat to flare of psoriasis, hence justifying treatment.

Evidence
A systematic review found no evidence to support the use of antibiotics in the management of established guttate psoriasis or in prevention of the development after a streptococcal sore throat. Antibiotics and tonsillectomy have not been shown to be beneficial for patients with recurrent guttate psoriasis or chronic plaque psoriasis [17] *Level M*

Acceptability to patient
Patients should be aware of common adverse reactions experienced with use of antibiotics. Koebner phenomenon, resulting in worsening of psoriasis, may be seen with severe drug rashes.

Follow up plan
Monthly or bimonthly visits to assess response.

Patient and caregiver information
No good evidence for its use.

LIFESTYLE
A beneficial effect is seen by:
- Reduction of stress – using psychological interventions
- Smoking cessation
- Dietary changes including fish oil supplementation and oral vitamin D
- Reduction of alcohol intake

RISKS/BENEFITS
Benefit: psychological interventions to reduce stress improve psoriasis activity scores slightly but significantly.

ACCEPTABILITY TO PATIENT
- Some patients may have difficulty accepting referral to psychologist
- Most find smoking cessation extremely hard

PATIENT AND CAREGIVER INFORMATION
Benefit from these interventions will take time to become apparent.

EFFICACY OF THERAPIES
Unfortunately, none of the treatments provide a cure and at best they produce an improvement for a limited time before relapse occurs. Some provide longer remittance periods than others, e.g. phototherapy, and some may maintain clearance as long as the drug is taken, e.g. methotrexate. These treatments tend to have adverse effects or limitations that require their eventual withdrawal.

Evidence
Topical therapies:
- Erythema, scaling, and itching may be improved in patients treated with capsaicin. There was significant heterogeneity in the trial results in this systematic review [2] *Level M*
- Combination treatment with lubricating base (oil-in-water type) plus UVB exposure may lead to a significant improvement in scaling, infiltration, and erythema [3] *Level P*
- Tar has been found to be more effective than emollient in improving disease activity scores [4] *Level P*
- Anthralin improves chronic plaque psoriasis when compared with placebo [5] *Level P*
- Calcipotriene has been found to have similar or better efficacy than other medications used for psoriasis (including tar, topical steroids, and dithranol short contact treatment); however, it may cause more skin irritation than potent topical corticosteroids [6] *Level M*
- Combination therapy with calcipotriene and topical steroids leads to better clearance and maintenance [5] *Level P*
- RCTs have shown temporary improvement in psoriatic lesions with the use of mid-to high-potency topical corticosteroids. Occlusive dressings enhance clinical activity [5] *Level P*
- Tazarotene is effective in the short-term management of chronic plaque psoriasis. When used in combination with topical corticosteroids, further benefit may be achieved [5] *Level P*

Oral medications:
- Evidence from RCTs suggests that pustular and erythrodermic psoriasis are more responsive to oral retinoids than plaque psoriasis [5] *Level P*
- Cyclosporine has been shown to effectively clear psoriasis in RCTs, especially at higher doses. There is a high incidence of adverse effects [5] *Level P*
- A small RCT reported that low-dose cyclosporine is effective for maintenance in palmoplantar pustular psoriasis [11] *Level P*
- The combination of retinoids and PUVA or UVB accelerates the clinical response and reduces the cumulative exposure of radiation and the dose of retinoids [5] *Level P*

Other therapies:
- Psoriasis may be improved and the use of routine treatment reduced after a 4-week course of heliotherapy [12] *Level P*
- A systematic review found no evidence to support the use of antibiotics in the management of established guttate psoriasis or in preventing the development after a streptococcal sore throat. Antibiotics and tonsillectomy have not been shown to be beneficial for patients with recurrent guttate psoriasis or chronic plaque psoriasis [17] *Level M*
- Stress reduction has been shown in RCTs to improve psoriasis [5] *Level P*
- The Ingram regimen may be as effective as PUVA in the management of patients with moderate to severe psoriasis. There is no evidence for the efficacy of the Goeckerman regimen [5]

Phototherapy:
- UVB phototherapy may be effective for maintenance when administered weekly to patients with cleared lesions [16] *Level P*

■ There is evidence from RCTs that PUVA is an effective treatment for chronic plaque psoriasis. There is a significant risk of developing cutaneous squamous cell carcinoma with long-term use of this treatment [5] *Level P*

PROGNOSIS

■ Course of disease is chronic and may be refractory to treatment
■ Often difficult to treat because of sporadic course
■ Guttate psoriasis may clear spontaneously if left untreated over a period of several months or may progress to chronic plaque psoriasis
■ Pustular psoriasis may persist for decades. Treatment is difficult – topical psoralen photochemotherapy and systemic retinoids are of most value
■ 8% of patients with psoriasis will develop psoriatic arthropathy

Clinical pearls

■ Psoriasis can be debilitating due to psychosocial impact
■ There are increased rates of alcoholism amongst psoriatics. Beyond usual concerns, this is particularly relevant when considering potentially hepatotoxic therapies such as methotrexate or retinoids

Therapeutic failure

If topical treatments are ineffective in improving psoriasis or the condition worsens despite treatment, referral should be made to a specialist for consideration of phototherapy or oral second-line medications such as oral retinoids, methotrexate, and cyclosporine.

Recurrence

Due to the nature of the condition, recurrence is inevitable. First-line treatments, either the same or different, may be used again or referral for specialist treatment is an option.

Deterioration

May deteriorate to the point where the patient becomes erythrodermic and systemically unwell. Admission is indicated at this point.

Terminal illness

Highly unlikely. Generalized pustular psoriasis and erythrodermic psoriasis may be life-threatening if untreated. Psychosocial impact can cause severely affected patients to become suicidal.

COMPLICATIONS

8% of patients with psoriasis may develop psoriatic arthropathy.

CONSIDER CONSULT

■ Referral may be indicated for phototherapy or decision to use second-line oral drugs

PREVENTION

- There are no effective preventive measures to be taken against the development of psoriasis
- Flare-ups may potentially be reduced by modification of risk factors; interventions have proved disappointing

RISK FACTORS

- Smoking: associated with palmoplantar pustular psoriasis; possibly a link with chronic plaque psoriasis
- Streptococcal infection: often precedes a diagnosis of guttate psoriasis
- Drugs: especially beta-blockers, lithium, antimalarials
- Alcohol: strong association between heavy drinking and development of psoriasis

MODIFY RISK FACTORS
Lifestyle and wellness
TOBACCO
Unfortunately there is no evidence that stopping smoking benefits palmoplantar pustular psoriasis.

ALCOHOL AND DRUGS
Continued drinking is associated with therapeutic failure and abstinence with remission.

DRUG HISTORY
Avoiding the use of beta-blockers, antimalarials, and lithium may improve the course of psoriasis.

CHEMOPROPHYLAXIS
- No evidence that giving antibiotics for streptococcal sore throat prevents the development of guttate psoriasis
- No evidence that treating psoriasis with antibiotics produces any improvement in the condition

PREVENT RECURRENCE
Smoking cessation will probably not influence recurrence. Alcohol reduction may prevent recurrence, as will avoidance of known precipitating drugs.

Reassess coexisting disease
INTERACTION ALERT
- Beta-blockers for hypertensives may cause a flare of psoriasis
- Lithium for prophylaxis of cluster headache may cause a flare of psoriasis, and an alternative should be used. Probably no choice in bipolar disorder

ASSOCIATIONS

PsoriasisNet – on-line patient education service of The American Academy of Dermatology
American Academy of Dermatology
930 N Meacham Road
Schaumburg, IL 60178
Tel: 847-330-0230
Fax: 847-330-0050
http://www.skincarephysicians.com

National Psoriasis Foundation
6600 SW 92nd Ave, Suite 300
Portland, OR 97223-7195
Tel: 503-244-7404 or 800-723-9166
Fax: 503-245-0626
http://www.psoriasis.org

KEY REFERENCES

- Collier J, Longmore M, Duncan Brown T. Oxford handbook of clinical specialties, 5th edn. New York: Oxford University Press, 1999
- Gupta G. Dermatology. In: Kalra PA, ed. Essential revision notes for MRCP. PasTest, 1999
- Ashcroft DM, Po AL, Williams HC, Griffiths CE. Systematic review of comparative efficacy and tolerability of calcipotriol in treating chronic plaque psoriasis. BMJ 2000;320:963–967
- Chalmers RJG, O'Sullivan T, Owen CM, Griffiths CEM. Interventions for guttate psoriasis (Cochrane Review) In: The Cochrane Library, 2, 2001. Oxford: Update Software
- Jones G ,Crotty M, Brooks P. Interventions for treating psoriatic arthritis (Cochrane review) In: The Cochrane Library, 2, 2001. Oxford: Update Software
- Owen CM, Chalmers RJG, O'Sullivan T, Griffiths CEM. Antistreptoccal interventions for guttate and chronic plaque psoriasis (Cochrane Review). In: The Cochrane Library, 2, 2001. Oxford: Update Software
- Chalmers RJG, Griffiths CEM, O'Sullivan T. Interventions for chronic palmoplantar pustular psoriasis (protocol) In: The Cochrane Database of Systemic Reviews. The Cochrane Library 2001
- Skin disorders. In: Clinical Evidence. London: BMJ Publishing Group, 2000
- Williams HC. Smoking and psoriasis. BMJ 1994;308:428–9

Evidence references

1 Zhang WY, Li Wan Po A. The effectiveness of topically applied capsaicin: a meta analysis. Eur J Clin Pharmacol 1994;46:517–522. Reviewed in: Clinical Evidence 2001;5:1150–1164
2 Volger BK, Ernst E. Aloe vera: a systematic review of its clinical effectiveness. Br J Gen Pract 1999;49:823–828. Reviewed in: Clinical Evidence 2001;5:1150–1164
3 Berne B, Blom I, Spangberg S. Enhanced response of psoriasis to UVB therapy after pretreatment with a lubricating base. Acta Derm Venereol 1990;70:474–477. Reviewed in: Clinical Evidence 2001;5:1150–1164
4 Kanzler MH, Gorsulowsky DC. Efficacy of topical 5% liquor carbonis detergens vs. its emollient base in the treatment of psoriasis. Br J Dermatol 1993;129:310–314. In Clinical Evidence 2001;5:1150–1164
5 Naldi L, Rzany B. Chronic plaque psoriasis: skin disorders. In: Clinical Evidence 2001;5:1150–1164. London: BMJ Publishing Group
6 Ashcroft DM, Li Wan Po A, Williams HC, Griffiths CE. Systematic review of comparative efficacy and tolerability of calcipotriol in treating chronic plaque psoriasis. BMJ 2000;320:963–967. Medline
7 Katz HI, Pawer SE, Medansky RS, et al. Intermittent corticosteroid maintenance treatment of psoriasis: a double-blind multicenter trial of augmented betamethasone diproprionate ointment in a pulse dose treatment regimen. Dermatologica 1991;183:269–274
8 Kragballe K, Jansen CT, Bjerke JR, et al. A double-blind comparison of acitretin and etretinate in the treatment of severe psoriasis. Results of a Nordic multicentre study. Acta Derm Venereol 1989;69:35–40. Reviewed in Clinical Evidence 2001;5:1150–1164
9 Wilkens RF, Williams HJ, Ward JR, et al. Randomized, double-blind, placebo controlled trial of low-dose pulse methotrexate in psoriatic arthritis. Arthritis Rheum 1984;27:376–381. Reviewed in Clinical Evidence 2001;5:1150–1164

10 Van Dooren-Greebe RJ, Kuijpers AL, Mulder J, et al. Methotrexate revisited: effects of long-term treatment of psoriasis. Br J Dermatol 1994;130:204–210. Reviewed in Clinical Evidence 2001;5:1150–1164

11 Erkko P, Granlund H, Remitz A, et al. Double-blind placebo-controlled study of long-term low-dose cyclosporine in the treatment of palmoplantar pustulosis. Br J Dermatol 1998;139:997–1004. Reviewed in Clinical Evidence 2001;5:1150–1164

12 Snellman E, Aromaa A, Jansen CT, et al. Supervised four-week heliotherapy alleviates the long-term course of psoriasis. Acta Derm Venereol 1993;73:388–92. In: Clinical Evidence 2001;5:1150–1164

13 Jerner B, Skogh M, Vahlquist A. A controlled trial of acupuncture in psoriasis: no convincing effect. Acta Derm Venereol 1997;77:154–156. Reviewed in: Clinical Evidence 2001;5:1150–1164

14 Boer J, Hermans J, Schothorst AA, Surmond D. Comparison of phototherapy (UVB) and photochemotherapy (PUVA) for clearing and maintenance therapy of psoriasis. Arch Dermatol 1984;120:52–57. Reviewed in: Clinical Evidence 2001;5:1150–1164

15 Gorgen PM, Diffey BL, Mathews JN, Farr PM. A randomized comparison of narrow-band TL-01 phototherapy for psoriasis. J Am Acad Dermatol 1999;41:728–732. Reviewed in: Clinical Evidence 2001;5:1150–1164

16 Stern RS, Armstrong RB, Anderson TF, et al. Effect of continued ultraviolet B phototherapy on the duration of remission of psoriasis: a randomized study. J Am Acad Dermatol 1986;15:546–552. Reviewed in: Clinical Evidence 2001;5:1150–1164

17 Owen CM, Chalmers RJG, O'Sullivan T, Griffiths CEM. Antistreptococcal interventions for guttate and chronic plaque psoriasis (Cochrane Review). In: The Cochrane Library, 4, 2001. Oxford: Update Software

FAQS
Question 1
Are my patient's family members at risk for developing psoriasis?

ANSWER 1
Psoriasis can be familial. If your patient developed psoriasis before the age of 40, family members are at increased risk. If psoriasis developed later in life, the increased risk is much reduced.

Question 2
What new therapies are being developed for psoriasis?

ANSWER 2
The hottest area of research at the moment is in compounds that interfere with T-cell activation or cytokines that promote inflammation. In particular, various proteins that block accessory molecules or cytokines from binding receptors are in various stages of development.

Question 3
Does psoriasis pose excessive risk of infection during surgery?

ANSWER 3
In general, the answer is, 'no'. There seems to be an increase in a variety of endogenous compounds with antimicrobial effects in the skin of psoriatics. This is in contrast to atopic dermatitis patients, whose skin harbors large quantities of staphylococci.

Question 4
Does stress cause psoriasis?

ANSWER 4
Although clearly stress is not the cause of psoriasis, it can exacerbate the disease. Conversely, psoriasis can induce significant amounts of stress.

CONTRIBUTORS
Randolph L Pearson, MD
Seth R Stevens, MD
Richard Averitte, MD

SQUAMOUS CELL CARCINOMA

SUMMARY INFORMATION

DESCRIPTION

- Second most common type of skin cancer
- The age-adjusted incidence among Caucasians is 1–1.5/1000 per year in the US
- Clinical presentation varies from scaly erythematous plaques or cutaneous horn to crusted ulcerated lesions
- Unlike basal cell carcinomas, squamous cell carcinomas are associated with a substantial risk of metastasis
- Chronic sun exposure is the strongest environmental risk factor
- Precancerous lesions associated with sun damage are strong risk factors
- Malignant tumor of malpighian cells of the epithelium
- Histology shows full-thickness, pleomorphic, atypical keratinocytes in the epidermis. Invasive squamous cell carcinomas also show dermal invasion

KEY! DON'T MISS!

- Biopsy any lesion that could be squamous cell carcinoma
- Early excision of small lesions can have excellent prognosis
- Late excision of deeper lesions has poorer prognosis, especially if metastasis has occurred

BACKGROUND

ICD9 CODE
173.9 Skin neoplasm, site unspecific

SYNONYMS
- SCC
- Skin cancer

CARDINAL FEATURES
- The age-adjusted incidence among Caucasians is 1–1.5/1000 per year in the US
- Clinical presentation varies from scaly erythematous plaques or cutaneous horn to crusted ulcerated lesions
- Unlike basal cell carcinomas, squamous cell carcinomas are associated with a substantial risk of metastasis
- Second most common type of skin cancer
- Chronic sun exposure is the strongest environmental risk factor
- Precancerous lesions associated with sun damage are strong risk factors
- Malignant tumor of malpighian cells of the epithelium
- Histology shows full-thickness, pleomorphic, atypical keratinocytes in the epidermis. Invasive squamous cell carcinomas also show dermal invasion

CAUSES
Common causes
- The cause of squamous cell carcinoma is multifactorial
- Chronic sun exposure is the strongest environmental risk factor: ultraviolet (UV) B (290–320nm) radiation is principally responsible, with UVA (320–400nm) radiation adding to the risk
- Outdoor occupations are at higher risk of squamous cell carcinoma, including farmers and sailors

Premalignant conditions that are confined to the epidermis predispose to squamous skin cancer, including solar keratoses (actinic keratoses)
- Patients with solar keratoses have a 10–15 times greater risk of developing squamous cell carcinoma than people with no solar keratoses
- Actinic cheilitis and some cutaneous horns are premalignant forms of squamous cell carcinoma
- Ionizing radiation, used for treatment of acne in the 1940s
- Bowen's disease is the most common form of squamous cell carcinoma in situ
- Immunosuppression can lead to squamous cell carcinoma – renal transplant patients are up to 65 times as likely to develop squamous cell carcinoma as age-matched control subjects
- HIV disease is associated with squamous cell carcinoma where the lesion is more aggressive

Rare causes
- Arsenic exposure may lead to premalignant lesions – arsenic keratoses – historic use in 'tonics' and medications
- Cyclic aromatic hydrocarbons in tar, soot, or shale may lead to premalignant conditions
- Squamous cell carcinoma can rarely arise from scars (e.g. burns, hidradenitis suppurativa, and lupus vulgaris)
- Infection with human papillomavirus types 6, 11, 16, and 18
- Xeroderma pigmentosa is a rare genetic disease that predisposes to cutaneous malignancy, including squamous cell carcinoma

Contributory or predisposing factors

- Cumulative exposure to sunlight (UVB radiation) is the most significant factor – most tumors arise on sun-exposed areas of the head and neck
- Incidence of these tumors increases with decreasing latitude
- Thinning of the protective ozone layer may increase the risk of squamous cell carcinoma
- Fair skin – Celtic skin and a tendency to sunburn easily have a three times greater risk of developing squamous cell carcinoma than other skin types
- Albinos are at high risk of developing squamous cell carcinoma in early adulthood due to the lack of melanin protection
- Squamous cell carcinoma incidence increases with age and male sex
- The risk of lip or oral squamous cell carcinoma increases with tobacco use
- Immunosuppression induced by disease and drugs can lead to increased risk of squamous cell carcinoma. In contrast to the general population, organ transplant patients are more likely to develop squamous cell carcinomas than basal cell carcinomas (squamous cell carcinoma/basal cell carcinoma ratio of 3:1)
- UVB light and human papillomaviruses may be cocarcinogens
- Squamous cell carcinoma can arise from long-standing skin diseases such as venous ulcers or in sinus tracts
- PUVA therapy for inflammatory dermatoses (e.g. psoriasis)

EPIDEMIOLOGY
Incidence and prevalence
INCIDENCE
The age-adjusted incidence among Caucasians is 1–1.5/1000 per year in the US.

Demographics
AGE
- Incidence increases with age
- Peak incidence is 66 years

GENDER
Male/female ratio 2:1.

RACE
Caucasian skin, especially fair Celtic skin, is most at risk if chronically exposed to UV radiation.

GENETICS
A few rare congenital diseases predispose to cutaneous malignancy.

GEOGRAPHY
- Incidence increases with decreasing latitude (e.g. southern US, Australia)
- Tumors are more common on the left side in the US and on the right side in England. This could be due to asymmetric exposure during driving
- In certain geographic locations, exposure to arsenic in well water or from industrial sources may significantly increase the risk of squamous cell carcinoma

SOCIOECONOMIC STATUS
Higher social classes may be financially well off to spend holidays in hot climates predisposing to skin cancer, including squamous cell carcinoma.

DIFFERENTIAL DIAGNOSIS
Solar keratosis
Also known as actinic keratosis. The main features of solar keratosis are as follows:

FEATURES
- Premalignant scaly lesions that are often more easily felt than seen
- Develop on skin damaged by UV radiation
- Normally occur on the scalp, forehead, neck, and back of hands
- Scaly erythematous macules or patches
- May itch or ulcerate
- Histology shows pleomorphic hyperchromatic keratinocytes in the lower epidermis and areas of parakeratosis
- Normally takes several years to transform to squamous cell carcinoma
- Solar keratoses are best treated by cauterization or cryotherapy
- Patients should be advised to avoid the sun and apply a topical sunscreen when sun exposure is unavoidable
- Patients with solar keratosis have a cumulative lifetime risk of having at least one invasive squamous cell carcinoma of 6–10%

Keratoacanthoma
Lesion that appears malignant but acts benign. The main features of keratoacanthoma are as follows:

FEATURES
- Lesion grows rapidly
- Within 6 weeks produces a large, indurated, dome–shaped papule
- Has a characteristic central crater filled with a keratinous plug
- Histology is often indistinguishable from squamous cell carcinoma
- Involutes spontaneously, leaving a depressed scar
- Treatment is by curettage and cautery at the base
- Rarely, it may metastasize

Verruca vulgaris
The main features of verruca vulgaris are as follows:

FEATURES
- Papules initially appear as flesh-colored and rough-surfaced; later develop a hyperkeratotic appearance with black dots on surface
- Papules are typically dome-shaped, usually 1cm in diameter
- Most frequently occurs in children and young adults

Seborrheic keratosis
The main features of seborrheic keratosis are as follows:

FEATURES
- Rough, sharp-bordered lesions
- May range in color from flesh to tan to dark brown
- Lesions usually have a 'stuck on' appearance, occur mainly on the trunk, and may have a greasy surface
- Lesions can be removed if they irritate or bleed

Bowen's disease

Squamous carcinoma in situ. The main features of Bowen's disease are as follows:

FEATURES
- Intraepidermal carcinoma
- Preinvasive stage
- Persistent, red, scaly plaque similar to psoriasis
- Characteristic histology with loss of epidermal polarity, large atypical cells, and frequent mitotic figures
- Few lesions become malignant
- Many cases are due to arsenic ingestion in 'tonics' and medication
- Excision is the preferred method of treatment

Basal cell carcinoma

Malignancy arising from epidermal basal cells. The main features of basal cell carcinoma are as follows:

FEATURES
- Most common type of malignancy in European-Americans
- Several clinical types of basal cell carcinoma
- Most common type is the noduloulcerative basal cell carcinoma that begins as a small pearly nodule and undergoes central ulceration
- Various amounts of melanin may be present in the tumor
- Tumors with heavier accumulation of melanin are referred to as pigmented basal cell carcinoma
- Risk factors include UV radiation, age, male gender, fair skin, and family history
- 85% of the tumors are found on the head and neck areas, with 30% found on the nose
- Commonly found on the trunk and extremities
- Superficial basal cell carcinoma may be treated with topical imiquimod or 5-fluorouracil
- Small tumors can be treated with electrodesiccation and curettage
- Larger, more aggressive tumors need complete excision
- Radiation therapy can be used where surgery is not an option
- The tumor rarely metastasizes but can cause extensive local tissue destruction
- Lasers have also been used to treat tumors

SIGNS & SYMPTOMS
Signs
- The clinical appearance is highly variable
- Usually the tumor presents as an ulcerated lesion with hard raised edges
- The tumor may be in the form of a hard plaque or a papule, often with an opalescent quality, with telangiectasia
- The tumor can lie below the level of the surrounding skin and eventually ulcerates and invades the underlying tissue
- The tumor commonly presents on sun-exposed areas (e.g. back of the hand, scalp, lip, and superior surface of pinna)
- On the lip, the tumor forms a small ulcer, which fails to heal and bleeds intermittently
- Evidence of chronic skin photodamage, such as multiple solar keratoses (actinic keratoses)
- The tumor grows relatively slowly
- Unlike basal cell carcinoma, squamous cell carcinoma has a substantial risk of metastasis
- Risk of metastasis is higher in squamous cell carcinoma arising in scars, on the lower lips or mucosa, and occurring in immunosuppressed patients. About one-third of lingual and mucosal tumors metastasize before diagnosis

Symptoms
- The lesion is often asymptomatic
- Ulcer or reddish skin plaque that is slow growing
- Intermittent bleeding from the tumor, especially on the lip

ASSOCIATED DISORDERS
- Malignancy occasionally arises in old scars, especially if from severe burns or lupus vulgaris or from sites of ionizing radiation
- Squamous cell carcinoma can arise in a long-standing venous ulcer, sinus tracts, and hidradenitis suppurativa
- Immunosuppression can lead to squamous cell carcinoma lesions that are more aggressive, including HIV disease, and renal transplant patients

KEY! DON'T MISS!
- Biopsy any lesion that could be squamous cell carcinoma
- Early excision of small lesions can have excellent prognosis
- Late excision of deeper lesions has poorer prognosis, especially if metastasis has occurred

CONSIDER CONSULT
- Referral to a dermatologist for biopsy of suspicious lesions is mandatory

INVESTIGATION OF THE PATIENT
Direct questions to patient
Q How long ago did you notice this lesion? Often the lesion has been present for a while before medical help is sought.

Q Do you have any other similar lesions? Look for evidence of sun-damaged skin due to chronic sun exposure, such as multiple solar keratoses (actinic keratoses), solar elastosis, or solar lentigines.

Q Have you been diagnosed with skin cancer before? Patients often have a history of cutaneous skin cancer, such as basal cell carcinoma.

Q Does the lesion bleed? Intermittent bleeding of the tumor is common, especially on the lip.

Q Where is the lesion? The tumor commonly presents on the back of the hand, scalp, lip, and superior surface of the pinna (sun-exposed sites).

Contributory or predisposing factors
Q Has the patient been chronically exposed to the sun or used tanning salons? Chronic sun exposure is the strongest environmental risk factor.

Q Does the patient have evidence of sun-damaged skin? Multiple solar keratoses (actinic keratoses) are evidence of sun damage, and patients with solar keratoses have a 10–15 times greater risk of developing squamous cell carcinoma than patients with no solar keratoses.

Q Does the patient have a history of Bowen's disease? This lesion is a superficial squamous cell carcinoma, in situ, and needs excision.

Q Does the patient suffer from xeroderma pigmentosa? This is a rare genetic disease that predisposes to cutaneous malignancy, leading to squamous cell carcinoma.

Q Does the patient suffer from immunosuppression due to disease or medication? This can lead to squamous cell carcinoma – renal transplant patients have up to 65-fold increased risk.

Q Did the patient receive radiation therapy for acne or internal malignancy?

Family history
Q Has anyone in your family been diagnosed with skin cancer? Cutaneous skin cancers can occur in families, especially those with congenital diseases such as xeroderma pigmentosa.

Examination

- **What is the appearance of the lesion?** The clinical appearance is highly variable, ranging from an ulcer to a plaque. All lesions should be biopsied because early diagnosis is important
- **Is there evidence that the lesion bleeds?** Ulcers on the lip that intermittently bleed are strongly diagnostic of squamous cell carcinoma
- **Where is the lesion?** The tumor commonly presents on the back of the hand, scalp, lip, and superior surface of the pinna
- **Is there evidence of sun-damaged skin?** Multiple solar keratoses suggest that the patient has had chronic exposure to UV radiation
- **Is the skin fair?** Celtic complexion that is exposed to sunlight is especially prone to cutaneous malignancies
- **Does the lesion arise in a scar?** Malignant skin lesions occasionally arise in old scars, particularly those due to severe burns or lupus vulgaris

Summary of investigative tests

- Biopsy of suspicious lesions is essential because small early lesions will have better prognosis
- Family practitioner guidelines state that pathologic examination of all skin biopsies is mandatory
- Early biopsy is essential with ulcers of the lip because up to one-third have metastasized at diagnosis

DIAGNOSTIC DECISION

Obviously benign lesions, such as classic seborrheic keratoses, need not be sampled. Any lesion about which uncertainty remains should be removed and examined pathologically by a dermatopathologist.

CLINICAL PEARLS

- Skin screening of asymptomatic patients should be performed as part of the routine physical examination, with particular attention to sun-exposed sites
- Consider the diagnosis of squamous cell carcinoma in recalcitrant 'warts'

THE TESTS
Biopsy
SKIN BIOPSY
Description

- A skin biopsy of the lesion is essential
- The patient may need to be referred to a dermatologist for this procedure
- The preferred type of biopsy for diagnosis is shave biopsy that goes through the upper papillary dermis of the lesion
- The lesion is then sent for histologic analysis using microscopy
- The mode of treatment will depend on the histology

Advantages/Disadvantages
Advantages:

- Biopsy is easy to obtain and quick to perform
- Diagnostic of squamous cell carcinoma
- High sensitivity and specificity

Disadvantages:

- Usual risks associated with minor surgery of bleeding, delayed wound healing, and infection
- The biopsy procedure is blind and may damage underlying structures such as blood vessels (use of a large volume of local anesthetic to distend the subcutaneous tissue reduces this risk)

Abnormal

Histology will show the following features:

- Grossly disorganized epidermis with pleomorphic full-thickness atypia
- Hyperkeratosis
- Parakeratosis
- Frequent mitotic figures
- May show invasion of the dermis by atypical keratinocytes

TREATMENT

CONSIDER CONSULT

- Squamous cell carcinoma is one of the most common reasons that patients are referred to dermatologists
- Due to the infiltrative growth pattern, surgical removal requires excision or electrodesiccation and curettage in most cases to a variable extent beyond the clinically apparent lesion. Refer when knowledge and technical skill are insufficient to remove the entire lesion
- Referral for X-ray therapy
- High-risk tumors should be referred for Mohs' micrographic surgery

PATIENT AND CAREGIVER ISSUES
Patient or caregiver request

- **Will this tumor spread?** This depends on the histology
- **How serious is the tumor?** This depends on the histology
- **Will the surgery scar?** The lesion will need to be removed completely with the borders free of tumor, which can cause a poor cosmetic result
- **Will I need further treatment?** The lesion should be removed in its entirety. Inadequate margins will require additional surgery. Repair of surgical defects should be performed. If metastasis has occurred, then irradiation and chemotherapy may be indicated

Health-seeking behavior
Has the patient tried to treat the lesion? The patient may have used topical medications on the lesion.

MANAGEMENT ISSUES
Goals

- Achieve a cure by eradicating local disease, including microinvasive disease
- Treat lymph node spread (by lymph node dissection and irradiation)
- Treat metastatic spread (chemotherapy is indicated)
- Prevent recurrence
- Reduce morbidity and mortality rates
- Heighten surveillance because patients with one squamous cell carcinoma are at increased risk for second cutaneous malignancies

Management in special circumstances

- Treatment regimens may need to be less intense in elderly patients, including X-ray therapy in patients who are not surgical candidates
- Perineural invasion (may manifest as facial paralysis); invasion to the subcutis; patient immunosuppression; lesion arising from within radiation sites, scars, or chronic ulcers; and poorly differentiated histology are poor prognostic signs and warrant more aggressive therapy

COEXISTING DISEASE

- Immunosuppression can lead to squamous cell carcinoma lesions, which are more aggressive, including tumors in HIV disease and renal transplant patients
- These tumors will need careful management to check for complete eradication

COEXISTING MEDICATION

- Immunosuppression medication can lead to squamous cell carcinoma lesions, which are more aggressive
- These tumors will need careful management to check for complete eradication

SPECIAL PATIENT GROUPS

Treatment regimens may need to be less intense in elderly patients with metastatic squamous cell carcinoma, especially if chemotherapy is indicated.

SUMMARY OF THERAPEUTIC OPTIONS
Choices

- The treatment of cutaneous squamous cell carcinoma should be based on an analysis of risk factors influencing the biologic behavior of the tumor. These include the size, location, and degree of histologic differentiation of the tumor and the age and physical condition of the patient
- Early diagnosis and excision are essential to avoid metastases
- Small tumors 1cm or less in diameter on the neck, trunk, arms, or legs can be treated by electrodesiccation and curettage, cryotherapy, or simple excision. The disadvantages of electrodesiccation and curettage and cryotherapy are lack of histologic confirmation and a higher recurrence rate
- Tumors >1cm in diameter that do not involve subcutaneous fat may be removed by excision or using Mohs' micrographic surgery. An advantage of Mohs' micrographic surgery is that it allows viewing of 100% of the peripheral and deep margins, leading to complete removal of the tumor in the most tissue-sparing way
- Metastatic disease is managed by local tumor removal, as well as radiation therapy (irradiation of tumor) and/or chemotherapy (13-cis-retinoic acid and interferon-2A). Chemotherapy or a biologic response modifier is required for metastatic squamous cell carcinoma and is used for curative and palliation therapy. The patient must be referred to an oncologist who should advise the correct regimen
- Lifestyle changes include avoiding sun exposure and wearing protective clothing

Guidelines

- The American College of Preventive Medicine has developed the following guidelines, also available at the National Guideline Clearinghouse. Skin protection from ultraviolet light exposure. [1]
- The American Academy of Family Physicians has produced the following: Jevant AF, Johnson JT, Sheridan CD, Caffrey TJ. Early detection and treatment of skin cancer. [2]

Clinical pearls

Prophylactic use of retinoids (isotretinoin or acitretin) may be useful in patients with a history of multiple squamous cell carcinomas.

Never

An uncommon variant of cutaneous squamous cell carcinoma is verrucous carcinoma. There are three subtypes with defining sites: epithelioma cuniculatum (feet), giant condyloma of Buschke and Löwenstein (anogenital), and florid oral papillomatosis (mouth). These should never be irradiated because that will greatly increase the risk of metastasis.

FOLLOW UP
Plan for review

- Follow up is needed on treatment and its compliance, especially for aggressive lesions and metastatic lesions
- Long-term follow up is required for the detection of recurrence, metastasis, and new skin cancers

Information for patient or caregiver

- Patients should be informed of the potential complications of both the diseases and treatment modalities
- Patients must be followed up, and this must be emphasized, especially because there is a high risk of recurrence of squamous cell lesions

DRUGS AND OTHER THERAPIES: DETAILS
Surgical therapy
ELECTRODESICCATION AND CURETTAGE

A procedure that destroys the tumor and a surrounding margin of clinically unaffected tissue by electrodesiccation, electrocoagulation, or electrocautery. The area is then scraped with a curet. The curettage is directed by the differential texture of diseased and normal tissue. This process is repeated several times to ensure complete removal of the tumor.

Efficacy

- Not as effective as surgical excision for lesions of the lip or ear
- Not effective for high-risk lesions
- Should be reserved for the treatment of small, uncomplicated primary lesions
- Effective for the treatment of actinic keratosis

Risks/benefits
Risks:

- Higher recurrence rate
- Wound will take 4–6 weeks to heal
- Leaves a hyperpigmented or hypertrophic, depressed scar
- Blind method of removal and thus provides no margins to ensure that the lesion is completely removed

Benefits:

- Requires training and experience in the technique but is easy to learn and perform
- The tissue should break down easily, thus confirming the clinical impression during the procedure
- Curettage can be used in combination with cryotherapy or as a first-stage debulking procedure in combination with other therapies
- Inexpensive and time-efficient

Acceptability to patient
Patients who want minimal time involvement in treatment often prefer this approach. Frustration may arise in patients who opt for this therapy in whom the tumor is found to extend into the subcutis because they will require some other form of therapy. Patients who desire a good cosmetic result may find this treatment unacceptable.

Follow up plan
The wound can take up to 6 weeks to heal and should be monitored over this period of time.

Patient and caregiver information
Patient should immediately report any sign of wound infection or recurrence of tumor at the site of therapy.

SIMPLE EXCISION
Surgical excision of the lesion, with a margin of macroscopically normal tissue.

Efficacy
- Useful for primary and recurrent tumors (although less effective for recurrent)
- Recurrence depends on the initial size, histology, and depth of the tumor and on the surgical margins achieved
- Effective for larger lesions
- The optimal margin for primary excision of tumors of 2cm or less is 4mm; for those of >2cm the optimal margin is 6mm

Risks/benefits
Risks:
- Complete excision with wide tumor margins is not always achieved because the procedure depends on clinical judgment
- Some normal tissue must be sacrificed
- Training for the procedure is required and is time-consuming
- May need to be performed as an inpatient under general anesthetic, depending on the size and location of the lesion and other patient factors

Benefits:
- Allows histologic examination of the tumor margins
- Can be used for large tumors with clearly defined borders
- Acceptable cosmetic result
- Faster healing than with other methods

Evidence
There is a lack of evidence defining the optimal surgical margin for squamous cell carcinomas [3]

Acceptability to patient
Generally well tolerated.

Follow up plan
Patients should be seen in the postoperative period for inspection of the wound and removal of sutures.

Patient and caregiver information
Patient should immediately report any sign of infection or recurrence of tumor at the site of therapy.

MOHS' MICROGRAPHIC SURGERY
- Technique used by which excised tissue is prepared and orientated by markers to display its entire cut surface for immediate histologic examination
- Used for primary tumors and recurrent tumors

Efficacy
- Permits the position of any residual tumor to be mapped out and excised without delay
- The optimal margin for primary excision of tumors of 2cm or less is 4mm; for those of >2cm the optimal margin is 6mm
- Reported to have a lower recurrence rate than other treatment options

Risks/benefits
Risk: The surgeon must be able to undertake the surgical excision and histologic interpretation

Benefits:
- One of the major advantages of this procedure for skin cancers of the head and neck is the complete removal of the tumor with maximal tissue conservation, leading to more cosmetically acceptable results
- Permits the position of any residual tumor to be mapped out and excised without delay

Evidence
There is a lack of good quality evidence comparing Mohs' surgery with standard surgery as the primary therapy [3]
- Mohs' micrographic surgery has been shown to have a reduced rate of recurrence (3%) compared with standard surgery (8%) in a review of case series. This evidence should be treated with caution due to the methods used [4]
- A comparison of efficacy depending on location found that Mohs' surgery had an improved recurrence rate for lesions of the lip and ear [4]

Acceptability to patient
All surgery has the risk of tissue destruction and scarring, particularly of vital structures such as eyelids, lip margins, and motor and sensory nerves.

Follow up plan
Follow up for sepsis and recurrence of the tumor is necessary.

Patient and caregiver information
- The cosmetic result may be distressing, with tissue destruction and scarring, though most well-trained Mohs' surgeons are excellent at cosmetically acceptable repairs
- Involvement of vital structures with malignancy can require their sacrifice, leading to loss of function, such as facial droop
- Reconstruction can often be performed immediately after Mohs' surgery at the same visit. If not, a delayed repair can usually be performed in a few days or weeks, minimizing long-term disfigurement
- Full consent is needed prior to surgery

Radiation therapy
- Radiation therapy and/or lymph node dissection is needed for tumors with regional metastasis
- Radiation can be used for incompletely excised tumors because the recurrence rates for these tumors are >50%

IRRADIATION OF TUMOR
A course of irradiation therapy to the tumor area is performed.

Efficacy
- Radiation can reduce the recurrence and metastatic potential of squamous cell carcinoma
- Metastatic potential of verrucous carcinomas is increased by radiation

Risks/benefits
Risks:
- Long-term scarring with postradiation depigmentation and gradual development of chronic radiodermatitis, including telangiectasia, thinning of the skin, and hyperkeratosis
- Rarely, nonhealing ulceration can occur
- Increased metastatic potential of verrucous carcinoma

Evidence
There is insufficient evidence that radiation after surgery affects local recurrence of squamous cell carcinoma [3].

Acceptability to patient
Long-term scarring with postradiation depigmentation and gradual development of chronic radiodermatitis, including telangiectasia, thinning of the skin, and hyperkeratosis.

Follow up plan
Follow up for recurrence of the tumor is necessary.

Patient and caregiver information
- Patients must be warned about the potential of long-term scarring due to radiation therapy
- Full consent is necessary

Chemotherapy
13-CIS-RETINOIC ACID AND INTERFERON-2A
Risks/benefits
Risks:
- Should only be administered under specialist supervision
- Use caution when administered to patients with suicidal tendencies
- Severe or fatal gastrointestinal hemorrhage has been reported in association with alfa-interferon therapy
- Caution should be exercised when administering interferon alfa-2a, recombinant to patients with myelosuppression or when interferon alfa-2a, recombinant is used in combination with other agents that are known to cause myelosuppression.

- Side effects include:
Central nervous system: depressive illness, suicidal behavior, fatigue, myalgia/arthralgia, flu-like symptom, fever, chills, asthenia, sweating, leg cramps, malaise, depression
Gastrointestinal: diarrhea, nausea, vomiting
Skin: injection site reaction, alopecia, rash

Interactions (other drugs):
- **Theophylline** (causing reduced clearance of theophylline)

Contraindications:
- **Known hypersensitivity to alfa interferon or any component of the product. The injectable solutions contain benzyl alcohol and are contraindicated in any individual with a known allergy to that preservative**
- **Pregnancy and breast-feeding**

Other therapies
CRYOTHERAPY
Cryotherapy destroys tissue by reducing the temperature of the lesion to tumoricidal levels. Liquid nitrogen is administered with a spray device or cryoprobe.

Efficacy
- May be effective for small, well-defined, in situ primary tumors
- Effective for the treatment of actinic keratosis

Risks/benefits

Risks:

- Contraindicated in patients with cold intolerance, cryoglobulinemia, cryofibrinogenemia, or platelet deficiency
- Pigment loss over the scar, hypertrophic scarring, and neuropathies are possible complications
- May have severe postoperative pain, and there may be swelling and blistering of the wound

Benefits:

- Useful when there are multiple lesions
- Useful in the elderly or patients with coexisting disease, where other forms of surgery may be contraindicated
- Anesthesia is not usually required for small lesions
- Inexpensive and time-efficient

Acceptability to patient

Patients who desire a good cosmetic result may not find this treatment acceptable.

Follow up plan

The patient should be followed up to ensure that there is adequate analgesia and wound healing.

Patient and caregiver information

- Patients should be informed that a wound may appear a few days after treatment
- The wound should be washed daily with soap and water
- Patients should immediately report any sign of infection or recurrence of tumor at the site of therapy

LIFESTYLE

- The patient must avoid sun exposure
- If sun exposure occurs, then the patient should wear protective clothing and use sunscreens with a high sun protection factor (SPF)

RISKS/BENEFITS

Benefit: prevents recurrence and the development of new tumors.

EFFICACY OF THERAPIES
Mohs' micrographic surgery has been reported to have a lower 5-year recurrence rate compared with other therapies.

Evidence
- There is insufficient evidence for the use of radiation therapy after surgery to prevent recurrence of squamous cell carcinoma [5]
- There is insufficient evidence that Mohs' micrographic surgery is superior to simple excision in terms of local recurrence rates [5]
- Significantly fewer solar keratoses were found with daily sunscreen vs placebo in a randomized controlled trial (RCT) of people with a history of solar keratoses. In this 7-month trial, there was a significantly greater chance of remission of lesions with sunscreen [6] *Level P*
- A 40% reduction in incidence of carcinoma was found with daily application of sunscreen to head, neck, arms, and hands compared with discretionary application in a 4.5-year RCT [3] *Level P*

Review period
6 months.

PROGNOSIS
- Survival is related to size, location, degree of differentiation, immunologic status of the patient, depth of invasion, and presence of metastases
- Metastases are more common in squamous cell carcinoma arising in scars, on the lower lips, and in immunosuppressed patients
- Tumors at the mucocutaneous junction are more difficult to cure
- Tumors of the scalp, forehead, nose, and lip carry a worse prognosis
- Metastatic rates were 11% for tumors on the ear and 14% for those on the lip, compared with an average for all sites of 5%
- Patients with a tumor that penetrates the dermis or exceeds 8mm in thickness are at higher risk of recurrence
- Lesions >2cm in diameter compared with lesions <2cm have more than twice the local recurrence rate (16% vs 6%)

Clinical pearls
- Consider the diagnosis of squamous cell carcinoma in patients with recalcitrant 'warts', particularly older patients and sun-exposed sites
- Continued surveillance for second cutaneous malignancy should occur in patients with squamous cell carcinoma

Therapeutic failure
- Further surgery, radiation, and chemotherapy are indicated for recurrence or metastases
- Referral to a dermatologist and, in the case of internal involvement, an oncologist is indicated

Recurrence
Lesions >2cm in diameter compared with lesions <2cm have more than twice the local recurrence rate (16% vs 6%) and three times the rate of metastasis (23% vs 8%).

Deterioration
- Further surgery, radiation, and chemotherapy are indicated for recurrence or metastases
- Referral to a dermatologist and an oncologist is indicated

CONSIDER CONSULT
- Referral to a dermatologist and an oncologist is indicated for recurrence or metastases

PREVENTION

RISK FACTORS

- UVB radiation from sun exposure: the patient must minimize sun exposure by using protective clothing, avoiding the midday sun, and liberally using sunscreen with a high SPF
- Precancerous and in-situ lesions: these require early treatment
- Tobacco: cigarette, cigar, and pipe smoking and smokeless tobacco use are related to squamous cell carcinoma of the lip and oral cavity
- Polycyclic hydrocarbons: protection against prolonged, frequent contact with these compounds was one of the first public health/occupational safety measures related to cancer prevention. UVB and polycyclic hydrocarbons synergistically induce squamous cell carcinoma

MODIFY RISK FACTORS

- Avoidance of sun exposure in early life prevents squamous cell carcinoma in later life
- Avoidance of tobacco products will reduce the risk of squamous cell carcinoma of the lip

Lifestyle and wellness

TOBACCO
Avoid.

ENVIRONMENT

- Avoidance of sun exposure is the most important preventive measure for squamous cell carcinoma
- Wearing protective clothing, liberally using sunscreens with high SPFs, avoiding tanning salons, and avoiding the midday sun (between 10 a.m. and 2 p.m.) all help in prevention

SCREENING

- Screening for premalignant lesions is important to prevent squamous cell carcinoma
- Solar keratoses imply sun-damaged skin and are treated by cryotherapy, electrodesiccation and curettage, or chemotherapy with topical 5-fluorouracil

PREVENT RECURRENCE

- Avoidance of UVB radiation is the strongest preventive measure
- Removal of premalignant lesion is important in preventing squamous cell carcinoma

Reassess coexisting disease

Careful regular follow up of squamous cell carcinoma is required because the recurrence rate is high, especially for patients with HIV disease or organ transplantation.

ASSOCIATIONS

American Cancer Society
1599 Clifton Road, NE
Atlanta, GA 30329
Tel: 800-ACS-2345
http://www.cancer.org

KEY REFERENCES

■ Alam M, Ratner D. Cutaneous squamous-cell carcinoma. N Engl J Med 2001;344:13 975–83

■ Lumps and bumps. In: Buxton P. ABC of dermatology. London: BMJ, 1991

■ Cross P. Is histological examination of tissue removed by GPs always necessary? even specialists get the clinical diagnosis wrong. BMJ 1998;316:778

■ Do sunscreens prevent skin cancer? Drug Ther Bull 1998;36(7):49–51

■ General Medical Services Committee. Minor surgery in general practice: guidelines. London: RCGP, 1996

■ Green A, Marks R. Squamous cell carcinoma of the skin: non-metastatic. Skin disorders. Clinical Evidence 2001;5:1190–1195. London: BMJ Publishing Group

■ Motley D. Dermatology surgery and the use of lasers. Medicine 1997;25(8):10–14

■ Padgett JK, Hendrix JD Jr. Cutaneous malignancies and their management. Otolaryngol Clin North Am 2001;34(3):523–53

Evidence references

1 The American College of Practice Medicine. Skin protection from ultraviolet light exposure. Am J Prev Med 1998;14:83–6

2 The American Academy of Family Physicians: Jevant AF, Johnson JT, Sheridan CD, Caffrery TJ. Early detection and treatment of skin cancer. American Family Physician, 2000.

3 Green A, Marks R. Squamous cell carcinoma of the skin: non-metastatic. Skin disorders. In: Clinical Evidence 2001;5:1190–1195. London: BMJ Publishing Group

4 Rowe DE, Carroll RJ, Day CL. Prognostic factors for local recurrence, metastasis, and survival rates in squamous cell carcinoma of the skin, ear, and lip. J Am Acad Dermatol 1992;26:976–990. Reviewed in Clinical Evidence 2001;5:1190–1195

5 Green A, Williams G, Neale R, et al. Daily sunscreen application and betacarotene supplementation in prevention of basal cell and squamous cell carcinomas of the skin: a randomised controlled trial. Lancet 1999;354:723–729. Reviewed in Clinical evidence 2001;5:1190–1195

6 Thompson SC, Jolley D, Marks R. Reduction of solar keratoses by regular sunscreen use. N Engl J Med 1993;329:1147–1151. Reviewed in Clinical evidence 2001;5:1190–1195

FAQS
Question 1
Do sunscreens increase or decrease the risk of skin cancer?

ANSWER 1
Sun avoidance is the best way to reduce the negative effects of sun exposure. There is controversy surrounding the role of sunscreens in skin cancer. This controversy revolves around the relative roles of UVA and UVB radiation in carcinogenesis vs the relative ability of sunscreens to protect in these portions of the UV spectrum. In particular, the question has been, 'Do sunscreens protect against sunburn (redness, pain, blistering) to a greater extent than against carcinogenesis?' thereby removing the natural signal to get out of the sun, causing increased exposure to sunlight and enhancing melanoma risk. The issue is greatly clouded by the evolution in sunscreen formulations over the past few decades, including the former use in Europe of psoralens as sunscreens, which form DNA adducts and are clearly mutagenic. More recently, broad-spectrum sunscreens have been and are being developed that protect against UVA (the so-called tanning rays) and UVB (the so-called burning rays). Currently, opinion leaders believe that broad-spectrum, high-SPF sunscreens are protective.

Question 2

What is SPF?

ANSWER 2

SPF – sun protection factor – is determined experimentally for sunscreens by exposing human subjects to simulated sunlight with and without sunscreen protection. The amount of light that induces redness (usually measured in seconds) in sunscreen-protected skin, divided by the amount of light that induces redness in unprotected skin, is the SPF. SPF is predominantly a measure of UVB protection. Thus a sunscreen with an SPF of 15 will delay the onset of sunburn in an individual who would otherwise burn in 10min to burn in 150min (2.5h). This sort of exposure is not uncommon.

Question 3

Is it worthwhile to treat actinic keratoses as a preventive measure against squamous cell carcinoma development?

ANSWER 3

Yes. Depending on the study, actinic keratoses become squamous cell carcinomas at the rate of 0.01–1%/lesion/year. Thus a patient who has several actinic keratoses for several years has a significant risk of developing squamous cell carcinoma. Furthermore, it can be difficult to identify an early squamous cell carcinoma in a sea of actinic keratoses, leading to a delay in definitive therapy.

Question 4

What is the relationship between squamous cell carcinoma, basal cell carcinomas, and melanomas?

ANSWER 4

Each are cancers of epidermal cells. They are all linked to UV light exposure. Development of melanoma is more closely linked to acute, blistering sunburns early in life, wheras the nonmelanoma skin cancers are associated more with chronic UV exposure.

CONTRIBUTORS

Fred F Ferri, MD, FACP
Seth R Stevens, MD
Christine C Lin, MD

TINEA VERSICOLOR

SUMMARY INFORMATION

DESCRIPTION

- Macular rash mainly on trunk
- Macules may be pale brown, pink, or hypopigmented
- Macules scale with scraping
- These scales contain the yeast fungus on microscopic examination

KEY! DON'T MISS!

Immunosuppression may be an underlying cause of tinea versicolor.

ICD9 CODE
111.0 Tinea versicolor

SYNONYMS
Pityriasis versicolor

CARDINAL FEATURES
- Eruption is usually asymptomatic
- Mild pruritus may be a feature
- Macular rash occurs mainly on trunk
- Facial lesions are more common in children
- Macules may be pale brown, pink, or hypopigmented
- Lesions become conspicuous on tanned skin
- The lesions may be hypopigmented on black skin
- Macules scale with scraping
- These scales contain the yeast fungus on microscopic examination
- High recurrence rate

CAUSES

Common causes
- The infection is caused by *Malassezia furfur*
- Lipophilic yeasts, *Pityrosporum orbiculare* (round form) and *Pityrosporum ovale* (oval form), are saprophytes
- These organisms are normal inhabitants of skin flora but change from the saprophytic form to the hyphae form of *Malassezia furfur*
- Depigmentation is due to the fungus producing azelaic acid, which inhibits tyrosinase activity, which in turn is involved in the process of normal melaninization

Contributory or predisposing factors
- Pregnancy
- Malnutrition
- Immunosuppression
- Oral contraception
- Excess heat and humidity (heavy clothing with perspiration)

EPIDEMIOLOGY
Incidence and prevalence
- Tinea versicolor is very common in the tropics
- Incidence in temperate climates has increased over the past three decades
- More prevalent in the summer due to lesions becoming more evident on tanned skin

INCIDENCE
Because this is a nonreportable infection, exact incidence and prevalence are not known.

Demographics
AGE
Adolescence and young adulthood.

GENDER
Female:male ratio 1:1.

GEOGRAPHY
High incidence of tinea versicolor in the tropics.

DIFFERENTIAL DIAGNOSIS
Vitiligo
Vitiligo is a common condition, in which completely white patches occur as a result of destruction of melanocytes. The acquired loss of epidermal pigmentation is characterized histologically by absence of epidermal melanocytes.

FEATURES
- Depigmented lesions over sun-exposed areas
- Areas around body orifices and fingertips are particularly affected
- Symmetric distribution
- Can affect hair, which may become white
- Autoimmune disease with circulating antimelanocyte antibodies

Secondary syphilis
Secondary syphilis is a sexually transmitted disease with characteristic skin lesions.

FEATURES
- Maculopapular lesions on palms and soles
- Widespread scaly erythematous lesions on trunk
- Mucocutaneous lesions
- Generalized lymphadenopathy
- Mucous patch lesion on oral and genital mucosa

Pityriasis rosea
Pityriasis rosea is a common self-limiting skin eruption.

FEATURES
- Herald patch lesion
- Followed more than one week later by eruptive phase
- Salmon-pink papules and plaques up to few hundred, mainly on the trunk, with 'Christmas tree' distribution
- Lesions have scaly border
- More frequent in the fall and spring

Seborrheic dermatitis
Seborrheic dermatitis is a skin inflammation characterized by scales and papules.

FEATURES
- Greasy scales and underlying erythematous patches or plaques
- Scalp, central face, presternal areas, and upper back are particularly affected
- Pruritus
- Secondary infection common

Pityriasis alba
Pityriasis alba is a form of eczema that leads to pale patches on the skin.

FEATURES
- Inflammation of skin
- Pruritus
- Pale patches of involved skin
- Children especially affected

SIGNS & SYMPTOMS
Signs
- Macular rash mainly on trunk
- Facial lesions more common in children
- Macules may be pale brown, pink, or hypopigmented
- Lesions become conspicuous on tan skin
- Lesions may be hypopigmented on black skin
- Lesions range from 4–5mm in diameter to large confluent areas
- Macules scale with scraping

Symptoms
- Eruption is usually asymptomatic
- Mild pruritus may be a feature

KEY! DON'T MISS!
Immunosuppression may be an underlying cause of tinea versicolor.

CONSIDER CONSULT
- If uncertain of diagnosis
- In cases of severe depigmentation

INVESTIGATION OF THE PATIENT
Direct questions to patient
Q **How long have you noticed the rash?** Tinea versicolor can be present for months.

Q **Are there any symptoms?** Tinea versicolor is usually asymptomatic.

Q **Which areas of your body are affected?** Trunk and face are commonly affected areas.

Q **Have you any other illnesses?** Any other condition that leads to immunocompromise increases the risk for tinea versicolor.

Q **Have you had a similar rash before?** Recurrence is common.

Contributory or predisposing factors
Q **Are you pregnant?** Pregnancy can increase the risk of tinea versicolor.

Q **Do you spend time in the tropics?** Hot humid conditions can predispose patients to tinea versicolor.

Q **Do you wear heavy clothing for work?** Areas prone to perspiration have increased risk for developing tinea versicolor.

Examination
- **Examine the trunk.** The trunk is the most common site for tinea versicolor; other sites include face, upper arm, and groin
- **Assess the color of the skin.** Tinea versicolor can vary in color from pink or brown, to hypopigmentation
- **Assess the size and form of the lesion.** Characteristic lesions are macular in nature and range from 4–5mm in diameter to large confluent areas
- **Scrape the lesion.** Tinea versicolor forms scales when scraped

Summary of investigative tests
- Diagnosis is primarily clinical and is confirmed by demonstrating the hyphae and spores of *Malassezia furfur* within skin scales removed by scraping (i.e. microscopic examination); 10% potassium hydroxide test will remove skin scales to reveal yeasts
- Culture is difficult and unnecessary

DIAGNOSTIC DECISION

Microscopic examination of skin scales using 10% potassium hydroxide will confirm diagnosis.

CLINICAL PEARLS

- Tinea versicolor is rarely depigmented. If complete depigmentation is seen, then vitiligo must be excluded
- Frequently recurrent

THE TESTS
Biopsy
MICROSCOPIC EXAMINATION OF THE SKIN
Description

- Scrape the lesion to remove scale
- Use 10% potassium hydroxide to remove skin scales
- Observe the large blunt hyphae and thick-walled budding spores forming a 'spaghetti and meatballs' appearance under the low-powered lens of a microscope

Advantages/Disadvantages
Advantages:

- Quick
- Easy to do
- Painless
- Noncontaminating
- Reliable in diagnosing fungal infections

Normal
No hyphae demonstrated.

Abnormal

- Large blunt hyphae and thick-walled round spores observed under low-powered lens
- Keep in mind the possibility of a falsely abnormal result

Cause of abnormal result
Conversion of normal nondermatophyte dimorphic fungal skin flora to a hyphal form, causing tinea versicolor.

CONSIDER CONSULT
- If underlying cause suspected (i.e. immunosuppression)

PATIENT AND CAREGIVER ISSUES
Patient or caregiver request
- **Will the lesions scar?** Once the fungus has been treated the skin should return to normal after several months
- **What causes the lesion?** A treatable fungal infection causes the lesion
- **How long will the treatment last?** It may take one month to eradicate the fungus
- **Will the treatment be harmful?** Most treatments are topical and have a low side effect profile
- **Is the lesion due to malignancy?** The lesion is completely benign
- **Is the lesion contagious?** The fungus is of low infectivity

Health-seeking behavior
- **Have you tried any over-the-counter creams or lotions?** Patients may self-medicate before presentation
- **Have you had increased sun exposure recently?** As skin tans, lesions can become more apparent

MANAGEMENT ISSUES
Goals
- To eradicate fungus infection from skin
- To maximize treatment compliance because it can take up to 4 weeks to eradicate the fungus infection
- To reduce recurrence

Management in special circumstances
SPECIAL PATIENT GROUPS
Pregnant patients will need special management because certain treatments are contraindicated.

PATIENT SATISFACTION/LIFESTYLE PRIORITIES
- Patients need to be warned that the treatment may need to be continued for up to 4 weeks
- Patients need to be informed that the hypopigmented areas will not disappear immediately on treatment
- It may take several months for the skin to regain the pigment

SUMMARY OF THERAPEUTIC OPTIONS
Choices
- Sunlight accelerates repigmentation of hypopigmented area
- Treatment with topical keratolytics (e.g. salicylic acid 1.46% applied daily for one week) results in a cure rate of up to 90%
- Topical antifungals (e.g. 2.5% selenium sulfide, miconazole, clotrimazole, and econazole) are effective if used twice daily for 2 weeks
- Oral imidazoles (e.g. itraconazole, ketoconazole, and fluconazole) can be given as either a 5-day regimen or as a single dose. Cure rates of >90% are achieved. This treatment should only be used in recalcitrant cases, because it is an expensive treatment
- Relapse is common whatever treatment is employed, but certain lifestyle measures may be instituted to help prevent recurrence

Clinical pearls
Ketoconazole is secreted in sweat, and therefore exercise (without washing) after taking the medication will improve efficacy.

Never

Never give large doses of oral antifungals without assessing the patient's renal, hepatic, and pregnancy status first.

FOLLOW UP

Careful follow up to check on treatment compliance is needed.

Plan for review

- The patient should be followed up weekly to check that the treatment is being used effectively
- Support and reassurance is needed because the skin may take several months to regain normal pigment

Information for patient or caregiver

- Treatment may need to be continued for up to 4 weeks
- Compliance needs to be optimal to improve eradication rates
- The skin may not regain its natural pigment for several months after successful eradication of the fungus
- Recurrence will occur in over 80% of previously cured cases over 2 years

DRUGS AND OTHER THERAPIES: DETAILS
Drugs
SALICYLIC ACID
Keratolytic.

Dose
Adult and child topical dose: apply once daily for one week.

Efficacy
Cure rates up to 90%.

Risks/benefits
Risks:
- Use with caution in children
- Avoid contact with mucous membranes, eyes, and surrounding normal skin

Side effects and adverse reactions
- Skin: irritation, sensitivity, dryness
- Systemic effects after long-term use (salicylism: dizziness, confusion, headache, tinnitus, hearing disturbances)

Interactions (other drugs)
- No known interactions

Contraindications
- Diabetes or other disorders with impaired blood circulation ■ Warts on mucous membranes, facial or genital areas ■ Warts with hairs growing from them
- Moles, birthmarks ■ Infected or irritated skin

Acceptability to patient
Although application of the agent is quite time-consuming, it is effective in up to 90% of cases (provided compliance is maintained), and thus should be quite acceptable. Moreover, only one week of application of the agent is required.

Follow up plan
Careful follow up is required to assess compliance with treatment.

Patient and caregiver information
Compliance is essential in ensuring success of therapy.

SELENIUM SULFIDE
Antifungal agent.

Dose
- Adult and child topical dose: apply from neck to waist daily and leave on for up to 15min for 7 days
- Repeat this treatment weekly for one month and then monthly for maintenance

Efficacy
- Results in a cure rate of up to 90%
- Relapses are common

Risks/benefits
Risks:
- Use caution in gastrointestinal disease, renal impairment, and inflamed skin
- Use with caution in infants
- Under ordinary circumstances selenium sulfide should not be used for the treatment of tinea versicolor in pregnant women

Side effects and adverse reactions
- Side effects should not occur at recommended doses
- Selenium toxicity: alopecia, dermatitis, diarrhea, fatigue, halitosis, irritability, metallic taste in mouth, nausea, vomiting

Interactions (other drugs)
- None listed

Contraindications
- Neonatal prematurity ▪ Benzyl alcohol hypersensitivity

Acceptability to patient
Although application of the agent is quite time consuming, it is effective in up to 90% of cases (provided compliance is maintained), and thus should be quite acceptable.

Follow up plan
Careful follow up is required to assess compliance with treatment.

Patient and caregiver information
- External use only: patient should avoid contact with eyes
- May damage jewelry: patient should remove before using
- Compliance is essential in ensuring success of therapy

IMIDAZOLES
Antifungal agents, including itraconazole, ketoconazole, and fluconazole.

Dose
Adult oral doses:
- Ketoconazole: 200mg every day for one week or 400mg in a single dose
- Itraconazole: 200mg every day for 5 days
- Fluconazole: 400mg in a single dose

Efficacy
- Approx. 90% cure rate
- Relapse is common
- Single dose not effective in a hot, humid climate

Risks/benefits
Risks:
- Drug-induced hepatitis may be caused. Thus, the risk must be weighed against the benefit (i.e. treatment of a completely benign condition)
- Ketoconazole: risk of fatal hepatotoxicity; use caution in renal and hepatic disease and in patients with sulfite sensitivity
- Itraconazole: use with caution in hepatic and renal disease; discontinue if peripheral neuropathy occurs
- Fluconazole: use with caution in hepatic and renal disease; has been associated with rare cases of serious hepatotoxicity, including fatalities, primarily in patients with serious underlying medical condition; risk of anaphylaxis (rare)

Side effects and adverse reactions
Ketoconazole:
- Central nervous system: headache, dizziness
- Gastrointestinal: nausea, vomiting, diarrhea, abdominal pain
- Hematologic: blood cell disorders
- Skin: rashes, urticaria, irritation, stinging

Itraconazole:
- Cardiovascular system: edema, hypertension
- Central nervous system: depression, dizziness, headache, fever, fatigue
- Gastrointestinal: vomiting, nausea, diarrhea, hepatitis, altered liver function, abdominal pain
- Genitourinary: sexual dysfunction
- Metabolic: hypokalemia
- Skin: rashes, pruritus

Fluconazole:
- Central nervous system: seizures, dizziness, headache
- Gastrointestinal: abdominal pain, diarrhea, hepatitis, altered liver function, vomiting, nausea
- Hypersensitivity: anaphylaxis
- Skin: exfoliation, Stevens–Johnson syndrome

Interactions (other drugs)
Ketoconazole:
- Alfentanil ■ Antacids ■ Antibiotics, such as erythromycin ■ Antimuscarinics ■ Antiulcer agents (cimetidine, famotidine, omeprazole, nizatidine) ■ Antivirals (amprenavir, didanosine, indinavir, ritonavir, nelfinavir, saquinavir) ■ Anxiolytics (buspirone, chlordiazepoxide) ■ Astemizole ■ Benzodiazepines ■ Calcium-channel blockers (dihydropyridines) ■ Cisapride ■ Corticosteroids ■ Cyclosporine ■ Estrogens ■ Ethanol ■ Isoniazid ■ Methadone ■ Oral anticoagulants ■ Phenytoin ■ Quinidine ■ Rifampin ■ Statins ■ Sucralfate ■ Sildenafil ■ Tacrolimus ■ Terfenadine ■ Tolteridine

Itraconazole:
- Antacids
- Antiulcer drugs (cimetidine, famotidine, lansoprazole, nizatidine, omeprazole, sucralfate)
- Antivirals (amprenavir, didanosine, indinavir, nelfinavir, ritonavir, saquinavir)
- Astemizole
- Benzodiazepines
- Buspirone
- Chlordiazepoxide
- Cyclosporine
- Digoxin
- Ethanol
- Felodipine
- Macrolide antibiotics
- Methadone
- Methylprednisolone
- Oral anticoagulants
- Phenytoin
- Pimozide
- Quinidine
- Rifampin
- Statins
- Tacrolimus
- Terfenadine
- Tolbutamide

Fluconazole:
- Antihistamines
- Antilipemic statins
- Benzodiazepines
- Buspirone
- Caffeine
- Celecoxib
- Cisapride
- Cyclosporine
- Felodipine
- Losartan
- Methadone
- Oral anticoagulants
- Phenytoin
- Pimozide
- Quinidine
- Rifampin
- Ritonavir
- Sulfonylureas
- Tacrolimus
- Theophylline
- Zidovudine

Contraindications
- Imidazoles in general are contraindicated in pregnancy and patients with significant liver damage

Ketoconazole:
- Hypersensitivity to ketoconazole
- Pregnancy and breast-feeding
- Fungal meningitis
- Ketoconazole tablets have not been systematically studied in children of any age, and essentially no information is available on children under 2 years. Ketoconazole tablets should not be used in pediatric patients unless the potential benefit outweighs the risks

Itraconazole:
- Hypersensitivity to itraconazole
- Pregnancy and breast-feeding
- Not recommended in children or the elderly
- Do not administer with pimozide, quinidine, triazolam, oral midazolam, or statins

Fluconazole:
- Pregnancy and breast-feeding

Acceptability to patient
The short treatment schedules are well accepted by patients.

Follow up plan
Careful follow up is required to assess compliance with treatment.

Patient and caregiver information
Compliance is essential in ensuring success of therapy.

TOPICAL ANTIFUNGALS
Topical antifungals include miconazole, clotrimazole, and econazole.

Dose
Topical application twice daily for up to 4 weeks.

Efficacy
- Up to 90% cure rate
- Relapse is common

Risks/benefits
Risk: discontinue drug if sensitization or irritation is reported during use.

Side effects and adverse reactions
- Gastrointestinal: nausea, abdominal pain (oral administration)
- Skin: burning, rash, urticaria, stinging
- Genitourinary: dyspareunia, urinary frequency

Interactions (other drugs)
- Cyclosporine ▪ Tacrolimus

Contraindications
- Known hypersensitivity ▪ Pregnancy and breast-feeding

Acceptability to patient
Generally well accepted, although prolonged treatment (4 weeks or more) is necessary.

Follow up plan
Careful follow up is required to assess compliance with treatment.

Patient and caregiver information
Compliance is essential in ensuring success of therapy.

LIFESTYLE
- Heavy clothing and perspiration are causal factors for tinea versicolor, and should be avoided if possible
- Improving hygiene may prevent recurrence

RISKS/BENEFITS
Benefit: reduced incidence/recurrence of tinea versicolor.

ACCEPTABILITY TO PATIENT
If occupation requires heavy clothing and exposure to hot, humid conditions, then the patient may not be able to comply.

EFFICACY OF THERAPIES

All of the mentioned therapies (salicylic acid, selenium sulfide, imidazoles, topical antifungals, and lifestyle measures) are effective. The point to remember is that the fungus resides in the stratum corneum of the epidermis, or the outermost layer of the skin, and it takes an average of 4 weeks to undergo the normal cycle of sloughing of the stratum corneum. This means that whatever treatment is utilized, it will still take 4 weeks to eliminate the fungus completely.

PROGNOSIS

- Correct application of treatment will result in good fungal eradication rates
- Recurrence is over 80% in 2 years

Clinical pearls

Application of 2.5% selenium sulfide once a month may minimize recurrence.

Therapeutic failure

- Changing the antifungal agent may be beneficial if recurrence occurs
- Recurrence rate is 80% in 2 years
- Maintenance topical treatment can reduce this recurrence rate

Recurrence

If repeated recurrence occurs and treatment compliance is optimal, then referral is indicated.

Deterioration

If deterioration occurs, referral is indicated because comorbidity needs to be excluded.

CONSIDER CONSULT

- Referral is indicated in the case of deterioration, for diagnosis/exclusion of comorbidity
- Referral should also be considered in the case of repeated recurrence where treatment compliance is optimal

RISK FACTORS
Causal factors of tinea versicolor include:
- Using oral contraceptives
- Pregnancy
- Poor hygiene: perspiration
- Excess heat and humidity
- Immunosuppression

MODIFY RISK FACTORS
Lifestyle and wellness
Good nutrition, hygiene, and a cool climate prevent tinea versicolor.

DIET
- Malnutrition can lead to tinea versicolor
- Good nutrition will prevent recurrence

PHYSICAL ACTIVITY
Excessive perspiration can lead to tinea versicolor.

ENVIRONMENT
Reduce the heat and humidity in the living environment to prevent recurrence.

DRUG HISTORY
- Oral contraceptives can cause tinea versicolor
- Other means of contraception may be indicated

CHEMOPROPHYLAXIS
Ketoconazole 400mg orally every 14 days or ketoconazole 200mg orally for three consecutive days per month.

PREVENT RECURRENCE
Recurrence rate is 80% in 2 years. Reducing the causal factors will lead to lower recurrence. Causal factors include:
- Using oral contraceptives
- Pregnancy
- Poor hygiene: perspiration
- Excess heat and humidity
- Immunosuppression

Reassess coexisting disease
Immunosuppression can lead to tinea versicolor.

INTERACTION ALERT
Oral contraceptives can cause recurrence.

RESOURCES

KEY REFERENCES

- Weatherall DJ, Ledingham JGG, Warnell DA, eds. Oxford textbook of medicine. Vol.1, 3rd edn. New York: Oxford University Press, 1996
- Tierney LM, McPhee SJ, Papadakis MA. Current medical diagnosis and treatment. Stamford, CT: Appleton and Lange, 1993
- Burton J. Essentials of dermatology. 3rd edn. Philadelphia, PA: Churchill Livingstone, 1990
- Thaler DT, Hope RA, Longmore JM, eds. Oxford handbook of clinical medicine. New York: Oxford University Press, 1995

FAQS
Question 1
What is the difference between tinea versicolor and tinea corporis?

ANSWER 1
Tinea corporis is due to a true dermatophyte, whereas tinea versicolor is caused by a yeast; thus, the term 'tinea' is inappropriately used in describing this condition.

CONTRIBUTORS
Fred F Ferri, MD, FACP
Seth R Stevens, MD
Elma D Baron, MD

VITILIGO

DESCRIPTION

- Hypopigmented and depigmented lesions
- Sun-exposed skin, body folds, and areas around body orifices are particularly affected
- Lesions tend to be bilateral and symmetrical
- Hair in affected areas may be white
- Exact cause of melanocyte destruction is unknown

ICD9 CODE
709.1 Vitiligo

SYNONYMS
- Trichrome vitiligo
- Marginal inflammatory vitiligo

CARDINAL FEATURES
- Hypopigmented and depigmented lesions
- Sun-exposed skin, body folds, and areas around body orifices are particularly affected
- Lesions tend to be bilateral and symmetrical
- Sites of trauma can be affected – Koebner's phenomenon
- Hair in affected areas may be white
- Exact cause of melanocyte destruction is unknown
- Ring of hyperpigmentation at margin of lesions – trichrome vitiligo
- Lesions can have raised borders – marginal inflammatory vitiligo
- A halo of vitiligo (Sutton's nevus) occurs around pigmented nevi

CAUSES
Common causes
- Precise cause is unknown. Cases occur due to combination of neurogenic, immunologic, and genetic factors
- Pathophysiologic theories include: autoantibodies against melanocytes; neurochemicals selectively destroy melanocytes; melanocytes destroyed by cytotoxic melanin precursors
- 30% of cases are familial; mode of genetic transmission is unknown (variable expression)

Contributory or predisposing factors
Antimelanocyte antibodies may be a causal agent.

EPIDEMIOLOGY
Incidence and prevalence
Relatively common.
PREVALENCE
10/1000 population.

Demographics
AGE
- Can occur at any age
- 50% of cases diagnosed in those under 20 years

RACE
Occurs in all races, but it is more obvious in those with darker skin.

GENETICS
Positive family history in 25–30% of cases.

DIFFERENTIAL DIAGNOSIS
Pityriasis alba
Pityriasis alba is a nonspecific dermatitis primarily affecting children.

FEATURES
- Pale patches on skin and mild eczema
- Hypopigmented not depigmented skin
- Round or oval lesions
- Face is most commonly affected site
- Scaling of lesions is a late feature

Pityriasis versicolor
Pityriasis versicolor is a fungal infection of the skin caused by yeast (*Malassezia furfur*). Adolescents and young adults are particularly affected.

FEATURES
- Macular rash
- Pale brown, pink, or depigmented lesions
- Lesions scale with scraping
- Yeast fungus contained in scale
- Relapse is common after treatment

Tuberous sclerosis
Tuberous sclerosis is an autosomal-dominant disease with cerebral sclerosis.

FEATURES
- Elliptical white macules on trunk
- Cerebral sclerosis
- Severe learning impairment
- Epilepsy
- Cutaneous angiofibromata producing pink papules around nasolabial folds
- Shagreen patch (connective tissue nevus)
- Fibromata emerge from nailfolds

Halo nevus
Halo nevus is a depigmented nevus causing skin and nevus to become paler.

FEATURES
- Skin around nevus becomes depigmented
- Antibodies to melanocytes
- Nonmalignant lesion with good prognosis
- Increased risk of developing vitiligo

Hansen's disease (leprosy)
Hansen's disease is a chronic granulomatous infection that primarily affects the skin and peripheral nerves.

FEATURES
- Skin lesion (which may be hypopigmented, hyperpigmented, or erythematous)
- Sensory loss, muscle atrophy, weakness
- Anhidrosis

- Palpable peripheral nerves
- Skin smears or skin biopsies of the affected site demonstrate acid-fast bacilli (*Mycobacterium leprae*)

Nevus anemicus
Nevus anemicus is a congenital lesion that is more common in females.

FEATURES
- Most commonly occurs on the chest or the back
- Well-defined white macule with an irregular border
- Multiple smaller lesions may surround the main lesion
- Histology is normal

SIGNS & SYMPTOMS
Signs
- Hypopigmented and depigmented lesions; in long-standing disease there should be depigmented lesions
- Sun–exposed skin, body folds, and areas around body orifices are particularly affected
- Lesions tend to be bilateral and symmetrical
- Sites of trauma can be affected – Koebner's phenomenon
- Hair in affected areas may be white
- Ring of hyperpigmentation at margin of lesions – trichrome vitiligo
- Lesions can have raised borders – marginal inflammatory vitiligo
- A halo of vitiligo (Sutton's nevus) may occur around pigmented nevi

Symptoms
- Usually asymptomatic
- Sun exposure can make lesions irritative
- Distress if vitiligo presents a serious cosmetic problem

ASSOCIATED DISORDERS
Vitiligo is associated with autoimmune diseases including:
- Alopecia areata
- Diabetes mellitus
- Hyperthyroidism
- Hypothyroidism
- Pernicious anemia
- Addison's disease

CONSIDER CONSULT
- A patient diagnosed with vitiligo or with an uncertain diagnosis should be referred to a dermatologist
- If an autoimmune disease is suspected, the patient should be referred to a dermatologist or rheumatologist

INVESTIGATION OF THE PATIENT
Direct questions to patient
Q **How long have you had these lesions?** Vitiligo is a chronic disease with onset under age 20 years in 50% of cases.
Q **Are the lesions irritative?** Usually lesions are asymptomatic but exposure to sunlight can cause irritation.
Q **Where are the lesions?** Lesions favor areas around body orifices, intertriginous areas, genitalia, and sun-exposed skin.

Contributory or predisposing factors

Q Do you have an autoimmune disease? Vitiligo is associated with a variety of autoimmune diseases including: alopecia areata, diabetes mellitus, hyperthyroidism, hypothyroidism, pernicious anemia, Addison's disease. Occasionally vitiligo is the presenting feature of an autoimmune diathesis. Thus, patients may have symptoms of these other diseases without knowledge of the diagnosis. Therefore, questions about signs and symptoms referable to these are appropriate.

Family history

Q Have any members of your family suffered similar symptoms? 25–30% of patients will have a positive family history.

Examination

- Are there hypopigmented and depigmented lesions? These are present in vitiligo
- Where are the lesions? Sun-exposed skin, body folds, and areas around body orifices are particularly affected
- What is the pattern of the lesions? Lesions tend to be bilateral and symmetrical
- Are the lesions over sites of trauma? Koebner's phenomenon can occur
- Is the hair affected? Early graying or patches of white hair in affected areas is a feature of vitiligo
- Are the borders of the lesions hyperpigmented? Trichrome vitiligo
- Do the lesions have raised borders? Marginal inflammatory vitiligo
- Are there halos (Sutton's nevi) around pigmented nevi? Can be present in vitiligo
- Does Wood's light make examining the lesions on the skin easier? Wood's light examination may enhance lesions in light-skinned individuals

Summary of investigative tests

- Complete blood test to detect pernicious anemia associated with vitiligo
- Fasting blood glucose to detect diabetes mellitus, which can be linked with vitiligo
- Thyroid function test to detect hyper- and hypothyroidism associated with vitiligo

DIAGNOSTIC DECISION

Clinical features of depigmentation around facial orifices and hands should prompt consideration of vitiligo. Biopsy sent to a dermatopathologist will demonstrate the absence of melanocytes, even in very lightly pigmented patients.

CLINICAL PEARLS

Although only hypopigmented macules may present in very early cases, truly depigmented macules are usually seen in cases of vitiligo.

THE TESTS
Body fluids

COMPLETE BLOOD COUNT
Description
Venous blood sample.

Advantages/Disadvantages
Advantage: quick, simple, cheap, and reliable.

Normal
- Hemoglobin: male 13.6–17.7g/dL (8.4–11.0mmol/L); female 12–15g/dL (7.4–9.3mmol/L)
- Mean corpuscular volume (MCV): 76–100fL

Abnormal
- Hemoglobin: male <13.6g/dL (8.4mmol/L); female <12g/dL (7.4mmol/L)
- MCV: >100fL
- Keep in mind the possibility of a false-positive result

Cause of abnormal result
Pernicious anemia associated with vitiligo.

FASTING BLOOD GLUCOSE
Description
Fasting venous blood sample.

Advantages/Disadvantages
Advantage: quick
Disadvantage: patient needs to fast

Normal
Fasting plasma glucose: 70–110mg/dL (700–1100mg/L).

Abnormal
- Fasting plasma glucose >110mg/dL (>1100mg/L)
- Keep in mind the possibility of a false positive result

Cause of abnormal result
Diabetes mellitus – can be linked with vitiligo.

THYROID FUNCTION TEST
Description
Venous blood sample.

Advantages/Disadvantages
Advantage: quick, simple, and reliable.

Normal
- Thyroid stimulating hormone: 2–11mU/L
- Thyroxine (T4): 4–11mcg/dL (40–110mcg/L)

Abnormal
- Thyroid stimulating hormone: <2 or >11mU/L
- Thyroxine (T4): <4 or >11mcg/dL (<40 or >110mcg/L)
- Keep in mind the possibility of a false positive result

Cause of abnormal result
- Thyroxine (T4) <4mcg/dL (<40mcg/L): hypothyroidism
- Thyroxine (T4) >11mcg/dL (>110mcg/L): hyperthyroidism
- Thyroid stimulating hormone <2mU/L: central hypothyroidism
- Thyroid stimulating hormone > 11mU/L: peripheral hypothyroidism

Drugs, disorders and other factors that may alter results
Thyroid disease.

TREATMENT

CONSIDER CONSULT

- Vitiligo is a condition whose evaluation and treatment generally requires specialized knowledge base. Unless the primary care physician has a special interest in vitiligo, patients with vitiligo should be referred to a dermatologist, in particular, when phototherapy with ultraviolet A (UVA) is indicated

PATIENT AND CAREGIVER ISSUES
Patient or caregiver request

- **What is vitiligo?** Patients may not know about this disease and an explanation is needed
- **Will it spread?** The patient may be worried that vitiligo will cause a serious cosmetic problem. Vitiligo typically spreads to sites of trauma. The final extent of disease, which can be very extensive, is highly variable and unpredictable
- **Can vitiligo be cured?** It is an incurable disease but there are treatments that restore some pigmentation to the affected areas. Spontaneous remission is not uncommon
- **Is it contagious?** Vitiligo is not contagious
- **Do I have cancer?** Vitiligo is a benign condition
- **Will my children inherit it?** There is a genetic link and up to 30% of cases have a positive family history

Health-seeking behavior

Have you sought any treatment up to now, e.g. from the pharmacist? Patient may have tried self-remedies to treat the lesions.

MANAGEMENT ISSUES
Goals

- To minimize impact of vitiligo; treatment is primarily for cosmetic purposes
- To provide patient with a good explanation of vitiligo
- To minimize sun exposure to the vitiligo lesions

Management in special circumstances

PATIENT SATISFACTION/LIFESTYLE PRIORITIES
Cosmetic treatments may reduce psychologic impact of vitiligo.

SUMMARY OF THERAPEUTIC OPTIONS
Choices

Treatment is indicated primarily for cosmetic purposes when depigmentation causes emotional and social distress. Depigmentation is more obvious in darker complexions. Strong motivation is required on the part of the patient for maximal compliance. Vitiligo is complex to treat but can respond to:

- Cosmetic masking agents, which can be very effective in reducing social and emotional distress
- Topical corticosteroids (e.g. 0.1% triamcinolone) for up to 4 months on a twice-daily regimen for localized disease (high-potency topical corticosteroids are the most effective therapy for localized vitiligo)
- Psoralens and ultraviolet application (PUVA) therapy – an oral or topical psoralen (usually methoxsalen) with UVA phototherapy has a good success rate; phototherapy usually requires referral to a specialist center
- Ultraviolet-B light therapy is the most effective therapy for generalized disease; phototherapy usually requires referral to a specialist center
- A psoralen (usually methoxsalen) and graded exposure to sunlight to prevent erythema can also be used

- Systemic corticosteroids (e.g. betamethasone) for up to 4 months
- Total depigmentation in extensive vitiligo with monobenzone: if this treatment is used, minimal sun exposure must be lifelong
- A variety of techniques for autologous melanocyte transfer have been reported, some with seemingly satisfactory results. If patients are highly motivated, referral to a center that performs this procedure may be appropriate
- Lifestyle measures: patients should avoid sun exposure and use a topical sunscreen at all times

Clinical Pearls
The treatment of vitiligo may be quite easy and spontaneous remission will occur while it is quite difficult in other cases. When spontaneous remission does not occur, only highly motivated patients are likely to be successfully treated. They must be willing to undergo frequent phototherapy for relatively extended periods of time.

FOLLOW UP
- Assess effectiveness of treatment
- Support patient through the treatment to ensure maximal compliance
- Explore different treatments if required
- Assess for associated other autoimmune diseases

Plan for review
Patient should initially be followed up weekly to check on treatment compliance and effectiveness.

Information for patient or caregiver
- The National Vitiligo Foundation can give advice to patient
- Vitiligo is a benign, noncontagious disease but it is not curable
- Cosmetic problems can be minimized by masking agents
- There is a genetic link and up to 30% of cases have a positive family history

DRUGS AND OTHER THERAPIES: DETAILS
Drugs
METHOXSALEN
Methoxsalen (psoralen) with UVA therapy can be used to repigment the skin.

Dose
- Adult oral dose: 20mg taken with milk or food up to 3 times weekly 2–4h before exposure to measured doses of UVA
- Adult topical dose: apply to lesions once weekly before exposure to measured doses of UVA
- 150–200 treatments are required over 1–2 years
- Not recommended for children under 12 years

Efficacy
Highly variable. One reason for this is that patients find it difficult to comply with a regimen requiring visits to the physician's office or to the hospital three times weekly for over a year. In general, the face responds better than do hands and feet, and adults respond better than do children. A reasonable rule of thumb is that 50% of patients will have 50% or greater repigmentation.

Risks/benefits
Risks:
- With topical use, serious burns from either UVA or sunlight (even through window glass) can result if the recommended dosage of the drug and/or exposure schedules are not followed

- Use caution with cardiac and hepatic disease
- Use caution with pregnancy and nursing mothers

Side effects and adverse reactions
- Central nervous system: dizziness, headache, depression
- Cardiovascular system: edema, hypotension
- Ears, eyes, nose, and throat: cataract formation
- Gastrointestinal: nausea
- Musculoskeletal: leg cramps
- Skin: cutaneous tenderness, erythema, pruritus, severe burns

Interactions (other drugs)
- **None listed**

Contraindications
Oral and topical prepaprations:
- Hypersensitivity to psoralens ▪ Melanoma ▪ Patients with invasive squamous cell carcinomas

Oral only:
- Safety in children has not been established ▪ Patients with aphakia, because of the significantly increased risk of retinal damage due to the absence of lenses

Topical only:
- Safety and effectiveness in children below the age of 12 years have not been established
- Patients with photosensitivity diseases such as porphyria, acute lupus erythematosus, xeroderma, and pigmentosum should not use topical methoxsalen

Acceptability to patient
Repigmentation may take 6–24 months.

Follow up plan
- Assess effectiveness of treatment
- Support patient through the treatment to ensure maximal compliance
- Explore different treatments if required

Patient and caregiver information
- Do not sunbathe 24h prior to and after methoxsalen and UVA exposure
- Wear wraparound sunglasses for 24h following ingestion of psoralens
- Repigmentation may require 6–9 months of treatment
- Depigmentation may recur

TRIAMCINOLONE (0.1%)
Topical midpotency steroid.

Dose
Adult topical dose: apply to affected area twice daily.

Efficacy
Highly variable. It is difficult to assess the treatment response to topical steroids given the possibility of spontaneous remission.

Risks/benefits
Risks:
- The potential for systemic absorption must be considered
- Use with caution in children

Side effects and adverse reactions
- Skin: rash,dermatitis, pruritus, atrophy, hypopigmentation, striae, xerosis, burning, stinging upon application, alopecia
- Eyes, ears, nose, and throat: conjunctivitis

Contraindications
- **Do not use on face, axilla, or groin**

Acceptability to patient
Easy to apply.

Follow up plan
- Assess effectiveness of treatment
- Support patient through the treatment to ensure maximal compliance
- Explore different treatments if required

BETAMETHASONE
- Systemic steroid
- This is an off-label indication

Dose
Adult oral dose: 5mg/day on two consecutive days weekly for 2–4 months.

Efficacy
Highly variable.

Risks/benefits
Risks:
- Long-term use of potent topical corticosteroids can result in permanent thinning of sensitive skin, telangiectasias, or redness
- Caution needed in long-term use (10 days or more); may lead to secondary ocular infections, glaucoma, optic nerve damage, cataract
- May mask signs of pre-existing or secondary ocular infection
- Caution needed in pregnancy and lactation
- Safe use in children has not been established
- Use caution in liver or renal disease, hypothyroidism, heart failure, or hypertension
- Use caution in diabetes mellitus, seizures or psychosis, myasthenia gravis
- Use caution in pre-existing coagulopathy or thromboembolic disease

Side effects and adverse reactions
- Gastrointestinal: dyspepsia, peptic ulceration, esophagitis, oral candidiasis, nausea, diarrhea
- Cardiovascular system: hypertension, thromboembolism
- Central nervous system: insomnia, euphoria, depression, psychosis
- Eyes, ears, nose, and throat: cataract, glaucoma, blurred vision
- Endocrine: adrenal suppression, impaired glucose tolerance, growth suppression in children, Cushing's syndrome
- Musculoskeletal: proximal myopathy, osteoporosis

- Skin: rash, dermatitis, pruritus, atrophy, hypopigmentation, striae, xerosis, burning, stinging upon application, alopecia, conjunctivitis. Cutaneous atrophy can occur after a few weeks. If applied over large surface areas, inhibition of the hypothalamic-pituitary-adrenal axis can occur. If used chronically (unlikely in these photodermatoses) in children, growth retardation can occur

Interactions (other drugs)
- Aldesleukin ▪ Aminoglutethimide ▪ Antibiotics ▪ Anticholinesterases ▪ Anticoagulants ▪ Antidiabetics ▪ Antifungals ▪ Barbiturates ▪ Bismuth subsalicylate ▪ Colestyramine ▪ Colestipol ▪ Diltiazem ▪ Ephedrine ▪ Estrogens ▪ Formoterol ▪ Imitanib mesylate ▪ Insulin ▪ Mifepristone ▪ Nondepolarizing muscle relaxants ▪ Oral contraceptives ▪ Phenytoin ▪ Rifabutin ▪ Rifampin ▪ Rifapentine ▪ Salicylates ▪ Troleandomycin ▪ Verpamil ▪ Xanthine derivatives

Contraindications
▪ Lack of a definite diagnosis ▪ Systemic infection ▪ Avoid live virus vaccines in those receiving immunosuppressive doses ▪ Poor circulation ▪ History of tuberculosis (intranasal preparation only) ▪ Cushing's syndrome ▪ Recent myocardial infarction

Acceptability to patient
Systemic preparation may be more attractive to patient.

Follow up plan
- Assess effectiveness of treatment
- Support the patient through the treatment to ensure maximal compliance
- Explore different treatments if required

MONOBENZONE
- Depigmentation agent
- Use only in extensive vitiligo on rare patch of residual normal pigmentation for complete depigmentation

Dose
Rub into pigmented areas two or three times daily.

Efficacy
- Depigmentation normally observed after 1–4 months
- Complete depigmentation may require 9–12 months

Risks/benefits
Risk: use caution in pregnancy and nursing mothers.

Side effects and adverse reactions
Skin: burning, dermatitis, irritation.

Contraindications
- Melanoma
- Pigmented nevi

Follow up plan

- Assess effectiveness of treatment
- Support patient through the treatment to ensure maximal compliance
- Explore different treatments if required

Patient and caregiver information

- This drug is not a mild cosmetic bleach
- Treated areas should not be exposed to sunlight
- Lifelong protection of skin with a topical sunscreen is required
- Only to be used in severe cases of vitiligo

LIFESTYLE

- Patients should avoid sun exposure as vitiligo lesions have no pigmentary protection and can be damaged by UV light
- Patients need to use a topical sunscreen at all times, even in normal daylight

EFFICACY OF THERAPIES

Treatments have highly variable results; thus, treatment modalities should be selected for maximum benefit and minimum risk, with consideration for the body surface area involved.

PROGNOSIS

- Vitiligo is not a curable condition
- Some lesions will repigment only to return years later
- Stabilization of the disease can occur after several months with the lesion number and size remaining constant

Clinical Pearls

Spontaneous remissions may occur.

Therapeutic failure

- Patient will need to be closely supervised when undergoing treatment for vitiligo
- If treatment is ineffective, alternative therapies should be instituted by a dermatologist

Recurrence

Referral to a dermatologist is indicated if there is recurrence of vitiligo.

Deterioration

Referral to a dermatologist is indicated if vitiligo patches on the skin increase.

CONSIDER CONSULT

- Referral to a dermatologist is indicated if vitiligo patches on the skin increase or recur

Vitiligo is not specifically preventable in the general population.

PREVENT RECURRENCE
- Avoid sunlight exposure, which will damage skin
- Use topical sunscreens at all times, even in normal daylight

Reassess coexisting disease
Treating autoimmune diseases associated with vitiligo may prevent deterioration of existing lesions: diabetes mellitus, hyperthyroidism, hypothyroidism, pernicious anemia, Addison's disease.

ASSOCIATIONS
National Vitiligo Foundation
611 South Fleishel Ave
Tyler, TX 75701
Tel: (903) 531-0074
Fax: (903) 525-1234
www.nvfi.org

KEY REFERENCES
- van Geel N, Ongenae K, Naeyaert JM. Surgical techniques for vitiligo: a review. Dermatology 2001;202:162–6
- Hope, et al. Oxford handbook of clinical medicine. New York: Oxford University Press, 1996
- Collier, et al. Oxford handbook of clinical specialties. New York: Oxford University Press, 1990
- Burton J. Essentials of dermatology, 3rd edn. New York: Churchill Livingstone, 1990, p34,125
- Rubenstein, et al. Lecture notes on clinical medicine, 4th edn. Malden (MA): Blackwell Scientific Publications: 1991, p168
- Fry, et al. Dermatology. Hingham (MA): MTP Press, 1995

FAQS
Question 1
Is vitiligo contagious?

ANSWER 1
No, but hypopigmented patches may be caused by tinea versicolor, a yeast infection of the skin in susceptible patients.

CONTRIBUTORS
Gregory J Raglow, MD, FAAFP
Seth R Stevens, MD
Richard Averitte, MD

Index

Index